"A GROUNDBREAKING WORK.

Dr. Kessler gives a clear path to having a strong, fit body for a lifetime. I hope this book is read by doctors as well as patients."
—MITCHELL GAYNOR, M.D.
Director of Medical Oncology,
Strang Cancer Prevention Center

"The Bone Density Program is packed with useful information. Dr. Kessler has successfully combined conventional and complementary therapies for preventing and treating osteoporosis."
—LEO GALLAND, M.D., F.A.C.P., F.A.C.N.
Author of *Power Healing*

"Intriguing advice . . . Worthwhile . . . This easy to follow guide tells why cutting down on salt and soft drinks and making other simple lifestyle changes can go a long way toward preventing osteoporosis."

—*Self*

"George Kessler's caring and reasonable voice comes through clearly in this wonderful book. It presents to the reader a truly integrative perspective on an important condition. I look forward to sharing this book with my patients, and think it will prove very helpful in my practice."
—BEN KLIGLER, M.D., M.P.H.
Medical Director
Beth Israel Center for Health and Healing

"This is a well-written, solid mainstream book on osteoporosis. It is reader-friendly and thoughtful in covering all the bases of the contemporary medical approach to bone health."
—ANNEMARIE COLBIN, C.H.E.S.
Author of *Food and Our Bones*

"The most complete yet, this invaluable handbook will guide you through tailoring your own best program for maintaining or increasing bone density."
—RUDOLPH BALLENTINE, M.D.
Author of *Radical Healing*

"An astonishingly simple diet and exercise program designed to help those who are suffering from osteoporosis or who are at risk of this bone disease. . . . The books reassuring tone and practical information make this a useful guide for anyone concerned about his or her bones."

—*Publishers Weekly*

The Bone Density Program

6 Weeks to Strong Bones and a Healthy Body

George J. Kessler, D.O., P.C.,
with Colleen Kapklein

Ballantine Books   New York

TO K.T. AND M.E.

I always told you that amino acids were very important and that your body was like a car and would only run well if you used good fuel. Since my life would not be complete without you, I am dedicating this work to both of you and to your healthy and happy futures. Life is what you make of it, and I am very proud of who you both are.

—GEORGE J. KESSLER

Matt, you've waited more than ten years for it: This one's for you.

Also, for my mother and grandmothers, who go this road before me, and for my daughter, Casey, for whom I hope the road is smooth.

—COLLEEN KAPKLEIN

Contents

Acknowledgments

There are many people without whom this undertaking would not even have begun, let alone been finished. I would like to specifically mention a few.

Janis Vallely and Meredith Bernstein showed me there was a book in my ideas and worked tirelessly to make the book a reality. Colleen Kapklein taught me how to put my ideas on paper. Colleen was also instrumental in enlarging those ideas and merging them with the research done to produce this book. I also wish to acknowledge and thank my editor, Maureen O'Neal, and Leslie Meredith, and the many people at Ballantine Books for believing in me and for providing the resources and wisdom needed for the completion of this project.

I would like to thank my friend and colleague, Dr. Mitchell Gaynor, who inspired me. He used very few words and spoke them softly, but he pushed very hard and not so quietly—and by his force has changed my life. I thank my children, Emily and Katie, for bringing joy and perspective to the mix. To my friends, Dave Genser and Mark Easton, who constitute my regular weekend golf and sanity outings, I thank you for your (wise) friendship and support.

I also thank my office staff, who make coming to work a

pleasure I look forward to. They have allowed me the time and peace with which to undertake and complete this book while still carrying out my usual duties.

I also wish to thank my colleagues at the Contemporary Healing Institute in New York City for sharing with me their wisdom and energy.

My brother, Robert, has helped me to focus my ideas and priorities and my sister-in-law, Debbie, has done a wonderful job of making this prescription for health not only easily achievable, but also delicious.

Abby Greenspun, M.S., R.D., has taken the food ideas and recipes and made sure that they conformed to the excellent nutritional standards we sought.

My thanks to Noah Hyman, P.T., Martin Barandes, M.D., Joseph Lane, M.D., Diana Lapiano, R.N., Theresa D. Galsworthy, R.N., O.N.C., and Gloria Hussell for their valuable contributions and assistance.

Lastly, I wish to give special thanks to my wife, Linda Diane Kessler, who has stood by me all these years and has encouraged and helped me to achieve my goals.

—GEORGE J. KESSLER

Of course, there would be no book if not for the expertise of George Kessler. He, our team of agents, and our editor and other backers at Ballantine provided the vision and support to bring this project to fruition.

Yoga instructors Alice Cassman and Shelly Greenberg allowed us to make our vision real—not to mention the much-needed respite Alice's class provided me.

Dr. Asa Hershoff generously gave his time and expertise, and Dr. Ed Klaiber and Dr. John Lee shared enlightening case histories, all of which I am grateful for.

Rick North of the Silver Spring YMCA has worked to educate Y members about the importance of bone health. He kindly accommodated my search for information, and several times pointed me in just the right direction.

Thanks also to the many members of the osteoporosis newsgroup *(sci.med.diseases.osteoporosis)* who graciously shared their perspectives.

Dale Valentine and Melissa Sabaka at the Children's Center provided warm and loving care for my daughter, allowing me to focus my energies on this book knowing she was in the best of hands.

My family and friends gave me space and time to get this done, provided help and advice when I needed it, and brightened my hours *not* spent in front of the computer, but those are only a few items on a very long list of reasons I'm grateful to be part of such a wide and wonderful circle.

Finally, special thanks to the many, many women who shared their own experiences, greatly enriching this book by providing human faces for the medical facts.

—Colleen Kapklein

Foreword

As director of the leading osteoporosis prevention program at a major academic hospital center, I speak—and listen—to thousands of people every year who are concerned about keeping their bones healthy. So I know there is a great thirst for information, and for cutting-edge information in particular, among the general public as well as patients following prevention or treatment plans. And while science is making great strides in understanding bone health, in diagnostic testing, and in the advancement of treatment options, most people focus on quality of life. They want to add life to their years—not just years to their lives. They want to stay healthy and vigorous throughout their lives.

The way to do that is prevention across the decades, beginning with children and continuing right on through the more seasoned years—for men as well as women. That's why I was so pleased to read *The Bone Density Diet*. By stressing a six-week plan that provides a range of prevention techniques for anyone, no matter what stage she or he is in right now, the information in this book will help minimize the need for bone-loss treatment strategies (which are also thoroughly explained in the book). Focusing on prevention and wellness, rather than illness, is the most effective strategy as well as the most positive one when it comes to maintaining strong, healthy bones—and therefore, strong, healthy bodies—over a lifetime.

The Bone Density Diet presents the widest range of approaches to building and maintaining strong bones. The most common prevention and treatment strategies are comprehensively explained, and the personal stories throughout show how they work for real people. "Alternative" approaches are also included for any readers uncomfortable with conventional approaches and for those who are trying to do as much as possible to support their bodies.

We still need much more information about the various alternatives presented here before we can know for certain how well they work compared to "conventional" therapies. There's more to learn about those conventional choices, too. There have been many authoritative studies done in that area, but questions still remain. Some early results on alternatives are promising, so when used responsibly—whether as adjuncts or as alternatives—these "complementary medicine" techniques are worth investigating with a health-care provider who can monitor your progress regularly.

This book also provides the key to how to use whatever approach you choose responsibly and with maximum effectiveness, and how to monitor your situation. Having your bone density measured—and remeasured, as appropriate—and tracking your rate of bone breakdown, as explained in this book, will allow you to make any necessary adjustments, according to how well what you're doing is working for you.

In my public speaking, I always include some of the alarming statistics about osteoporosis: one out of every two Americans over age 70 will suffer a bone fracture as a result of osteoporosis—with 1 in 5 diagnoses being in men (this is *not* only a "woman's disease"). Women over 50 are more likely to get osteoporosis than breast cancer, heart disease, and ovarian cancer *combined*. Over a million people every year will have a hip or spinal fracture. In the case of hip fractures, one-third of those patients die of complications within a year, and another third never return to independent living.

These are depressing and very real statistics, but the human story represents the devastation of this disease. The many men and women I see in hospital corridors or on the city streets who suffer from osteoporosis struggle daily. The spinal deformity, or "dowager's hump," resulting from fractures can affect all systems, from decreased self-image and consequent depression to altered visual ability, breathing difficulties, poor digestion, vulnerability because of changes in balance, and, most profound, chronic pain. Osteoporosis is a debilitating disease. Many people suffering from it are unable to continue with the chores of daily life and become socially isolated.

I take this kind of "scared straight" approach because I want to underline the importance of taking action right now to prevent all these effects. But osteoporosis is a "silent" disease. It sneaks up on people because it doesn't produce symptoms until the first unexpected fracture occurs—and because for a long time, osteoporosis was thought to be an inevitable part of aging. What this means in real life is that 77 percent of women who have osteoporosis don't know they have it—and so aren't doing anything about it. Men have been screened less often than women, but with newly emerging interest in osteoporosis in men, I suspect many more men are at risk than we previously realized.

In a positive light, it is thought that osteoporosis is generally a preventable disease. We know how to avoid low bone density, and the answers, at least as far as prevention goes, are simple. Good eating and exercise habits (as explained in this book) will take you most of the way there—and for a lot of people, that is all that will be required to stack the odds of a long, strong, healthy life in their favor.

The truth is that *everyone* will benefit from the most basic preventive strategies. By their early 20s, both men and women have acquired about 98 percent of the skeletal mass they will ever have. So anyone older than that should be working to prevent bone loss and maintain that maximum, and anyone younger should be working to make the maximum as high as possible before bone loss begins. Most people need to understand that they are at risk (without any outward sign) before they are truly motivated to make any changes. That's why I emphasize the urgent need to take action to ensure a vigorous lifestyle through the decades.

Today there is a lot of optimism in the field. Since 1998, federal law ensures that Medicare will pay for bone-density testing nationwide, and many insurance companies are following suit. The technology for measuring bone mass is constantly improving, and before long we should be able to measure not just the amount of bone but the quality as well. Early results of clinical trials of medications that will directly stimulate the cells that build new bone look promising. We're improving our understanding of how and why to measure how fast bone is breaking down, and while you can get a test in your doctor's office now, you may soon be able to buy an at-home test kit for easier monitoring of your condition. An experimental surgical technique for correcting and stabilizing spinal fractures appears to give immediate pain relief for fractures identified early enough, and in time this technique will become more widely available. Studies continue to help us better understand the role of exercise—and which kinds are most effective for strengthening individual bones, keeping muscles strong, and preventing falls.

The best news of all, though, is that with what we already know, right now, we can prevent fractures even if bone density is low. It's never too early or too late to begin protecting your bones. The recommendations here, particularly about nutrition and exercise, are designed with your bones in mind—but they will also provide wide-ranging, long-lasting benefits to your overall health.

This book will put readers in control of their own health. Well-informed patients are prepared to participate as equal members of their health-care team and constructively talk over any issues with their health-care providers. I know from my work at the hospital that educated patients are more likely to follow through on health-related plans—and are more optimistic about the outcome. I've dedicated my career to getting the information that makes all that possible into patients' hands, and now *The Bone Density Diet* takes up the cause. It's a good thing, too: if we don't do better at prevention, according to what we already know, it is projected that the medical costs for osteoporosis will be over $64 billion in the year 2040.

But I foresee a very different future. I see a world where all men and women stand straight and tall throughout their lives, strong and healthy and active. By the time we reach the estimated $64 billion question, I believe low bone density will no longer be a common problem. That's assuming all people have access to thorough, reliable, and cutting-edge information, as found in *The Bone Density Diet*. And now they do.

This book should be a call to action for readers determined to stay healthy, as well as for health-care professionals and scientists working on improving our options for doing just that. Readers who make the six-week commitment to learning all they need to keep their bones healthy and strong, and to creating the habits they need to put that knowledge to use, will see encouraging results. Even those who can reach just one goal right now will be headed in the right direction—and if they monitor their progress as described in this book, they'll know if what they are doing is enough. Everyone should find something here that fits her or his needs.

The Bone Density Diet also points out where the gaps in our knowledge are, and as the public becomes more educated about the importance of bone health, the outcry for scientific progress— and the financial support for this necessary work—should grow. I've no doubt that the future will hold still more choices. In the meantime, it is wonderful to have many options in place, all of our options leading us toward the day when low bone density will be a rarity.

—Theresa Galsworthy, R.N., O.N.C.
New York, New York

The Bone Density Program

Chapter 1

The Importance of Being Dense

Maria always watches what she eats, but she's concerned more with nutritional quality than with calories. Until recently, she never had to pay attention to her weight, but ever since she passed 40, it seems to creep up on her if she's not careful. She's probably out buying organic baby spinach and portobello mushrooms and free-range chicken for dinner tonight—if she's done with her three-mile walk—and picking the right wine to go with it. She took a multivitamin this morning that also contains several trace minerals, and before bed tonight she'll take a calcium and magnesium capsule. Her new doctor helped her cut down on the amount of thyroid hormone she was taking to counteract her underactive gland—and her energy level redoubled. Her colleagues at the university are always saying they would mistake her for a student if they didn't know better, and although she always dismisses that as pure flattery, inside she feels no different from how she did in her younger days. Last weekend she wallpapered the nursery at her very pregnant younger sister's house, then went hiking with her old graduate school buddies.

Sheila finally kicked a long-standing fatty-food habit a few years back, after taking a good look at the photos from her surprise 50th-birthday party. She remains a confirmed red-meat eater, but now with smaller servings only a couple of times a week. Just don't ask her to give up cheese! Once she cut out most of the sugary snacks she used to live on, she no longer felt lethargic after she ate, and she never got the uncomfortable sense of fullness that had taken away some of the pleasure of a nice piece of steak. Petite and "fine boned" (as her mother, who gave her daughter her peaches-and-cream complexion, always said), Sheila certainly stands out among many of the employees (who tend to be male and muscular) at the construction firm she founded. She was a devoted jogger for years when that was all the rage, but these days she prefers her ballet classes or swimming laps, even though some days she just can't get to either. But it's not like her company can run itself!

Althea, an African-American accountant—and grandmother of three—recently reached a personal best on the chest press machine at the gym, and was delighted to watch the man following her take the weight down a notch. She became a vegetarian many years ago, partly to keep her large frame healthy despite what the actuarial tables say is a few too many pounds for a woman of her height. These days, she is eating more vegan meals, though she does occasionally eat fish. After she switched from dairy milk to soymilk (calcium fortified)—except in her coffee, where nothing but cream will do—she noticed her on-and-off bouts of indigestion were more off than on. Then she read in a magazine about the heart-healthy and estrogenic effects of soy products, and began to think that maybe all those tofu stir-fries had something to do with her low cholesterol levels and why she never had menopausal symptoms. That's when she got some of that soy protein powder from the gourmet/organic food store in her neighborhood. She liked that store, even though the produce can't really compare with what she grows in her own large garden.

WHAT DOES A HEALTHY WOMAN LOOK LIKE?

Just like you. We are told so often and so much about "female problems" and the many ways women's bodies break down, especially as they age, that sometimes we lose sight of the fact that being healthy should be the norm—in fact, *is* the norm. The vibrant, dynamic women described above are all at different stages of their lives—early 40s, perimenopausal with no symptoms; early 50s, experiencing menopause with no symptoms; and mid-60s, finished with menopause and none the worse for wear.

Each has strong, healthy bones providing the foundation for strong, healthy lives and can expect to keep them. As health-conscious women and intelligent consumers, they are aware of the dangers of osteoporosis—literally "porous bones" (bones with holes) so brittle they can fracture from the force of nothing more than a sneeze—and the associated conditions of osteomalacia (soft bones) and osteopenia (low bone mass). But they haven't surrendered to the hype that makes it seem like a coming plague from which there is no escape (except for the salvation of harsh chemicals), nor the complacency that this simply, inevitably, is a part of growing older. Rather, they've put their energy into strategies much like the ones recommended in this book and have radiant health to show for it.

None of it is an accident. There may be some benefit from "good genes," but each of these women is health conscious and aware of her body and its needs, and takes care to do what is good for it and what feels good. But none has taken quite the same approach to wellness, and not all of them follow a specific plan. They've each made changes and adjustments, particularly at times of shifting hormones, but mostly they are busy living their lives, enjoying their work and their families, their homes and their friends, playing and resting and juggling many demands.

Just like you. Whatever your current situation, whatever your age, whatever your bones look like right now, if you know the right things to do for your body, you too can have the same healthy, active lifestyle as any of these women—and keep it for the rest of your life. You may need to do something differently from what they have, and you may want to try things they haven't. Your body may react differently to whatever tack you do take. But you can learn from them, and the people whose stories are told throughout this book, as well as from the facts and figures laid out here, and work out strategies for yourself to get and keep your bones strong for a lifetime.

USE WHAT WORKS

To do that, you'll want to access every variety of medicine, traditional and "alternative," preventive and therapeutic, pharmacologic and physiologic, cutting-edge and tried-and-true. That's just the wide spectrum I've brought to this book, and the six-week program walks you through all of them so you won't get lost in a tangle of conflicting information, but rather will leave with the best each has to offer.

As an osteopathic physician (more on just what that means in a minute), it's my life's work to integrate all these areas into one system of total wellness, uprooting any problems at their source, rather than focusing on fighting disease or reducing symptoms. In my practice, I work closely with a variety of practitioners, from orthopedic surgeons, endocrinologists, and neurologists to nutritionists, qi gong instructors, herbalists, acupuncturists, stress-reduction counselors, and physical therapists. I didn't learn much in medical school about nutrition or exercise, and certainly nothing about the benefits of tai chi or acupuncture or meditation. But now that I've learned—from colleagues and patients—how to integrate all these methods into my practice, I see my patients getting better and stronger in every way.

This integrative approach means that everything you do with and to your body has a role in how your body feels and performs on a day-to-day basis. What you eat (and don't eat), how you sleep, how and how much you move and which parts of your body you use, what work you do, which people you spend time with—all this makes a profound difference in your health. There is no magic bullet or prescription for a pill you can take to "fix" your bones. Too many doctors are pushing hormone replacement therapy or one of the new pharmacological "cures" for osteoporosis, without even mentioning the proven effects of noninvasive, all-natural approaches like eating foods rich in calcium and getting enough exercise that places demands on your bones, thereby stimulating growth.

The latest drugs the labs are turning out have a valuable place in the arsenal against excessive bone loss, but they should be no one's first choice. My goal with this book is to make sure you never get to the point where you need them. Nonetheless, it's nice to know they're there if you ever do. No matter how effective they are, and no matter how many even better and safer and more potent options emerge in the coming months and years, they are only an adjunct to the essential basics of nutrition, exercise, and hormone balance.

The 6-Week Bone Density Program puts together all the basics on bone density, so that at the end you have a simple, straightforward system of diet, exercise, supplements, and lifestyle *that can save your life*. If you follow the steps laid out here, you'll gradually create a revolution in the way you live that will serve you well for the rest of your life. It's not six weeks and—bam!—you have dense bones forever and ever, amen. It's a way of life, not a time-limited plan. But six weeks is all you need to learn what you need to know, gather all the relevant information, lay in supplies, get used to new things, and put everything in place. Six weeks is all you need to form good habits. Once you do, what right now seems like a deluge of information and advice will become second nature, and you'll no longer have to think consciously about each component of bone health. You'll just be *doing* it, without having to think about it.

There are no easy answers and no instant solutions. But there are plenty of things anyone can do, starting today, no matter what your particular situation or age, that will give you the healthy lifestyle your bones require to maintain peak mass. Plus, there are some altogether pleasant components, like sweatless workouts, relaxation techniques, and mandatory snacks.

IT'S UP TO YOU

Prevention, wellness, and low-tech body wisdom have never been mainstream medicine's strong points. On top of that, for years "women's diseases"—osteoporosis primary among them—have been largely overlooked, or assumed to be the same as in men, or, worse still, unquestioningly tolerated. That tide is finally turning. But as our awareness peaks, we need to make responsible choices. If you take a stroll down the aisles of your local health food store—or even your regular drugstore or grocery store—

you'll be bombarded with products claiming to build your bones or balance your hormones or give you all the calcium you could ever need. Suddenly, bone health is in the air, and the folks on Madison Avenue and in Product Development are clearly going to milk our newfound awareness for all its worth. You can't get all the way through a morning news show, or a woman's magazine, without seeing an ad for a new product (or an improved or en-riched old faithful) that offers the same kind of fountain-of-youth promises. But no matter what the packages promise, there are no magic bullets that go straight to your bones.

This book will sort through the clutter of commercial junk dreamed up by trend-spotting marketers and give you the first complete, integrated program to ensure the health of your bones. We start with a thorough assessment of your level of risk (before you shell out for a bone density scan or even make an appoint-ment for a general checkup). Once you know where you stand, there are no quick fixes, but the holistic program you'll find here is the real deal:

- Foods to eat and foods to avoid to support bone health (or, why kale is better than spinach), the best ways to get cal-cium into your diet and into your bones (and why that isn't enough), and complete menus and recipes to successfully launch you into a new way of eating.
- The nutrients you absolutely need—and how to get them in the proper combinations *and* in the minimum number of pills each day if you choose to use supplements to back up your occasionally imperfect diet.
- The truth about hormones—both "natural" and synthetic—and which ones you need and when, and when you should pass them up altogether, no matter what your gynecolo-gist says.
- The exercises proven to build your bones, and the bone benefits of kinder, gentler forms of movement.

With a comprehensive four-part prevention plan based in these areas, you're unlikely to ever need the chapters on treatment, but if you've already had significant bone loss, which can occur as early as your late 30s, the same areas are crucial to restoring density, strength, and resilience to your bones. As long as you adhere to the 6-Week Bone Density Program, the prescription drugs available for treatment—and some natural options as well—will have their maximum effect. Whatever stage you are at, this book puts all the pieces together into one easy-to-use plan, with help from (among other things):

- Checklists to help you keep track of what medical tests you need—and will probably have to specifically ask for in order to get—and when.
- "Best of" Lists sprinkled through the book give key information at a glance, like the top five easy high-calcium snacks or herbs that aid in digestion or the top ten flavors to try in a creamy tofu spread/dip.
- Action Plans at the end of each week to get you into action.
- Things to Think About to keep you on your toes.
- Fun with Computers tips to point you in the right direction on the information superhighway, where there's a wealth of information and support—and even more advertisements, snake-oil peddlers, outdated or biased information, and well-meaning but ill-informed surfers eager to give their two cents to anyone who will listen.
- Bone Boosters throughout the book give you quick tips to put into practice right away to jump-start your journey to a strong, tall, healthy you.

HYPE AND HOPE

You might like them as an occasional treat, but otherwise you're going to find no place here for so-called energy bars or nutrient shakes that contain way more sugar and fat than calcium or plant chemicals with beneficial hormonal properties. Some new products are more useful than others (like, say, calcium-fortified orange juice or soy milk), but mocha-chip-swirl-whatever is birthday cake, not a serious effort at guaranteeing long-term health and longevity.

The explosion of products may be inevitable in our consumer economy, and it is beneficial in one important way: all the hoopla is putting a crucial health issue that's been overlooked for far too long into the mainstream.

Amid the hubbub, there are also some real advances emerging in bone health. We'll look at the cutting-edge science that explodes some myths and illuminates new truths about bones and how to keep them healthy, whether it's natural hormone supplements without the possible increase in cancer risk, or the latest research on increasing bone density through a simple set of exercises, or the latest pharmacological drug now available for the first time. *But as wonderful as the rapid changes in our understanding are, they are just an adjunct to the most essential information in this book:* the basics of food, exercise, nutritional supplements, and hormones that can give you a lifestyle that prevents the possible devastation of low bone density or restores you to bone health even if you've already experienced loss.

THINGS TO THINK ABOUT

In early tribal hunter-gatherer societies, the end of the child-bearing years freed women to help care for others' children, which made the whole group more efficient survivors. That crucial collective benefit may seem hazier in our modern lives. But we all know women who have hit their own strides after child-rearing is behind them, and the strength and wisdom that come from experience shines through. Facing this transition with a positive outlook founded in the knowledge that the last third of your life consists of much, much more than some kind of chronic estrogen-deficiency disease is the first step to a healthy and happy outcome. Even though challenges may occur, your body is offering you a gift of renewed focus and energy at the start of a new journey.

MY JOURNEY INTO HOLISTIC HEALTH

I knew when I was 5 years old that I would be a doctor, though I couldn't say how that idea got in my head in the first place. As I grew older, my own pediatrician was my inspiration—and the only doctor I knew. He encouraged my interest from an early age, allowing me to come on hospital rounds with him before I had even finished high school. He taught me the most important lesson I ever learned about medicine. As we walked into a patient's room, he paused and told me to pay attention to what I smelled, and listed for me what it might indicate. Just which disease he was teaching me about that day is long gone from my memory, but I've always remembered that moment because suddenly I understood that part of becoming a doctor was learning to use all your senses—and developing a sixth sense, a kind of medical intuition. Medicine was more than science.

That was still very much on my mind when it came time to apply to medical school. Though I applied and was accepted to both traditional and osteopathic programs, where almost all of the coursework and clinical training are identical, in the end I chose osteopathy, which does require extensive additional work focusing on the musculoskeletal system, including bone health. To me the big difference was that osteopathy stressed taking care of the whole person, rather than a specific set of symptoms or a certain group of organs or a particular disease. When I read the passionate works of Andrew Taylor Still, the founder of osteopathic medicine, particularly about the connections among the body, mind, and spirit (a more revolutionary stance at that time), I knew there was no other choice for me. I knew that to really take care of my future patients, I'd need the latest medical research, and cutting-edge technology, and an understanding of the biochemistry that makes the human body work. But I also knew it would be equally important to integrate all aspects of a person's life and health into the hard, cold science. What I saw in holistic medicine that was missing from strictly traditional training was the core belief that a patient is much more than a collection of symptoms.

Even so, my medical training did not feature a course on

"Patients Are People, Too," or "Alternative Medicine, Open-mindedness and You," or "Why a Thorough Physical Takes More than 15 Minutes." Many of the specific details of providing a broad range of quality care I've picked up over the years from colleagues I admire, my own reading, and very often my patients themselves.

CHOOSING THE RIGHT PRACTITIONER

To assemble the right health care team to ensure you get the best overall care, you must act as coordinator to make sure each practitioner has all the relevant information, and that they communicate with each other as necessary. You must tell each professional who else you are working with and what strategies you are using. If you don't tell your cardiologist you've been seeing a homeopath, you won't be able to maximize either approach. If your homeopath tries to convince you homeopathic remedies are all you need, and that whatever your cardiologist advises will only interfere with the treatment, you need a different homeopath. Likewise, if your cardiologist has a blanket "quackery" response for any suggestion of complementary methods, you need a different cardiologist. Otherwise, you have many lenses working on your behalf, but they are all looking at their own little piece and never merging into one view. That's certainly not integrative or complementary or holistic, and you won't reap all the benefits of coordinated health care.

Conventional medicine has brought us many wonderful medicines and technologies. I wouldn't want to diagnose or treat low bone density without access to DEXA machines and pharmaceutical options like raloxifene. But I wouldn't want to do without qi gong or nutritional supplements, either. Both conventional and "alternative" therapies have their limits, and using them in true complementary fashion—according to their strengths and your beliefs and preferences—is the only way to achieve optimal health care and optimal health.

But from the start I was steeped in an atmosphere that focused on preventing illness, which was the only sensible way I could see to approach anything called "health care." I usually spend about half an hour with each patient, talking about diet, stress, exercise, his or her childhood, what the individual did this weekend and what I did this weekend—and then maybe what brought that person in that particular day. I ask patients coming into my practice for the first time to allow an hour and a half for our first consultation. It takes time for me to get to know the people I care for, and for them to get to know and trust me.

As a physician, I see my job as providing patients with all the information they need to make their own decisions. Patients have a duty, then, to learn as much as they can about keeping themselves healthy, and to work *with* their doctors to find strategies and solutions that are right for them. This book will work the same way. I'll give you all the knowledge you need to build and protect the strength of your bones. Your job is to take that ball and run with it. I've laid out a very specific plan of diet, exercise, and nutritional supplements—and conventional and complementary treatments, if that becomes necessary—that will keep you standing tall and strong for the rest of your life. Only you can say which approaches will work for you, which options you want to pursue, and how to incorporate my program into the rest of your life.

THINGS TO THINK ABOUT

Osteoporosis, like menopausal symptoms in general, falls into a kind of no-doctor's-land. The usual choices are gynecologist, internist, or endocrinologist. None specializes in osteoporosis by general training. You'll need to talk with anyone you seek out and get to know a bit about his or her treatment philosophy before you can tell who will work best with you.

My Story: Evelyn

*W*hen a bone scan showed I had bone loss that was serious, but not yet osteoporosis, my family physician referred me to a menopause clinic with a whole team of care providers. I saw an endocrinologist, a pharmacologist, a breast health nurse, and a nutritionist. Everyone was very knowledgeable and supportive, and wanted to help me take steps that would fit in with my life. If you don't like the idea of one pill, they have ten other options to tell you about. The information I got was very individualized, and by the time I went back to my regular doctor, I felt confident in the plan I had in place. For me, that meant weight lifting, aerobic walking, calcium supplements, and Fosamax. HRT hadn't agreed with me, so I was surprised and relieved at how many other ways I could protect my bones.

Women have big choices to make about how to care for their bones, and I can't say enough about what it meant to me to have a network of people pulling together on my behalf, knowing I had the best information in each area available to help me decide what was right for me.

EVERYTHING I NEEDED TO KNOW
I *DIDN'T* LEARN IN MEDICAL SCHOOL

Even with all my training, the women in my life have taught me much I needed to know about health and health care. A few years ago, my older daughter wrote her senior research project on women's medical issues, focusing on how the entire medical system is *not* geared toward humans of the female persuasion. Of course, I was pleased and proud she was showing an interest in medicine, but I teased her at first about being up on her soapbox. It's not like I took a course on how *not* to treat women, I told her, and except for whatever handful of male chauvinist doctors were out there (unfortunate, but unavoidable), I felt sure women received medical care on a par with men. But as she researched, and I thought about the stories my patients brought to me, and we talked, she showed me she was right.

HOW *NOT* TO BE A STATISTIC

- At least 25 million Americans have osteoporosis, and another 34 million people have bone density low enough to be at increased risk of fractures. *Almost all of these cases could have been prevented.*

- At least a third of American women who have been through menopause—and half of women over 65—have osteoporosis. By age 75, the proportion of women with osteoporosis goes up to 89 percent. Up to 18 percent of women ages 25 to 34 already have low bone density—during the years when bones should be at their peak. *Simple steps, starting young, would put all these percentages close to zero.*

- One in two postmenopausal women will break a bone (or bones) as a result of low bone density. *With good bone mass, you may have to worry about your bones if you have a dramatic skiing accident or something of the sort, but tripping over a loose electrical cord will be only annoying, not dangerous.*

- More women have osteoporosis than have heart disease, strokes, diabetes, or arthritis. A woman's risk of having a hip fracture is higher than the combined risk of developing breast, uterine, or ovarian cancer. *Genetics and other factors beyond your control play the largest role in determining whether you get the other diseases, but you have the power to avoid low bone density altogether— and you're holding it in your hand right now.*

- Osteoporosis is a leading cause of death in elderly women. Some studies show a death rate as high as 50 percent within a year after a hip fracture. The rate of death remains higher than otherwise expected for *years* after a hip fracture, even in patients who seem to have made a full recovery. *This easy preventive program can literally save your life.*

- About half of people who fracture a hip are permanently unable to walk unassisted, and never regain their accustomed level of social activity. *Keeping bones healthy and strong keeps you healthy and strong, living the life you choose, no matter how long the run.*

Around this same time, as my wife was going into peri-menopause, she had her first bone density measurement. She came home to report that the radiologist just said that everything was fine. But when a copy of the report arrived in the mail, I saw that it actually showed significant bone loss. At her routine visit to the gynecologist, the doctor didn't comment on the bone scan (which she had received a copy of), but did suggest calcium, exercise, and hormone replacement therapy (HRT), which, aside from the calcium, my wife declined. And so, with just one approach mentioned—and major components rejected—with no "Plan B," no plan for follow-up, no discussion of protective eating strategies or types of exercise or alternatives to standard HRT my wife might find more appealing, these doctors were satisfied to let the whole matter go, without even explaining the potential for serious trouble ahead! Once it hit this close to home, I finally realized the extent of the problem my daughter had pointed out to me. And nowhere was it more extreme than when it came to osteoporosis.

Until recently, bone fragility has been more or less shrugged off as an inevitable part of aging—and basically a woman's lot. Though this is a *totally preventable* disease, the incidence of osteoporosis has been increasing because it hasn't been properly addressed. As some new drugs were approved that provided a real treatment for low bone density for the first time, and I began to get visits from sales reps bearing information on the extent of osteoporosis among women, it became clear just how ignored this health issue had been. Most insurance companies wouldn't even pay for screening tests, and I saw too many of my patients do without the scans that could have given them crucial information for preserving their health and lifestyle, simply because they couldn't afford them. My practice was aging right along with Boomer me, and the topic was coming up more and more often. In talking with my patients with a sharper focus on bone health, I also realized how little information on the topic was available for women. Most patients, even those who could rattle off fat grams and recommended heart rates for aerobic exercise, knew precious little about how to correctly protect their bones—or even of the necessity of doing so. So began my crusade. If the ideal doctor-patient relationship is a true partnership, I saw I was going to have to educate myself *and* my patients if we were going to be able to promote the strongest possible bones.

STEER YOUR OWN SHIP

As I said, every patient has to be the captain of her or his own ship, and that includes my wife. But every captain needs a good first mate, and I was shocked at how little information, counsel, and support my wife was getting from her doctor in that role. I stand by hormone replacement therapy starting just before menopause as an excellent way for most women to protect their bones. But I know there are many reasons, both medical and personal, a woman might not want to use it. So if a case like my wife's came up in my office, I'd have made the same suggestion, HRT, as her doctor did. But first I would explain about bone loss and why, particularly before menopause, it is a serious danger sign. I would also detail what's been proved about how diet, nutritional supplements, and exercise can stop, prevent, or even reverse bone loss. I'd talk with her about how stress can worsen bone loss—and how stress reduction can alleviate it. I'd check her health history, and her family history, to see if she had additional risk factors she should be aware of. Only then would I talk about supplemental hormones, including the many different forms of HRT, as well as "natural" hormones and, in more advanced cases, the best prescription options we have to stop bone loss. If a patient didn't want or didn't need drug treatment, she'd still have all the information she needed to take a proactive approach to her health.

This book takes the same holistic approach to your life and health. Staying strong isn't just a matter of taking hormones, or working out with weights twice a week, or popping calcium pills left and right. In the right combination, those things will help, but bone density is an overall lifestyle issue. You need general good health to maximize bone density. Conversely, maximum bone density will enhance general good health. That's why I'm laying out all you need to know about what you eat, how you exercise, and what you take that affects your bone density (nutritional supplements,

> **DID YOU KNOW?**
>
> Medically, menopause is defined as having no period for a year. The average age for that to happen is 51, with 45 to 55 being the normal range. Perimenopause—the period leading up to menopause during which the ovaries start winding down—covers, on average, four to five years before your periods finally stop.

hormones, prescription drugs, and "alternative" treatments). This book describes all the risk factors you should eliminate or fight, so you can pinpoint your level of risk and tailor your program to your specific needs.

BUILDING A STRONG FOUNDATION

New breakthroughs about bone health are happening every day. There's always some cutting-edge technology described in the medical journals. There are loads of lab tests and diagnostic criteria and better treatments under development, and some of them will no doubt revolutionize the way we care for low bone density. The demand for these advances is high (every baby boom woman has a vested interest), so there's plenty of money in it for those who do the best work. By all means keep up with the news, which will inevitably outpace even an up-to-date book like this one, and choose the best new options to maximize your health.

But this book is not about high technology and cutting-edge science. *This book is about* not *needing treatment.* It's about *not* getting to that point in the first place. It's about avoiding a national health crisis. While I've included as many up-to-the-minute advances as having a deadline allows, I had to admit to myself that things change—and change rapidly—and no matter when the book was finished, I'd hear about something new the next week. *This book is about things that will never change because human bodies and metabolism aren't changing.* This book is about using the best resources available from the full spectrum of options. *This book is about intelligent care of our own bodies.*

Strong, healthy bones are literally the framework for a strong, healthy body. In fact, healthy bones are a necessary foundation for a healthy body, mind, and spirit. (The reverse is also true: a healthy mind and spirit contributes to a healthy body—and so to healthy bones.) Maintaining a natural healthy state that allows healing to occur quickly if illness does strike depends on many factors, of course, but good bones are critical. That's why I'm so concerned that weakened, soft, or brittle bones have reached epic proportions in this country, and that the ages of the people osteoporosis affects seem to be reaching new lows. The fortysome-things I see in my practice are worried. And they should be. Fortunately, *osteoporosis is 100 percent preventable—if* you know what to do.

Low bone density affects your health, longevity, and, perhaps most important, the quality of your life. The worst-case outcome of low bone density is osteoporosis—literally "porous bones." The worst-case outcome of osteoporosis is a combination of sponta-neous fractures, loss of height, deformity, bone pain, decreased mobility, and more. Osteoporosis increases your risk of death, of requiring a nursing home or around-the-clock care, of be-coming bedridden or confined to a wheelchair, and of living with chronic pain.

Fortunately, we now know what to do to keep everyone's bones healthy, and the answer is simple, especially for today's health-conscious woman: proper diet and exercise. That means eating enough protein to allow optimum calcium absorption, but not so much that it requires calcium to be leached from your bones to process it. It means avoiding the insulin burst that comes with eating simple carbohydrates and sugars that can interfere with proper bone metabolism, focusing instead on balancing complex carbohydrates with protein, vegetables and fruits, and heart-healthy fats. It means avoiding the very few foods that negatively impact your bones (sodas being enemy #1), and making sure you get enough of the many foods that help build strong bones, espe-cially the "beans and greens" too many people overlook. And it means moving your muscles against the resistance of your bones to build up strength in both places, as well as more contemplative forms of movement that emphasize flexibility and balance and stress reduction. With smart use of nutritional supplements, and prescription and/or "alternative" approaches as necessary, this six-week program takes you step by step to a lifetime commitment to healthy bones.

We are discovering more about how bone works every day; developments in this field are coming fast and furious. The technology of mainstream Western medicine provides many options for diagnosis and treatment of osteoporosis, and various labs will no doubt be making big breakthroughs as we move forward. But we are also coming to understand more about what "alternative" health traditions have to offer, and in combining these two ways of healing we have a broad enough spectrum of choices to find the right approach for every individual. What everyone agrees on is that what you put in your mouth, and how—and how much—you move your body are essential to healthy bones. This bone density program lays out the smartest strategies for you. It is never too early—or too late—to start. This book shows you how. And it shows you how to evaluate your specific situation and personalize the techniques accordingly. Take care of your bones now, and they will keep you walking tall for a lifetime.

Chapter 2

Healthy Bones, Healthy Body

M eet your bones. I bet you think of them—*if* you think of them at all—as solid like stone, strung together somehow to hold up the rest of you. ("The head bone's connected to the neck bone, the neck bone's connected to the . . .") Most people don't pay any attention to their skeletons unless they've broken something. But bone is living, growing, constantly changing tissue, and will benefit as much from TLC as your heart, muscles, waistline, or other body parts do. Properly cared for, your bones, *all 206 of them*, will give you health, longevity, and quality of life.

To understand the consequences of low bone density, and how to prevent and treat it, it helps to know a little bit about how bones work. So before we get to the nuts and bolts of what to eat and how to move and what to take to keep your bones healthy in the six-week program, here's a very brief physiology lesson. Hang in there with me, and I'll try to make this as painless as possible. Your bones will thank you later.

HOW BONE GROWS

Bone is constructed from calcium and other minerals crystallized on a soft *matrix* (a sort of 3-D frame) of collagen and other proteins. The combination of organic and inorganic materials makes bone both rigid and strong. (Unlike calcium alone—think of how easy it is to snap a piece of chalk, which is made primarily of calcium, in half.) Blood vessels run throughout bone. In the center of each bone you find marrow, where blood cells are made.

Your skeleton is made of two kinds of bone. About 80 percent of it is *cortical bone*, which is hard, dense, and stiff. It makes up the outer shell of most bones, and the long bones in your arms and legs, and most of your hip bones. It is designed to withstand quite a bit of stress. Spongy *trabecular bone* is found inside of cortical casings, in the vertebrae, at the ends of the long bones in your limbs, and in parts of your hips.

> ### THINGS TO THINK ABOUT
>
> Because calcium is vital to all essential functions of the body, Mother Nature makes sure you always have access to it. When you're lacking it anywhere in your system, your body will always take some from Mother Nature's calcium warehouse: the bones.

As bones age, cells called *osteoclasts* seek out old or damaged parts of the bone and dissolve them, which is called *resorption*. Resorption dissolves crystallized calcium and other minerals in your bones, returning them to the blood. This leaves small spaces, and cells called *osteoblasts* create new bone to fill them in. In forming new bone, calcium and other minerals are taken from the blood and crystallized in the bone. The continuous cycle of formation and breakdown is known as *bone remodeling*. When all goes well, this is a constant tit-for-tat for many years, with the osteoblasts (builders) staying just ahead of the osteoclasts (dissolvers) to produce bone that is growing and getting denser—or maintaining good density.

You lose and gain bone this way throughout your lifetime. Remodeling is orchestrated by various hormones, and in later chapters you will see how important maintaining natural levels of hormones is to the health of your bones. Throughout childhood and into young adulthood, bone formation outpaces resorption, so you get taller as your bones get longer, for one thing, and your bones also get wider and denser. But the neat teamwork of osteoblasts and osteoclasts comes uncoupled somewhere around age 35, and bone breakdown can then outpace bone formation—and that's the rub. If the osteoclasts are busier dissolving bone than the osteoblasts are busy making it, your bones actually get holes in them. That's *osteoporosis*—literally, porous bones. Thin bones like that are brittle and fragile, so they fracture easily. Osteoporotic fractures can cause disfiguration, chronic pain, immobility, and even death.

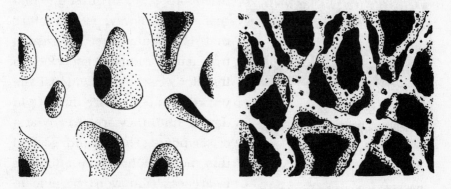

Left. Normal bone (thick bone matrix). Right. Osteoporotic bone (thin and porous bone matrix)

Officially, osteoporosis is divided into two categories. Type I, which is postmenopausal osteoporosis, mainly affects women between 50 and 65, and usually involves trabecular bone more than cortical bone. Type II, which is "age-associated," and the bane of older people, typically involves loss of cortical bone equal to that of trabecular. Osteoporosis known to be caused by a medication or disease (see Chapter 5) is known as secondary osteoporosis.

Osteomalacia, or soft bones, known as rickets in children, is a related concern, occurring when minerals don't crystallize on the bone matrix properly (often due to lack of vitamin D, which you need to make use of the calcium, phosphorus, and magnesium—not to mention vitamins A and E). With osteomalacia, you don't have enough calcium and phosphorus forming into bone, but that alone is not the same as osteoporosis. Osteoporosis involves lack of other minerals as well, along with a decrease in bone matrix.

For healthy bones, both bone mass and bone quality are key. Osteomalacia can be a precursor of osteoporosis.

Another precursor is *osteopenia*, which means simply low bone mass: density that is lower than normal, but not low enough to lead to fractures. This is a warning sign that osteoporosis—which does lead to a high rate of fractures—is on its way unless you take action.

> ### THINGS TO THINK ABOUT
>
> The Rule of 100:
> - 100% of the population is at risk for osteoporosis.
> - 100% of cases of osteoporosis are preventable.
> - 100% of cases of osteoporosis are treatable.
>
> But there is no cure. Prevention is always easier and more effective than treatment.

Far too often, the first sign of osteoporosis (or the first one that gets read, anyway) is a fracture that is spontaneous or results from a minor impact, especially in the hip, wrist, or spine. Most victims don't even realize they are in danger until they are already at a crisis point. The second goal of this book, after prevention, is awareness. You won't be able to protect yourself and keep yourself healthy unless you know you are at risk.

If you know their significance, there are other signs that your bones are already in trouble. Bad back pain, especially in the lower back, or other bone pain, is a common symptom, as is a decrease in height. Deformity is also a signal, particularly kyphosis—dowager's hump or hunchback—resulting from multiple fractures in the vertebrae that cause the vertebrate to become wedged together and the spine to collapse. Several other signs, especially if clustered together, may be pointing toward osteoporosis: leg and foot cramps, especially at night, extreme fatigue, large amounts of plaque on the teeth, periodontal disease, loss of teeth, brittle or soft fingernails, premature graying, and heart palpitations. Especially in the case of these more amorphous associations, you should rule out everything else before you pin the cause on osteoporosis or low bone density. Don't panic because you need your teeth cleaned more than every six months: you might just have a super-conscientious dentist, or need a better brushing/flossing routine, or you just have a lot of plaque.

HEALTHY BONES

You can wind up with low bone density two different ways. One, you could have an *accelerated loss of bone mass*, which is what happens to women at menopause. Or you could have *slowed bone growth*. The latter is currently harder to deal with. We are better at slowing loss than spurring new growth, though new developments in this area are coming fast and furious.

Resorption itself isn't the enemy. Destroying old or weak bone cells to make way for stronger new bone is crucial for healthy bones. Without remodeling, even dense bone wouldn't be healthy bone. In fact, many people who suffer fractures as a result of minor trauma have bones with normal density—but poor bone quality. The strategies presented in this book are specifically aimed at creating and maintaining good bone density, but will also give you generally healthy bones (as well as overall good health). The goal is not to stop bone breakdown but to foster the appropriate interrelationship between resorption and formation, making it as close to how it works in healthy young people as possible.

The breakdown of bone takes place relatively quickly, and the better part of each 120-day remodeling cycle is devoted to synthesizing new bone (making the proteins for the matrix as well as assembling the minerals that crystallize on it). Many chemicals in your body signal the starting and stopping of resorption and formation, including thyroid and parathyroid hormones, growth hormone, estrogen and testosterone, and others. The rate at which bone is made and broken down is also affected by calcium intake and your body's usage of it once it has it (which is in turn regulated by a series of hormones), and the amount of stress placed on the bone (such as from weight-bearing exercise).

When your body gets too many green lights for remodeling, you may get a quickening of the pace at which bone is formed, but it won't be enough to keep up with the increase in breakdown.

That's just what happens with the drop in estrogen in menopause, or with any condition that entails an imbalance of hormones (like hyper- or hypothyroidism, for example). Lack of calcium, too, can signal bone remodeling, perhaps prematurely. In addition, rapid turnover of bone cells usually yields bone of low quality, even if the quantity is normal. That's why, once again, this book is designed not just to build bone but to build and maintain healthy bone.

BONE LOSS

Over the course of your life, you go through four phases of bone development. For the first part of your life, you build bone. You then have a relatively short plateau phase, when you're maintaining the bone mass you've built up at basically peak levels. As you age, resorption overtakes formation, giving you a third phase, this one of bone *loss*. The fourth stage is also one of loss, but with the additional complication of formation and deposition slowing down (as well as breakdown picking up).

Throughout infancy and childhood and into young adulthood, your bones are growing longer, wider, and thicker, and getting denser *(phase one)*. Adolescence is a particularly busy time for your bones, as the sex hormones that drive puberty also spur bone growth. Half of all bone is made during the teen years. Even after you stop growing taller (and your bones stop growing longer), bone mass still increases as long as formation stays ahead of resorption. By the time you are 20, 90 percent of your bone mass is set. You still build, slowly, for a few more years, and reach peak bone density in your mid to late 20s. You generally stay there for about a decade *(phase two)*.

But by age 35 or so, you start *phase three*. Just about everyone begins to experience a slow decline in bone mass—0.5 to 1 percent a year—as resorption proceeds faster than deposition. For women, there is a drastic increase in the rate of bone loss for the first five to ten years after menopause—jumping to 3 to 5 percent lost each year—because of the decrease in estrogen (for women not taking hormone replacement therapy) and progesterone. Postmenopausal osteoporosis shows up in women between the ages of 50 and 65, generally. It is no surprise that the fracture rate accelerates greatly ten to fifteen years after menopause.

Women who undergo surgical menopause (having their ovaries removed) lose twice as much bone as other women at menopause, because even after menopause the ovary produces a small amount of estrogen, along with other hormones important to bone health. Women who have a hysterectomy but keep their ovaries also lose bone at an accelerated rate (though not as quickly as women with no ovaries), probably because the uterus makes vitamin D, which is necessary for healthy bones. Rapid bone loss may begin a year or two before your period actually stops, especially in the spine (and other trabecular bone). In fact, the rate of hip fractures rises dramatically for women in their early 40s, well before the average age of menopause. Over a third of premenopausal women lose bone faster than even the expected rate of loss, and for them, taking action is particularly important.

Men, too, have an acceleration in bone loss, but not until much later, around ages 60 to 65, probably connected to the decrease in testosterone. Without additional complications, they never lose as much as women do in menopause, but still, losing 1 percent of bone mass a year really adds up.

Eventually, the rate of loss slows again (for women) to about 1 percent a year throughout the rest of their lives, putting men and women on an equal footing by that point. But now you have an additional problem (phase four): your rate of bone formation is slowing down too, so you have more to contend with than just overenthusiastic bone breakdown. We absorb less calcium as we get older and make less vitamin D, meaning that bodies have less in the way of raw material to work with in building bone. On top of that, the older we get, the poorer our overall diets tend to be, for a variety of reasons. Combined with lower than optimal levels of hormones, low bone density becomes a serious risk.

Over an average lifetime, a woman loses 30 to 40 percent of her total bone mass, and a man about 20 to 30 percent. By age 80, many women have lost two-thirds of their skeletons. Because trabecular (spongy) bone is softer to begin with, most bone loss begins there. Loss in the spine begins as early as the 20s. Cortical bone is denser to begin with, and loss there generally doesn't occur at all until after age 50. Overall, more trabecular bone than cortical bone is lost. In the years just after menopause when the most bone is lost, women lose about 10 percent of their cortical mass and 25 percent of their trabecular bone mass, before the rate of loss slows again, and end up with a lifetime decrease of about 35 percent of cortical bone and 50 percent of trabecular. It is the dramatic decrease in trabecular bone (predominant in the spine) that causes women to shrink—losing up to 6 inches of height by the time they are 80. Men lose about 25 percent of the total of both kinds of bone over their lifetimes.

After bone loss starts, each decade increases your risk of fracture about one and a half times. A high rate of bone turnover puts you at increased risk regardless of your bone density, and low bone density most certainly ups your risk. The younger you are when your bone loss begins or quickens, the higher your risk of fractures will be later in life. That's just another way to say it's never too early to start on the 6-Week Bone Density Program. It is also never too late.

Chapter 3

Your Family and Bone Density

Most of this book is aimed at women in perimenopause and beyond, because they are most at risk—and most likely to know they are at risk—for low bone density. But the 6-Week Bone Density Program works for everyone—any age, both sexes—who wants to create a healthy foundation for a healthy life. I've already mentioned that it is never too early or too late to get or keep your bones healthy. We need to raise our awareness that men are definitely at risk, too, which is why I wanted to take some time out to address the male of the species here. For women reading this chapter, the take-home message is: this book *isn't* just for you. Your parents, children, partners, and friends need healthy bones, too, and the strategies here will work for all of them.

Most important—for both sexes—is the fact that the very best way to avoid low bone density is to reach the point when your body naturally starts to lose bone mass with the healthiest, densest bones possible. You can do this only while you are young. Very young. This book is predicated on the fact that you can make or keep your bones healthy at any age, but the fact of the matter is you get only one opportunity to create maximum bone density naturally. That window is wide open from birth through adolescence and into young adulthood. Once it closes, though, there are no "do-overs." You'll still have many effective options for protecting your bones, but you'll be fielding a team of second-string players, truth be told. The first-round draft picks are reserved for kids.

For the first quarter-century or so of your life, bone formation outpaces breakdown. Infants' bones rapidly grow longer and wider, adding calcium at a terrific rate. Lengthening and widening continues through childhood, while density and thickness also increase. The process speeds up still more during adolescence. Teenage growth spurts (between 11 and 15 for girls and 12 and 17 for boys) are a result of peak bone growth rates, and a fifth of full adult height is generally added during those times. Bone mass keeps building even after teens are no longer growing taller, and by the age of 20, 90 percent of total bone density is set.

Myth: Osteoporosis is something only menopausal women have to worry about.

Fact: Low bone density affects both men and women, and the best time to prevent it is before you're old enough to legally buy a beer.

If you want to give your children a gift that truly keeps on giving, help them develop healthy habits early. The best way to prevent low bone density and all its attendant problems is through good nutrition, adequate calcium intake, and plenty of exercise in childhood and adolescence. If you teach them well, not only will you help them build up all the bone density their genetic potential calls for, but you will also start them out with the kind of healthy lifestyle that will serve them well for a hundred reasons throughout their entire lives.

Genetics is holding most of the cards when it comes to determining peak bone mass. But the outcome of the game is by no means a foregone conclusion. One study of identical twins ages 6–14 showed that the twin given 1,800 mg of calcium a day up to puberty had bones 5 percent more dense than the other twin, given 900 mg a day. That 5 percent increase translates into a 40 percent drop in the risk of fracture later in life. Proper diet is your ace in the hole for reaching the genetic potential for bone density. Children need basically what adults need—which is laid out in the later part of this book. But I want to point out here some of their unique requirements in regard to calcium, and give you some hints for encouraging good habits in those who don't, say, share your enthusiasm for green leafy vegetables.

The average American child does not get enough calcium. Worse still, intake is generally falling. The typical child's diet now contains only about half the calcium it did fifty years ago. Most kids get only about 75 percent of the RDA for calcium. Girls in particular shortchange themselves after reaching the double digits, when weight concerns become common, and they tend not to eat enough nutritious food. They tend to cut back on "fattening" milk and dairy products, and "diet" primarily by drinking a lot of diet sodas. That's disastrous for any bones, but especially for growing bones.

For the first 6 months of life, babies should be getting 400 mg of calcium daily. As long as babies are exclusively drinking breast milk or formula, they will get basically what they need, but as you begin introducing solid food, you should be sure to include a variety of dairy products (and other good sources of calcium) as soon as your pediatrician OKs them. (All breast-fed babies do need liquid vitamin D supplements to make sure they can use the calcium they get.) From 6 to 12 months, infants need 600 mg a day, so it is best if they have several calcium-rich foods in their repertoires. After the first birthday, the calcium requirement goes up to 800 mg and increases again at age 6 to between 800 and 1,200 mg. Eleven-year-olds need 1,200–1,500 mg, and everyone should keep that up through age 24. (That's 5 cups of milk a day, to give you some perspective.) For girls, the period just before puberty brings the highest demand for calcium of any age, and bone builds at its fastest pace through about four years after the first period.

Studies have linked eating a wealth of dairy products—and so calcium—in childhood with greater bone density in adulthood. It is best to get calcium from food as much as possible, using fortified food and supplements if backup is needed. Dairy products will be the first choice for most children. Kids younger than 6

HOW MUCH CALCIUM DO KIDS NEED?	
Age	**Daily Amount**
Birth–1 year	600 mg
1–5	800 mg
6–10	800–1,200 mg
11–24	1,200–1,500 mg

need 3 cups of milk (or the equivalent—there are 300 or so mg of calcium in 1 cup) every day, pushing the tally up to 4 cups for those 6 and older and 5 cups for teenagers. That's got to mean serving milk with every meal and snack. (Hint: There's nothing wrong with mixing in a bit of chocolate syrup to entice reluctant milk drinkers.) Using low- or nonfat products for everyone over 2 will protect their hearts and weight while providing a smidge more calcium than whole milk. For bonus points, if you see one of those milk mustache ads with a celebrity your child thinks is "the coolest," point it out.

Even the straightforward solution of simply getting enough glasses of milk or cups of yogurt can be a tough goal for kids, just as it is for adults. Especially for girls, or nonmilk drinkers, a calcium supplement may be the way to go. More and more children's chewable vitamins are including calcium these days, though you'll have to read the label carefully to determine just how much is in the pills labeled "Extra Calcium!," since some are better sources than others. The levels are still pretty low in the multivitamins, so you might want to choose a separate supplement. Try a liquid or chewable form, or a flavored antacid (making sure you get the kind without any aluminum). See Chapter 9 on calcium for details about the best way to use calcium supplements, just keeping in mind the appropriate dose for your children's ages (see above).

Kids, too, need vitamin D to help their bodies use the calcium they get. Studies show that children who don't consume enough products fortified with vitamin D have inadequate calcium absorption and slowed bone formation, particularly during winter.

We already know our children watch too many hours of television, but here's another result of that you may not have considered: by being glued to the tube, they are spending too much time indoors and don't get enough sunlight to allow their bodies to make the vitamin D they need (see Chapter 10 on supplements).

After lack of calcium, the other biggest hurdle to good bone development in young people is how much soda they drink. Sound like any adults you know? Sodas contain lots of phosphorus, which interferes with bone formation (see Chapter 6). The caffeine in many sodas also contributes to the problem by increasing the excretion of calcium (taking it out of the body, rather than it going into the bones). Anyone who drinks an excessive number of sodas will have parathyroid hormone levels that are constantly at the highest end of the normal range, which is enough to slow the rate at which new bone cells are deposited where they are needed. Encourage your child to choose drinks wisely, and set a good example yourself. Unless you have a most unusual kid, you'll never get away with "Do as I say and not as I do." Actions speak louder than words.

You have complete control over your children's diet for only a short time. This is a good time to teach them to love wholesome, nutritious foods before they even discover the plethora of junk food out there in the wider world. You can't make them eat or not eat any particular food, so your best bet is to prepare them to make their own smart choices. The habits formed in the earliest years—whether good or bad—are hard to shake. Even children as young as 9 will make informed decisions about taking care of their health—*if* they have the information. They may be getting some lessons at school, but you can't count on that (or on what exactly they are taught), so you'll have to take an active role. At any rate, studies show that the teenagers with the healthiest diets have parents who are educated about and concerned with health issues. Despite the latest vogue for the notion that peers have more influence on kids than their parents do, that's proof that children absorb a huge amount both from what their parents themselves do and from what parents say to them.

I'm not giving away any secrets by telling you it is a tough job to get teenagers to change their ways. That's one more reason that the earlier kids learn good health habits, the better it is for them. Don't try to dictate to adolescents what they put into their bodies. It didn't work when getting pierced was at issue, and it won't work when milk vs. soda is the topic. Teenagers need space to practice making their own decisions, asserting themselves, and standing up to peer pressure—with a lot of support from the adults in their lives, particularly their parents. Girls especially also need to develop a strong positive body image and a sense of their own control over their lives, their health, and their bodies. By age 20, young adults should be more open to taking charge of their health. By then your job as a parent/nutrition counselor is mostly done—and so is the task of building up bone.

So don't sit back and wait for them to be ready to educate themselves. Encourage them as much as you can. You'll have to use every trick in the book. No one knows your kids better than you, and different strategies work better at different ages, so you'll have to map out your own course.

TIPS AND TRICKS FOR GETTING CALCIUM INTO KIDS

Here are a few things to try (you may like them too!):

- Try flavoring milk with a little bit of vanilla extract (or whatever other flavor your child likes), or, if you can't get away without the sugar, use a bit of flavored syrup. Even better, at the health food store, look for the herb stevia in a powdered form. Stevia is many times sweeter than sugar, but is extremely low in calories. Sprinkle some of the powder in milk or yogurt instead of sugar, honey, or syrup.

- Yogurts marketed for kids, especially, are nothing more than desserts, with sprinkles and candies and all kinds of "mix-ins." That may be fun for a treat, but it isn't particularly healthy if they are eating one every day. Try to keep it simple. Some kids will eat plain yogurt spruced up with a drop or two of food coloring, or some fruit—avoiding the huge dose of sugar that comes with the packaged kinds. Or let them mix their own with jelly or jam (try the all-fruit varieties)—they'll still get less sugar than what's in the prepared containers.

- Have grated Parmesan cheese as a regular condiment on your table. It is relatively low in fat—for cheese—and adds a nice bit of flavor to a lot more than a plate of spaghetti (though of course it is good there, too). It's a much better choice than butter on steamed vegetables, for example, or on a baked potato or rice. And you'll be sprinkling on a bit of calcium each time you use it.

- Let your children cook with you. If they are ever going to eat kale, the odds are greater they'll try it if they worked to make it.

- Even kids who don't like vegetables might eat "cream of . . ." soups. Make them yourself with low-fat dairy products paired with a high-calcium vegetable. You can't do much better nutritionally than homemade cream of broccoli soup.

- Pack shelf-stable milk-in-a-box instead of juice boxes for lunch. Half the fun is in poking the little straw through the hole anyway, so what is inside may matter less than you think even to a finicky child.

- Explore the limits of macaroni and cheese. I've yet to meet a kid who didn't like the dish, and he or she might be willing to expand beyond the bright yellow boxed variety. Try mixing part-skim ricotta and grated Parmesan with a little of the pasta cooking water to make a sauce, and toss with the drained noodles. Or make your own baked mac and cheese—old-fashioned comfort food that is also rich in calcium (you'll have to watch the fat content).

- Pizza! With vegetable toppings, this reliable favorite is a reasonable choice because of the calcium in the mozzarella. Try making your own, and you can go the Olde Pizza Shoppe one better by using nonfat or low-fat cheese. When you're in a hurry, the English muffin pizza will be a hit.

- Bean burritos—assemble your own—are as healthy as they are popular, since both beans and cheese will give you calcium. Use low-fat or nonfat cheese and refried beans to keep the calorie and fat counts down. Try a calcium triple play by including some steamed greens in your tortilla.

- Use less water when reconstituting powdered milk, or stir some of the powder into regular nonfat milk, to increase the amount of protein and calcium you get in a glass. Or try adding dried milk to smoothies, milk shakes, baked goods, pancake and waffle batter, or milk-based soups and sauces.

- Try serving cottage cheese, yogurt, or salmon salad (from canned salmon, bones in) in an ice cream cone for a fun—and calcium-rich—lunch.

- Provide a small cookie cutter along with a slice of cheese, and let your child create fun shapes to eat.

- Experiment with different combinations of milk, calcium-fortified soy milk, yogurt, ice, and fruit to perfect the smoothie. For a double shot of calcium, you can mimic an Orange Julius by mixing frozen calcium-fortified orange juice concentrate, milk or calcium-fortified soymilk—plain or vanilla—ice cubes, and (the secret ingredient) a splash of vanilla extract in the blender.

- Try freezing regular flavored yogurt to serve instead of commercial frozen yogurt. As I've said, packaged yogurt is often more like a dessert anyway, but it is still more nutritious than what they do sell as dessert. If it is too hard for your taste once frozen (though it can be fun to shave it down bit by bit with your spoon), try freezing it in an ice cube tray, then crushing the cubes in a blender or food processor to get a consistency more like that of soft ice cream.

- Above all, eat right yourself. Try new things. Your kids are watching.

MEN AND BONE DENSITY

Osteoporosis has been thought of as a woman's disease. National statistics show that 5 million men in this country have osteoporosis—and 20 million women. Less conservative ways of looking at it still indicate that men are only half as likely to get osteoporosis as women. Of the whopping annual bill for all the health care costs

KIDS ON THE MOVE

Besides eating right, kids need exercise, just like adults. There are ways you can help in this area, too:

- Set a good example. Let your child see you committed to fitness—and enjoying exercise.
- Exercise together. Ride bikes as a family. Invite your child to go jogging with you. Spend a Saturday hiking a nearby nature trail or mountain. Sign up for a parent/child dance or martial arts class. Make a weekly date to do an exercise video together. Learn how to in-line skate together. Whatever kind of movement you get excited about, share it. And let your child's enthusiasm be contagious.
- Encourage your children's interest in whatever sports catch their fancy. Resist the urge to focus on winning, and remember the joy of the game and the satisfaction of playing as well as you can. Don't force your children into a sport (or to continue in a sport). Let them find what suits them.
- Fitness and exercise is something kids need to do with their friends, too, not just a parent. It has to be *fun*, and something they'll want to do on their own. By all means, spend active time together, but also encourage their independent pursuits.
- Make it a point to spend time together outside every day, or at least every weekend day, and *move*. Play catch or tag, chase squirrels, shoot hoops, walk to the playground, pretend you are kangaroos and HOP . . . now, that's quality time.

racked up by low bone density patients, about 20 percent is for men.

The medical community is twenty years behind in evaluating men for bone density, just as it is only in the last twenty years that women have begun to be screened, diagnosed, and counseled on prevention (though many people can remember similar symptoms for generations back in their own families). As more men are screened, more will be diagnosed, and the total number of people with osteoporosis will be higher, as will the proportion of male patients.

Even before men will be in the unenviable position of having "caught up" to women, don't make the mistake of taking the "more women than men" outlook to mean that small numbers of men are affected. Best estimates are that between 4 and 9 million American men have low bone density. Bone loss severe enough to have health consequences plagues half of men over 75. Under 65, more women than men are affected—though surely not by as wide a margin as official numbers dictate, since we don't really screen men for low bone density. After age 65, the rates equalize.

Men take longer to show the symptoms of extremely low bone density, but once they do, they fare even worse than women in similar circumstances. For example, one study showed that half of men who break a hip leave the hospital only to go to a nursing home—and the vast majority of them are still there a year later. Far fewer than half ever regain the full level of ability they had before the fracture.

Men have heavier body frames than women, generally weigh more and have more muscle mass, and tend to be more physically active, so they build up more bone density to begin with (about 30 percent more, according to best estimates). Their diets are higher in calories on average, so they are more likely to get enough calcium. Hormones play an important

> **DID YOU KNOW?**
>
> One in five men over 65 will break a bone (or bones) as a result of low bone density.

> **THINGS TO THINK ABOUT**
>
> More Americans die from fractures related to osteoporosis each year than from heart attacks related to high cholesterol. Yet cholesterol checks are a routine part of a standard checkup, while many insurance companies still won't cover the cost of basic bone density screening—and many doctors still don't see a reason to insist on it.

Case in Point: Bob

Bob was only in his mid-50s when he came to see me. He'd had scoliosis for years, and was already developing a "hunchback" appearance. He got little exercise and ate a generally poor diet. Stress was his middle name. The x-rays to monitor his scoliosis showed small fractures in his vertebrae, which accounted for the forward curve in his upper back. A DEXA scan then showed his bone density was 18 percent below ideal levels in the spine and 34 percent lower than it should have been at the hip. Bob was a walking accident-waiting-to-happen. Even if good luck and balance kept him upright and unharmed, I knew the curve of his back could cause compression fractures in the spine that would be painful and debilitating and lead to even more pronounced scoliosis.

I encouraged Bob to commit to an exercise program—one that would minimize risk of injury until his bones were stronger—and he began attending a daily class that combined nonimpact weight-bearing movements and stretching (sort of an informal tai chi). He also made significant changes in his diet, and began taking supplements that filled in the gaps in what he ate.

But Bob's bone loss was already so significant he couldn't rely on diet and exercise alone to restore it, so I prescribed alendronate (see Chapter 20). Within several weeks, Bob reported that he felt great, which was probably the improved diet and exercise kicking in. After a year, his bones had regained five percentage points of lost bone mass, and his risk of fracture was greatly decreased. Assuming he sticks with eating right and getting enough exercise, Bob should get his bones back up to normal density within a few years. But if he and his doctors had been aware of his increased degree of risk—despite being young and male—due to scoliosis, he could have taken preventive measures sooner and spared himself all of this.

role in all bone growth, and for men it is their dominant sex hormone—testosterone—that promotes healthy bones. Testosterone levels in men do drop as they age, but not as early or as steeply as estrogen does in women. For men, bone loss doesn't accelerate until ten years or more after it does for women, and then proceeds at a slower rate, around 1 percent a year. Men also don't live as long as women, so they just plain don't have as much time to add up bone losses—on average. In all, men lose just two-thirds the amount of bone women do. But that is still more than enough to lead to serious trouble.

Men share all the same risks as women, and I don't want to see any more men have the first sign of any trouble with their bone density be a life-threatening hip fracture. Any men with significant risk factors as outlined in the upcoming chapters—and all men over 65—need to be every bit as concerned as women already are. The bone density diet will be good for any skeleton, male or female, and men should follow all the same guidelines as women. The one exception: for much of their lives, men's calcium requirement is slightly different (lower) than women's. They should get 1,000 mg a day after 25 and before 65. After that, men and women are even in calcium needs as well as low bone density risk, and should increase their intake to 1,500 mg a day. During the time everyone is building up bone mass to peak levels (before age 25), the recommendations for males and females are also the same.

Culturally, we just haven't considered bone density to be something that concerns men. Doctors don't ask men about it or talk to them about prevention; women talk among themselves about taking calcium and lifting weights, but don't discuss osteoporosis with the men in their lives; health-savvy adult children broach the topic with their aging mothers but not their fathers; men don't have the awareness they need to avoid this completely preventable condition. It is past time we all did.

Case in Point: Albert

Albert, in his 70s, had been undergoing thyroid treatment for years, and came to me for back pain and stiffness, complaining he could no longer play golf. I ordered x-rays to evaluate his postural problems and found his bones to be "see-through"—not an uncommon finding for someone taking synthetic thyroid hormone for so long. For the bone loss to be clear on an x-ray, I knew it was severe, and a bone density scan revealed that, indeed, his bone density was 15 percent below normal for his age at the hip. (Fifteen percent may not sound alarming, but the average for a man in his 70s is already very low.)

Albert had seen doctors a couple of times a year for decades prior to these x-rays, but he had never been advised to take preventive steps to protect his bone density. His primary care physician had asked an endocrinologist well known for treating osteoporosis to consult on the thyroid treatment, but neither doctor had looked for early signs of osteoporosis or explained precautionary measures like diet, exercise, or testing that could have made all the difference in the world. Too many doctors are still operating under the false assumption that osteoporosis is something only women get.

Albert's back pain cleared up after a few visits to my office for osteopathic manipulation, and for continuing treatment of his osteoporosis he went back to his usual doctor for prescription medication to stop his bone loss as quickly as possible. There are a lot of good options available to him now, but simply knowing about the proactive measures as soon as he started thyroid treatment could have kept him out of my office indefinitely. I'm always pleased to lose a patient that way.

FIND OUT WHERE
YOU'RE STARTING FROM

Before you can use a map to get somewhere, you have to know where you are starting from. Only once you find the "You Are Here" sign can you (1) make sure you have the right map, and (2) orient yourself and make a plan. So the first week of the program is designed to put you on the map. Your first assignment is just to get the lay of the land.

This and every week, you'll read a few chapters to give you the background information you need in order to choose what is right for you. At the end of the section, an Action Plan will guide you through the specific steps you need to take to start maximizing your bone health.

At Week 1, start with the quiz in Chapter 4 to assess your level of risk. In the next two chapters, you'll walk through the risks in more detail, to learn how to make the best of what you're stuck with and avoid as many of the hazards as you can. With the final chapter on the screening tests—and deciding which ones you'll need—you'll be ready to meet with your doctor and get baseline measurements as you start on your bone-building plan. "Decade Planners" help you keep track of which tests are the most helpful at each stage of life.

At the end of this section—and each of the other five weeks of the program—there's an Action Plan to help you on your way. With specific steps to get you on the road to strong healthy bones, and questions and reviews to help you pull out and organize the information relevant to your particular situation, you'll have everything you need to put what you're learning to work for you—and your bones—right away.

I'm going to give you a head start on this week's projects by telling you the first assignment now: get out a blank notebook. Because there's a lot of detailed and crucial information throughout this book, I encourage you to keep track of what's most important to you as you go along. Start by recording your score on the quiz in the next chapter, and the problem areas the following two chapters point up for you.

As you follow the plan you've personalized for yourself, and as your bone density improves, you'll periodically need to re-establish your goals. So keep your notebook, and revise as needed. The program you start out with will not necessarily be the same one for your entire life.

Chapter 4

Rate Your Risk

Before you spring into action for prevention or treatment of low bone density, I want you to find out just what your own status is. The self-test in this chapter can't tell you whether you have osteoporosis, but it can help you add up and weigh your personal risks. That way, by the time you appear in the doctor's office, you'll have a handle on the situation and will be able to intelligently discuss your concerns and options. And, as you move farther into this book, you'll know which sections need your closest attention.

The good news is that whatever your potential risk, you *can* reverse it. Two full chapters of the various risks—many of them rampant throughout the United States—follow this one, but don't panic, or worse, give up. You *should* feel a bit scared about what bone loss can do to you. It's been shrugged off for too long as an inevitable part of aging. Now that we know better, for you to needlessly experience the serious health consequences of bone loss would be a tragedy. And a little fear is probably good for your motivation to make the necessary changes in your life.

But don't lose sight of the main point: It is never too late. No matter what your current situation, no matter your age, no matter how many points you rack up below or how many mental check marks you put next to items in the next two chapters, no matter how much you dislike drinking milk or how inept you feel in aerobics class, there are ways you can preserve—and even rebuild—your bone density. Ideally, you start young with healthy habits that build the strongest bone possible before your rate of bone breakdown matches or surpasses your rate of bone formation. If you're 45 and looking back at a lifetime of junk-food days and couch-potato nights, you'll obviously have more work to do than someone who was a charter member of the health food co-op with a long-standing jogging habit. But even if you're an 80-year-old woman who never even considered hormone replacement therapy and has a checkered past when it comes to diet and exercise, you'll be able to build up your bones enough to give you a good shot at avoiding any future trouble. The older you are and the less prepared your past leaves your bones, the more aggressive you'll have to be. Some people will need treatment as well as prevention. *Everyone* will benefit from preventive measures.

FUN WITH COMPUTERS

At *www.agingresearch.com*, you can get your life expectancy estimated by answering a short series of questions about your health habits covering everything from eating vegetables to flossing to taking selenium to being a couch potato. The calculation isn't aimed at bone density directly, but living to 100 in excellent health (the goal of the researchers behind the site) will certainly require strong bones. Here, you can get a good idea of how long a journey you're going to need your bones for and—if you don't like the first answer it gives you—what changes you need to make to get you there.

The following quiz, adapted and expanded from a self-evaluation put together by Michael T. Murray, M.D., will help you see just where you stand—and what you need to do to get to where you *want* to stand. Just working through the items will give you a good idea of what the risks are, though the next two chapters will explain them in more detail. The point system weights the importance of each positive and negative step relative to the other factors listed. You'll learn which things should cause you the most concern and therefore which things you should work first and hardest to change. You'll also see that you don't have to follow the diet laid out in this book to perfection in order to have perfectly healthy bones for a lifetime. Doing 80 percent of what is recommended would be enough to keep most people's skeletons strong. So if you just can't give up that double espresso after lunch, if you do reasonably well with the other points, I say, don't sweat it.

RATE YOUR RISK OF LOW BONE DENSITY

Part I: Things You Can't Change

	Points
Frame (choose one)	
Small-boned; petite	10
Medium or large frame; lean	5
Medium frame; heavy or average weight	0
Ethnicity (choose one if applicable)	
Caucasian	10
Asian	10
General Health (choose as many as apply)	
Woman postmenopausal	30
Man over 65	20
Hypogonadism (in men): low levels of testosterone	20
Family history of osteoporosis, or of losing height, dowager's hump, or frequent fractures	20
Long-term use of corticosteroids	20
Long-term use of anticonvulsant	20
Long-term treatment for hypothyroidism	20
Long-term hyperthyroidism	15
Surgical removal of ovaries or premature menopause	10
Never bore children (for women)	10
Pregnancy without taking calcium, vitamin D, and other nutritional supplements	10
Breastfeeding without taking calcium, vitamin D, and other nutritional supplements	10

Chemotherapy	10
Type I diabetes	10
Long-term, frequent use of antacids containing aluminum	10
Poor diet through childhood, adolescence, and/or young adulthood	10
Poor exercise habits through childhood, adolescence, and/or young adulthood	10
Former smoker	5–10

Part II: Things You Can Change

General Health *(choose as many as apply)*

Drink more than 3 alcoholic beverages per week	20
Smoke 10 or more cigarettes a day	20
Smoke fewer than 10 cigarettes a day	10
Drink more than 1 cup of caffeinated coffee per day	10
Seldom get outside in sun and don't take vitamin D supplement	10
Take hormone replacement therapy	−20
Use of natural progesterone perimenopausally	−20

Diet *(choose as many as apply)*

Drink more than 1 soda daily (including club soda, but not seltzer)	10–20
Long-term consumption of more than 12 oz. of meat daily	20
Eat more than 4 oz. of meat daily	10
High-protein weight control plan for more than a year	10
Consume 3–5 servings of vegetables per day	−10
Consume at least 1 cup of green leafy vegetables each day (in *addition* to the 3–5 servings above)	−10
Consume a vegetarian diet (with proper supplementation if strictly vegetarian, or vegan)	−10
Include large serving of soy foods in diet daily	−10
Consume NIH-recommended level of calcium for your age (see page 144) each day, through food and/or supplements	−20

Exercise *(choose one)*

How often do you do at least 30 minutes of weight-bearing exercise (working your muscles against gravity) like walking briskly, dancing, doing yoga or tai chi, or weight lifting?

Seldom or never	30

Once a week	20
Twice a week	10
Three or 4 times a week	0
Five or more times a week	−10

HOW'D YOU DO?

If your score is higher than 50 points, you may be at increased risk of low bone density. Review your answers in Part II to see where you can improve: cutting out harmful behavior or adding healthy habits. If your score is below 50 points, you are ahead of the game. Keep up the good work, and try incorporating or stepping up any health-promoting activities mentioned in Part II of the quiz to give yourself extra insurance. The eating and exercise plans later in the book will give you detailed guidance.

Generally speaking, the higher your points, the greater your risk. The lower your age is, the more risk is attached to a high or even moderately high score. That is, if you are 25 years old and score 50 points—just at the time you should be at your peak bone mass—you should be concerned. If you are a postmenopausal woman not taking hormone replacement and you score 50, you should be patting yourself on the back for the good care you've taken of your bones—and promising yourself to stay on that track. In any case, 40 is better than 50 and 50 is better than 70. There's always room for improvement, and your whole body will thank you for each improvement by functioning more smoothly for longer.

> **THINGS TO THINK ABOUT**
>
> One study (using a much more basic list of risk factors than the detailed compilation we're working from here) showed that people who had more than five major risk factors had *nine times* the risk of hip fracture compared to people with two or fewer risk factors.

And now for the fine print: this list is intended as a screening questionnaire only. The point system is not to be used to diagnose osteoporosis, but to demonstrate the potential risk of developing it. There is no one number above which one will definitely develop osteoporosis and no one number below which risk disappears.

This list focuses on the most common and most important relevant factors. Not all the risks covered in the next two chapters show up here, like amenorrhea, eating disorders, scoliosis, long-term use of antibiotics, and lactose intolerance, among others. Some things that may lessen your risk, such as taking hormone replacement therapy (but not continuing it indefinitely), are also not accounted for in this list. You'll have to adjust your score accordingly if you have any of these additional risks. This isn't an exact science: if you have just one or two additional considerations, the adjustment would be small; the more you have, the more significant the cumulative effect will be. The best thing for everyone is to assume you are at risk—and then find out specifically whether or not your bones are acceptably dense.

There are tremendously effective treatments available for people with osteoporosis (as described in Weeks 5 and 6) that are not factored in here. If this test and thorough medical screening (see Chapter 7) show you have dangerously low bone density, discuss treatment options with your doctor.

Taking this quiz should allow you to see, objectively, without emotional bias or conflict, where your strengths and weaknesses lie. It gives you a chance to be honest in your evaluation. What you learn should, in turn, allow you to better customize a program for yourself.

Chapter 5

Risks You Can't Avoid

We all have our baggage. When it comes to your bones, you're probably hauling around at least a few pieces of luggage that could potentially harm you, as the previous quiz no doubt pointed out. This chapter lays out the risks you're pretty much stuck with, to give you a sense of where you're starting from and how long or trying a journey you should pack for. Most of what you'll find here comes to you thanks either to genetics or as a result of past actions you can't very well go back and undo now.

Though what's done is done, remember that no matter which or how many of these situations you find yourself in, there are always steps you can take to preserve and improve your bone density and so your health. You'll find the specifics on how to do that in the rest of the book, though I will briefly mention some of the strategies particular to certain risk factors here. Once you understand the many and varied risks associated with low bone density and osteoporosis (in this chapter and the following one on risks you *can* avoid), you can choose your prevention strategies accordingly.

> **DID YOU KNOW?**
>
> 200 million people around the world have osteoporosis.

GENDER

Women have generally been considered to be at higher risk for bone loss and osteoporosis than men. And it is true that the average woman's peak bone mass isn't quite as high as the average man's, and that bone loss generally starts earlier in women than men because of menopause. But as we get better at understanding and diagnosing low bone density, I think we'll start finding that many more men would benefit from building or maintaining bone mass. After all, the risks listed in this chapter, in the main, don't discriminate based on sex. Right now, we don't generally look for osteoporosis in men; as we do start looking, I believe we will (unfortunately) find it. The good news is that once we find osteoporosis—or increased risk of it—we now know what to do about it in order to preserve not just life, but also life*style*.

AGE

The older you are, the more likely you are to have already lost bone. But drastic bone loss is by no means a foregone conclusion if your diet and exercise habits have been sound over the course of your life, and, if you are a woman, you began taking HRT as you entered menopause. The biggest age-related jump in risk for women is menopause, during which bone loss accelerates for several years before settling down to a slower pace. For men, the rate of change doesn't pick up until around age 65. For both men and women, after ages 30 to 40, bone for the most part isn't being built up, it is slipping away.

BODY SIZE AND FRAME

At last, a health reason to *not* wish for the flattest of abs and the narrowest of hips: being "small-boned" and thin increases your risk of low bone density and osteoporosis. (One definition of "small," for the purposes of bone density risk, is weighing 127 pounds or less, though that obviously doesn't take height into account. Those 127 pounds on someone 5 feet high is a whole different ballgame from a 127-pound, 5-foot-10-inch supermodel

---

DID YOU KNOW?

Good news for those who have put on a few pounds over the years: one study showed that women who got heavier after the age of 25 *lowered* their risks—and that women who weigh less later in life than they did at 25 *increased* their risk of fracture.

---

pretender.) Even on a medium or large frame, being very lean ups the risk. The luckiest roll of the genetic dice in this case is a medium frame bearing average weight (or even being on the heavy side, although the other health risks of being seriously overweight are well known). Studies show that women in the lowest quarter of the population by weight are more likely to suffer a fracture.

Being very lean interferes with hormone formation and so, eventually, bone formation. The body makes and stores estrogen in fat tissue, so a little padding boosts your estrogen, which helps build bone. Heavier women have higher estrogen levels after menopause, which offers some protection against bone loss. In addition, low body weight means your bones aren't stressed as much by just the ordinary movements of everyday living, and (as we'll see in Chapter 15 on exercise) stressing your bones is actually key to strengthening them. Finally, the less you weigh, the less you generally eat and so the lower your nutrient intake, on average. Light eaters should be as capable as anyone of getting at least most of what they need from a well-balanced diet, but they will have to choose their foods wisely and studiously avoid empty calories.

Of course, you will want to maintain a reasonable weight for overall good health. But please, let this put the idea of the sexiness of "waifs" out of your head once and for all! Healthy women are three-dimensional.

ETHNICITY

Until very recently, the party line was that from the perspective of bone density, Caucasians and Asians get the short end of the stick compared to African-American, Hispanic and Polynesian people. I was taught that thanks to gene pool differences, and a greater tendency to have small frames, white and Asian people have a significantly higher risk of losing too much bone mass, developing arthritis and suffering fractures. But I recently learned from Dr. Juanita Archer, a metabolic bone specialist at Howard University, that the most recent studies indicate that African-Americans have the same risk as Caucasians. Historically, black people were presumed not to be much at risk for osteoporosis and so by and large weren't screened for it until there was already a fracture. When doctors challenged the assumptions they'd been working under, and started looking for low bone density in black women at random, they found it was prevalent in them, too. We don't have the data yet, but I'm guessing that when we begin to look at other ethnic groups, we'll discover the same risks.

FAMILY HISTORY

Your grandmother probably gave you many wonderful things both tangible and intangible, but if she had osteoporosis, good bones isn't one of them. One of the primary warnings you will have that you are at higher risk of low bone density is a history of osteoporosis in your family. If your mother, father, sibling, or grandparent suffered from it (or lost height; or had a dowager's hump or a hunchback; or got frequent fractures or fractures from minor trauma), you'll need to pay particular attention to your own plan to avoid a similar fate.

DIET AND EXERCISE HISTORY

A poor diet in childhood through young adulthood means you start at a disadvantage because your body may not have had everything it needed to maximize your bone density during the periods of most intense growth. The same goes for lack of exercise early in life. If you played for Team Couch Potato as a child, teenager, or young adult, that's a strike against you, too, since those are the key years for bone growth. Just remember, it is never too late to take action.

One Patient's Story:
Nana, Grandma, Mom, Me, and Rose

I watched my grandmother die an awful death. She'd been shrinking for years, and eventually started to hunch forward dramatically. When I was a kid, of course, I was so proud to grow taller than her. But after I stopped growing and still seemed to have to lean over farther and farther to kiss her each time I saw her, it was just sad. She was never officially diagnosed with osteoporosis, but it was obvious what was happening long before she finally broke her hip. Just like her mother before her—my nana—Grandma never even came home from the hospital. She struggled through some painful physical therapy, but died within a few months. I remember her telling me a long time ago that it was a shame that her own mother had to suffer so long in the hospital after breaking her hip before she died, though it had given Grandma a chance to adjust to the loss. It didn't bring me much comfort now.

As my mother went into menopause, she started to worry about following in her mother's and grandmother's footsteps. Her doctor recommended hormone replacement—which my grandmother certainly never had—and supplements of calcium, vitamin D, and magnesium. She experiments with hand weights, though she hasn't found a routine she likes well enough to make it a twice-a-week habit, and otherwise gets most of her exercise walking up and down the stairs to her fifth-floor apartment and occasional sessions on the treadmill in the study. She's generally careful about what she eats, but as a single person running her own very busy business, her meals are often catch-as-catch-can.

Nonetheless, the combination appears to be working. A DEXA scan almost five years into menopause showed her bones to be well within the normal range for the average 30-year-old! Even with "bad genes" (her father's mother also had a few too-easy fractures in the years just before she died), a few simple measures have saved my mother's life.

My mom has inspired me to take the necessary steps to protect my bones. I've seen and heard too much of what happens if you don't. I know my bones are as dense right now as they ever will be (I'm 30), and I want to keep them that way. Throughout my childhood a milk allergy *meant I ate no dairy products, so I worry that I'm starting with a disadvantage. I've taken calcium supplements since I graduated from college—and religiously while I was pregnant and breastfeeding. I started doing two circuits a week on the weight machines at the gym after I read about how strength training helps build bone—a whole-body workout that takes about half an hour. I take a once-a-week yoga class, and usually either swim or ride the stationary bike twice. I also walk about two miles a day, taking my daughter to and from school.*

But the most important changes of all may be the ones I made for my daughter Rose. She's still small enough that I control most of what she eats, so I make sure she gets a vitamin with extra calcium, some cottage cheese made with extra calcium, and a glass of calcium-fortified orange juice every day. She's never been much of a milk drinker—aside from on her cereal—and I've been known to bribe her by stirring in some chocolate syrup. She does like broccoli and beans, though, and we eat one or the other just about every day. The whole family eats vegetarian about half the time, with chicken or fish a few dinners a week, so Rose gets small amounts of meat protein. I'm hoping these good habits will be well ingrained by the time she makes her own decisions about what to eat. And I'm glad she'll never have to see her grandmother go through what mine did. Or her mother, either.

MEDICATIONS

A long list of medications negatively affect your bones, so if you use any of the problematic ones (below) over the long term, be sure to consult with your doctor about how to protect your bone density. Pay particular attention to diet, exercise, and calcium supplements, and make bone density evaluation a regular part of your medical follow-up. If you are a women near or past menopause, think long and hard about the risks and benefits of HRT.

Many of these medications cause rapid bone loss at the outset, and the rate slows over time, so it pays to think about prevention as early in your treatment as possible, preferably before you take your first dose. It is never too late to take action, even if you've been taking something for years, unaware of the potential harm to your skeleton. If you get to work now, you can stop any further loss and build back much of what is already gone.

Steroids—corticosteroids or adrenal corticosteroids, officially— are among the leading offenders because they interfere with calcium absorption, block calcium from being deposited into bone, and increase the amount of calcium you excrete. All this results in bone loss, primarily from decreased bone formation (as opposed to increased breakdown). This group includes prednisone, commonly used for asthma and arthritis, cortisone, and many other drugs commonly used to treat asthma, psoriasis, rheumatoid arthritis, lupus, Crohn's disease, ulcerative colitis, and multiple sclerosis, among others, and sometimes given along with chemotherapy for cancer and to people receiving an organ transplant.

You should consider getting a bone density scan before starting long-term treatment with a steroid drug, with a follow-up six months or a year later. In patients on oral or systemic cortisone, and especially in children, dramatic bone changes develop within three months. If you take it for longer than three months, or if your bone density drops more than 5 percent, you should adjust your dosage if possible, follow a serious bone-density boosting nutrition and exercise program, and consider adding a drug treatment like alendronate, calcitonin or risedronate (see Chapter 20) preventively.

Some studies suggest some inhaled corticosteroids may cause less harm than others. When they are more targeted to specific parts of the body, as with nasal cortisone for allergies, for example, you don't get the same interference with your adrenal glands and your metabolism. However, more investigation is needed before we can simply switch to the inhaled form and rest easy. Again, let me stress that every improvement helps.

Taking *thyroid hormone* is another risk factor for low bone mass. Hypothyroidism (not making enough thyroid hormone) is a common—and probably underdiagnosed—condition. Despite the problems associated with the treatment (which you'll see in a minute), it is a condition you want to address. The thyroid helps balance the calcium level in your blood and assists in bone formation, so you want to be assured of having enough of it. Once diagnosed with hypothyroidism, the standard treatment of taking

---

Case in Point: Kate

K ate was diagnosed with Graves' disease, a common cause of hyper-thyroidism, a decade ago, but often didn't take the medication prescribed to control it because she generally felt fine. When she made an appointment to see my good friend and colleague Martin Baran-des, an endocrinologist specializing in thyroid disease, he sent her for a bone density scan, even though she was only in her mid-30s, as part of the workup. The results showed she had osteopenia, and Kate was alarmed at the fact that her bones were 15 percent lower in density than expected for her age—at a time when her bones should have been at their peak!

The most important thing for Kate, besides eating well and getting exercise, was to have her thyroid medication adjusted properly—and then take it regularly. Having been caught off guard by the proven bone loss, she was motivated to stick with the pills now, and to maintain the lifestyle changes she made in the interest of her bones. Her bone loss soon slowed to a stop.

---

supplements of the hormone (like Synthroid) is quite effective. But if you don't strike just the right balance, it can quicken bone breakdown. If your body makes too much thyroid hormone on its own—hyperthyroidism—you've got the same problem.

The thyroid is normally involved in bone remodeling, so an overactive thyroid means overeager bone turnover. Be sure your doctor tests your blood regularly and adjusts your prescription until you find the lowest dose that works for you and keeps blood levels of the hormone in the normal range. From the perspective of your bones, most doctors wait too long to treat for low thyroid levels: thyroid stimulating hormone (TSH) levels up to 4 are considered normal, which is when most doctors would become concerned, but I recommend treatment if it is over 2.5–3. Another common mistake is to treat too aggressively, pushing TSH levels as low as possible. Though the low end of normal is considered to be just .4, the lowest levels are associated with bone loss, so I try to help my patients stay in the 1 to 2 range.

TALK TO YOUR DOCTOR

Taking thyroid hormone—for the common and probably underdiagnosed condition called hypothyroidism—puts you at increased risk for low bone mass, especially if you're using more than the absolute minimum dose your body requires.

Do not suddenly stop taking thyroid hormone, but try cutting down gradually, with your doctor's supervision, spending a few weeks at each new level before deciding whether to go lower still. If you deal with thyroid disease with natural remedies, even better! Norwegian kelp is sometimes recommended, as is the yoga shoulder stand (which is said to stimulate the thyroid), among other things. If your original diagnosis is far in the past, a thorough new evaluation is in order to make sure you in fact still need the hormonal supplement. Either way, if properly controlled, thyroid conditions won't negatively impact the bones, but if not handled properly, are a common contributor to low bone density.

Antacids containing aluminum are another area of concern. Long-term, frequent use can cause bone loss because aluminum combines with phosphorus and calcium and prevents them from being absorbed. Aluminum, on the other hand, can also be absorbed into the bones, causing osteomalacia. Antacids are a very common source of aluminum, but no matter where the aluminum comes from (polluted air or water, for example, or soda cans, or the pots and pans your food is cooked in, or other medications), it is hazardous. Even low levels of aluminum can step up the loss of calcium. The combination of osteomalacia and bone pain has been observed in people using this kind of antacid over a long period of time, so the importance of avoiding them is clear.

The newest antacid medicines, like Zantac, Tagamet, Pepcid, and Axid, which you take to prevent too much acid (as opposed to neutralizing what is already there) can be even worse. They work by

Case in Point: Rita

O ne of my patients, in her mid-60s, had severe gastro-esophageal reflux disease as well as osteoporosis. Rita took supplements of calcium, vitamin D, and a range of other important vitamins, minerals, and trace elements along with alendronate to stop the bone loss—a fairly aggressive approach. But at the same time, she frequently used one of the new antacid medications you take before you eat to stop acid production.

A year after beginning treatment for low bone density, when you would expect to see enough improvement to erase the increased fracture risk, a repeat bone scan showed no improvement in bone density. At least she wasn't losing any more bone, but the antacid medication seemed to be interfering with the alendronate's ability to increase bone density, and it was certainly preventing her body from absorbing and using all the nutrients she was taking to support her bones.

Rita stopped taking the medication to calm her reflux symptoms, and focused instead on controlling the condition with careful diet (and some of the other techniques described in Chapter 12). She also switched to Miacalcin and agreed to start on HRT. The improved use of calcium and other nutrients alone should help her build bone, lower her fracture risk, and help keep her healthy and active for years to come.

preventing stomach acid from being made, which interferes with digestion and absorption of all nutrients, including calcium.

Some antacids, like Alka-Seltzer and Tums, have little or no aluminum, so they are your best option if you must use an antacid. The best tactic is to improve your diet and digestion so you don't need antacids at all, and to rely on natural alternatives when you do need relief (see Chapter 12 on digestion for details). In any case, always read the label of any antacid (any medicine, actually) so you know exactly what you are getting.

Many *chemotherapy* drugs—toxic as they generally are—can damage your bones. In addition, many patients undergoing chemotherapy are inactive, which isn't good for bones. Many patients

TALK TO YOUR DOCTOR

Though diuretics generally increase calcium loss and therefore risk of low bone density and fracture, one particular class (thiazides) actually seems to offer some protection against hip fractures because it helps retain calcium despite the increase in urine output. It isn't a treatment for osteoporosis, or for fracture prevention, but it would be the best choice (as long as it is otherwise appropriate) if you need to take a diuretic. Thiazides are generally prescribed as diuretics, but are also sometimes used for mood disorders or sedation.

also have less of an appetite than they normally do, and if they don't eat enough, they won't get the nutrients their bones need. There are some options to relieve nausea and boost your appetite, and you should seek out appealing, nutritious foods, and be sure to resume exercising when you feel up to it. Cancer treatment is always difficult emotionally, and often difficult physically, but don't forget that preserving your general health is important, too, and bone density is an important aspect of that.

Diuretics used to treat high blood pressure, edema, and congestive heart failure are another danger because the increased urine output means an increase in the nutrients excreted, including calcium.

Anticonvulsants, including phenytoin and barbiturates, taken to prevent seizures or for any other reason, can damage bone over time. This includes medicines to treat epilepsy.

If you have to take a long-term course of *antibiotics*, including tetracycline, or if you take them often, you will excrete more calcium—calcium that then won't be available for your bones. Antibiotics can interfere with absorption of nutrients in general. Make sure you really need antibiotics before you take them; resist pestering your doctor for a prescription on the off chance your colds are actually bacterial (almost all are viral, and antibiotics won't do anything good for them). Sometimes you *do* really need

TALK TO YOUR DOCTOR

The pain medications Diclofenac (Cataflam, Voltaren) and naproxen, and the diuretic and antihypertensive hydrochlorothiazide *may help slow or stop bone loss.* They are not osteoporosis treatments, but you should consider them if you need to take something of the kind.

them, and then of course you should take them—antibiotics are one of the most beneficial discoveries in the entire history of medicine. But if you use them a lot over time, you must take the necessary steps to protect your bones, including exercise, diet, and supplements.

Other drugs that interfere with bone remodeling include cholestyramine, cyclosporin A (for organ transplants), and gonadotropin-releasing hormone analogues and agonists. You should also be concerned about methotrexate (for arthritis, cancer, psoriasis, and immune disorders); anticoagulants, including heparin and warfarin (Coumadin); lithium (and other drugs that treat bipolar disorder); benzodiazepines; warfarin; and other drugs. There are no doubt many more that impact on bone density, only we don't know it yet.

TALK TO YOUR DOCTOR

Anyone who takes multiple medications has an increased risk of falling and thus an increased risk of fractures, no matter how dense the bones and no matter what the specific medications are. A host of other quality-of-life issues are involved anytime you use combinations of medicines, so make sure your doctor is aware of everything you take (including supplements and herbs) and regularly evaluates all of them for effectiveness and potential interactions.

MEDICATIONS THAT CAN DAMAGE BONE DENSITY

Medications	Common Conditions Treated
Steroids (corticosteroids and adrenal corticosteroids)	Asthma, arthritis, psoriasis, rheumatoid arthritis, lupus, Crohn's disease, ulcerative colitis, multiple sclerosis, chemotherapy, organ transplant
Thyroid hormone	Hypothyroidism
Antacids with aluminum	Heartburn, indigestion, "excess stomach acid," or as a calcium supplement
Chemotherapy	Cancer
Diuretics	High blood pressure, edema, congestive heart failure
Anticonvulsants (including phenytoin and barbituates)	Seizures, epilepsy
Antibiotics (long-term or frequently, including tetracycline)	Bacterial infections (or "prevention" or misused for viral infections)
Cholestyramine, cyclosporin A	Organ transplants
Gonadotropin-releasing hormone analogues and agonists	To regulate levels of male sex hormones
Methotrexate	Arthritis, cancer, psoriasis, immune disorders
Anticoagulants, including heparin and Coumadin	Atrial fibrillation (irregular heartbeat), phlebitis, after some strokes and heart attacks, some heart conditions, polycythemia
Lithium	Bipolar disorder ("manic depression")
Benzodiazepines (including Valium, Librium, and Xanax)	For sedation, stress reduction, sleep, or tranquilization

MEDICAL CONDITIONS

Many chronic medical conditions can contribute to drastically low bone density. Some interfere with bone metabolism directly. Some impair your ability to absorb and use the nutrients you need for healthy bones. Some require medication that can damage your bones even as it addresses your other concerns (see section on medications).

Anorexia and other *eating disorders* increase your risk of low bone density, no matter what your age. For one thing, anorexia almost always has amenorrhea (no periods)—meaning low estrogen levels—associated with it. For another, taking in too few calories means by definition that you are not getting enough of the nutrients that are so important to bone health. Finally, anorexia is most common in girls and young women during the years when bone growth should be its fastest, meaning there's a strong likelihood peak bone density will never be reached. That is, when women who had eating disorders early in life go into the accelerated bone loss of menopause, they will be starting with a sizable disadvantage.

Case in Point: Shawna

*S*hawna had been struggling with bulimia for a long time when she went to my colleague, endocrinologist Dr. Ed Klaiber, because she hadn't had a period for over three years. Fair and small-boned to begin with, Shawna now had almost no body fat. When she had her estrogen levels tested, they were very low. Among other things, that put her bones at risk. Unfortunately, a bone density scan confirmed her doctors' fears: 25-year-old Shawna had the bones of a 65-year-old woman.

Working with her regular doctor, she finally seemed to be getting her eating disorder under control at this point. Following Dr. Klaiber's advice, she also began taking Fosamax and estrogen. Combining therapies in this way was unorthodox at the time, though studies now confirm that various drugs in combination provide increased responses over any one alone. It surely worked for Shawna: she's gotten back 18 percent of her bone in one year.

Anorexia and eating disorders are complicated to treat and potentially life-threatening. One component of treatment you might consider is taking birth control pills to supply the estrogen your body isn't making (think of it as a form of hormone replacement therapy).

High blood sugar levels, as in *diabetes*, inhibits the absorption of calcium, and long-term uncontrolled diabetes increases your risk of osteoporosis. It may be that insulin has a role in bone breakdown that contributes to that increase in risk. Diabetics have, on average, bone mass 10 percent lower than you would otherwise expect.

Other *endocrine diseases*, including Cushing's syndrome, hyperparathyroidism, hyperthyroidism, and thyrotoxicosis, are major culprits—and the treatment can also be problematic. Anything that lowers your sex hormones *(hypogonadism)*—for men or women—will also raise your risk of osteoporosis. Increased risk of osteoporosis and fractures also accompanies chronic *irritable bowel syndrome, celiac disease, scoliosis, jaundice, hypertension* (high blood pressure), *rheumatoid arthritis, cirrhosis, hypercortisolism, removal of the small colon, chronic lung disease*, and *removal of part or all of the stomach*. All these conditions change your metabolism, and so alter your body's nutritional requirements and demands and interfere with absorption of nutrients. You then may either have a higher requirement for calcium and other key nutrients for bone health that you are not meeting, and/or you may not be absorbing and using what you do take in.

Some people with *kidney stones* seem to be at higher risk for low bone density. If the stones contain calcium, the usual recommendation is to decrease the amount of calcium in your diet in order to lower the levels in your urine. But along with hindering stone formation, less calcium will also hinder bone formation. Sometimes diet changes do not affect how much calcium is excreted, and that indicates a different kind of problem. It is a sign of calcium imbalance, which your body addresses by taking calcium out of the bones to meet its needs. That's obviously not good for your bones, and if, on top of that, you are restricting your calcium intake, your risk of osteoporosis climbs higher still.

Being *bedridden* for an extended time, or spending a long period of time getting all your *nutrients through a tube or IV*, for any reason, causes excess bone loss. Complete inactivity over time doubles the amount of calcium you excrete.

BONE BOOSTERS

After bed rest of a week or more, taking 2,000 mg of calcium a day for seven times as long as you were in bed will help replace the bone you lost.

And anything that gives you *impaired balance or coordination*, making you more likely to fall or have some other sort of accident (for instance, the very common "postural hypotension"— light-headedness as you stand up as the result of a sudden drop in blood pressure), increases your risk of fractures, no matter what the status of your bones. *Dementia* is also a risk factor, probably because it affects the way you eat and increases the risk of falling.

Be sure to talk to your doctor about any steps you can take to avoid or counteract any negative impact on your bones. Generally, if you are dealing with any of these issues, you should be screened earlier than the average recommendation, and medical follow-ups should include bone density monitoring (see Chapter 7). Good diet and exercise habits and calcium supplements—as described later in this book—will be even more important for you than they are for people without these additional complications.

PREGNANCY

In pregnancy, if you're not taking in enough calcium, some will be withdrawn from your bones to nourish the growing baby. Bearing a large number of children multiplies your risk, as does carrying a single multiple pregnancy (eating for three—or more—is even more difficult than eating for two). Pregnancy later in life may pose more of a problem, since you'll have less time (and lower ability) to make up for any loss. The key to protecting yourself will be to take supplements, particularly calcium and vitamin D, in

Case in Point: Emily

*E*mily was first diagnosed with scoliosis in childhood, and suffered with anorexia for about a year in her late teens. She confessed she still was constantly dieting. She is otherwise a basically healthy, very petite, 40-year-old woman, and has no family history of low bone density. Recently, she had a bone density measurement done. She had no symptoms (most people don't until they break a bone), but she was concerned about the effects the scoliosis, anorexia, and continual dieting might have had on her bones.

Sure enough, Emily's DEXA scan revealed she already had osteoporosis in the vertebrae of her lower back. Her density was about 25 percent lower than average peak bone density. She had osteoporosis at a time when she should still have been at just about peak bone density. With her suspicions confirmed, she had tests of her NTX, vitamin D, parathyroid, and thyroid levels to determine the best way to stop any further loss and strengthen her spine.

I told her she'll be a prime candidate for HRT when the time comes, but she's not there yet. After I laid out the treatment options that exist, she decided to try calcitonin, since she recognized the hard fact that for her, with no treatment, the worst was yet to come. At menopause she could be losing even more bone density unless she took drastic action now—and she had probably ten years of loss at her current rate before she even got that far.

The aggressive approach she took consisted of improving her diet and exercise habits—like eating yogurt and soybeans at least once a day, starting strength training, and using supplements of calcium and other nutrients. Still she feared that might not be enough to keep her from shrinking and risking fractures and bone pain since her loss had become so advanced so early. With the calcitonin, her bone density was out of the danger zone within two years.

addition to a prenatal vitamin, during pregnancy, and eat a variety of foods rich in those nutrients to guarantee adequate intake for both (or all) of you.

Never having borne a child also increases your risk of low bone density, though the reasons are not well understood.

BREAST-FEEDING

The benefits of nursing your baby are well documented, but you will need to take precautions to make sure it doesn't leave you with softer bones. In order to make sure your breast milk has sufficient calcium for your child, nature has arranged it so that calcium from *your* bones will be added to it if enough isn't otherwise available. Some studies show that mothers breastfeeding their infants may drop up to 5 percent of their bone mass (although there is disagreement on this point). Bone density seems to be regained quickly once the children are weaned, but the moral of the story is that taking calcium and vitamin D supplements (in addition to continuing the "prenatal" vitamin your doctor prescribed) to ensure you get as much calcium as your body needs is a wise move, in addition to including in your diet many foods rich in these nutrients. Mothers young enough to still be building up to their peak bone mass should be extra careful, as should mothers old enough to be closing in on menopause (which is no longer particularly uncommon).

ANTE UP

In some of the "unchangeable" risk factors covered in this chapter, you actually have at least a modicum of control (i.e., you can't escape a diabetes diagnosis, but you can keep the condition well managed). Others you're just plain stuck with. (No matter what you tell *People* magazine when they call to interview you, your chronological age is immutable.) But it is always up to you how to play whatever hand you've been dealt. It is more than worthwhile to learn to play wisely, and well, because the jackpot is the most precious one imaginable: your life and your health.

Chapter 6

Things You Can Change

Now that you know what strikes you're stuck with, this chapter explains the factors *you* control. Nature and experience have packed one bag for you, but you are allowed two pieces of carry-on luggage and the contents of the second one are all up to you. To have a safe and pleasant journey all the way to the end of the line, be sure to bring enough of what you need and leave behind the stuff that just weighs you down.

DECREASED ESTROGEN

For women, one of the largest factors in overall bone health is estrogen. Anything that significantly cuts down on estrogen can have a negative effect on women's bones, since estrogen is so important to maintaining bone density. You can't always control the amount of estrogen your body produces (menopause comes whether or not it gets an engraved invitation from you), but there are several ways to make up for low levels of the hormone. Sometimes you do have some control: if you've exercised yourself to the point of stopping menstruation, for example, you can back off enough to restore your normal cycles (and therefore your estrogen). Or you can make sure you've exhausted other treatment options before having a hysterectomy.

The most obvious case of getting less estrogen than is optimal for your skeleton is *menopause*, when estrogen levels drop dramatically. Without so much estrogen, bone loss picks up dramatically for the first five years or so after the last period, and you might lose as much as 5 percent of your total bone mass *each year*.

Early menopause (before age 45), or "surgical menopause" like a hysterectomy or removal of the ovaries, increases your risk further still, since your body faces the same challenges as with menopause, but years earlier. Women who have their ovaries removed lose bone faster than do older women at menopause. Women who have had a hysterectomy but have both ovaries (which actually make estrogen) still show an increased risk. Even just experiencing menopause at a relatively young age (but still within the normal range) ratchets up the stakes for you, since every drop of estrogen you can come by naturally (without having to tally up potential risks and side effects from hormone replacement) is crucial.

> ### THINGS TO THINK ABOUT
>
> By the time you have night sweats or mood changes, your bone density is no longer optimal.

This is why HRT is such an important consideration whenever you enter menopause. Another way to protect yourself is with natural progesterone (see Chapter 19), which is particularly worth learning about if you are wary of or unable to take estrogen.

Some women experience low levels of estrogen well before menopause (upping the ante still more, especially if it occurs in girls and young women who should be in their peak bone-building years). *Amenorrhea* (loss of periods) or very infrequent and irregular periods are the most common ways this occurs. It happens to intensely active athletes, especially in sports where low body weight and extremely low body fat are advantageous and common (e.g., marathon runners, ballerinas, and gymnasts). Delayed onset of menstruation and interrupted periods have similar effects. For every year with few or no periods, you may lose about 2 percent of your bone mass.

Before menopause, normal menstrual cycles are best for you

for many reasons, bone health among them. Stress, poor nutrition, excessive exercise, and lack of exposure to natural light can all disrupt your menstrual cycle, interfering with hormonal reactions and so contributing to bone loss. Irregular periods and irregular ovulation put you at higher risk for osteoporosis. If your periods are irregular, consider using birth control pills, or natural progesterone (see Chapter 19) to restore them, as well as addressing

---

Case in Point: Daphne

*T*hough estrogen was what I recommended first, Daphne was opposed to taking HRT. When she was 55 and a few years into menopause, she had a bone density screening that showed she had moderate to severe bone loss. She had been taking medication to control her thyroid for many years, which probably accelerated her bone loss well before her body's estrogen levels dropped off and she had her last period. Daphne had also struggled with anxiety and depression, and although there are no double-blind, placebo-controlled studies proving a direct link between those conditions and bone density, I believe continual stress of any kind—especially something as severe as chronic emotional disruption—is hard on your bones (see Chapter 21). There are plenty of gold-standard studies demonstrating a crucial connection between the health of your mind and your body generally, and I see no reason why your skeleton would be exempt.

The good news for Daphne was that a simple lab test that assesses fracture risk and rate of progression of bone loss—independent of current bone density (see information on NTX in Chapter 7)—was smack in the middle of the normal range. With a reasonably low risk of fracture and a reasonably slow rate of loss, then, she had a chance to improve her general health along the lines of the program outlined later in this book, and find out if that would help her bones sufficiently, before she reached a crisis point. She decided to take alendronate (see Chapter 18) to make sure her situation wouldn't deteriorate, and she showed excellent improvement very quickly. So Daphne was able to remain committed to helping herself without using supplemental hormones.

the underlying causes so your body can get back to properly regulating itself. In fact, the pill can prevent bone loss—and perhaps even increase density—in any premenopausal woman, which you should factor into your decision about what contraceptive to use (on balance with the other attendant risks and side effects, of course). Your goals should be to maintain your physiology as close to Mother Nature's recipe as possible.

LACK OF EXERCISE

Poor diet and little exercise would be neck-and-neck for first place in a contest to see what can damage bones the most. A sedentary lifestyle significantly boosts your risk of having low bone density. Even generally active people might be shortchanging their bones if they don't get enough of the right kinds of exercise. Weight-bearing exercise is the key, as you'll see in Chapter 15 on exercise, and you should be doing it three times a week *minimum* to protect your bones. More is better (within reason), but anything is better than nothing.

POOR DIET

Calcium is the single most important ingredient in healthy, dense bone (though it cannot act alone), and lack of calcium is probably the most common *completely reversible* risk factor for low bone density. Without sufficient quantities *early in life* you won't reach your maximum potential bone mass, and after that the deficiency will leave you unable to maintain density or stave off loss. The best way to get any nutrient is through your diet whenever possible, but calcium is so crucial, and most people get so much less than ideal levels, that everyone should consider taking a supplement.

Without enough vitamin D through diet, supplements, and sun exposure combined (see Chapter 10), your body will not be able to absorb and use the calcium you get to make bone, another leading *preventable* risk factor.

A diet without a variety of vegetables, fruits, and whole grains will probably be missing critical nutrients for the complex task of

---

DID YOU KNOW?

Osteoporosis causes 1.5 million fractures each year in this country, at tremendous personal and societal costs, including $38 million in medical costs (not including time lost at work). A full 1.1 percent of all money spent on health care is on osteoporosis treatment: almost $14 billion each year.

---

bone remodeling, and so is another component increasing your risk of low bone density. (Eating a lot of fruits and veggies will also help you maintain a low level of saturated fat in your diet, which is just generally good for you.) Bonus: eating soybeans and other soy products and other items with *phytoestrogens* (estrogenlike chemicals found in plants) will help you build bone and avoid bone loss much the way estrogen does.

Inefficient digestion decreases your body's ability to absorb crucial nutrients, which raises your risk of low bone density. Calcium is difficult for many people to digest in the first place, and general digestion difficulties quickly compound the problem. As you age, your level of stomach acid general decreases, again making nutrients in general—and calcium in particular—difficult to absorb. Simple strategies such as those given in Chapter 12 can help you counteract this problem.

Lactose intolerance is a problem for many people, especially as they get older. Avoiding dairy products makes it even tougher to get the calcium you need (while *not* avoiding them can wreak havoc with your digestion). Check out milk and other products that have enzymes added to break down the parts your body has trouble with—there are plenty of options now on the market. The process by which yogurt is made does the same thing, so even sensitive people should have no problem eating yogurt. (The processing involved in making commercial frozen yogurt kills most of the natural bacteria that help digest lactose, so you may get a reaction to it.)

SODAS (PHOSPHORUS)

The balance between calcium and phosphorus is paramount—and precarious. Phosphorus is beneficial, generally speaking, working with calcium to form bones and teeth. We all get enough from the high-protein foods (many of which are also high in phosphorus) and processed foods (many of which have phosphorus added) in our diets. In fact, far too many Americans get *too much* phosphorus. The usual suspect? Sodas. (Can you remember when they used to be called "phosphates"?) Too much of the stuff throws the balance between calcium and phosphorus out of whack, which eventually leads to calcium deficiency and inefficient use of whatever does manage to get absorbed.

The relationship between the two elements is as complicated and sensitive as it is important. If you get too much phosphorus, it enters the blood and binds with calcium. Then your body is unaware of how much calcium it actually has in the bloodstream and, in the interests of preserving calcium levels within a narrow normal range, will draw calcium out of bones and into the blood. Even if calcium intake increases along with phosphorus, the phosphorus will end up getting absorbed better than the calcium, leading right back to imbalance. So you can't make up for too much phosphorus by upping the number of supplement pills you take. It won't work, for one thing, and it'll just aggravate the imbalance further. Getting too little calcium can also cause a problem, even if your levels of phosphorus are otherwise appropriate, because it will upset the delicate balance between the two nutrients.

As you can see, it is a vicious circle, once started, so the best thing to do is keep the two in proportion. All that requires is limiting the number of sodas you drink to one a day. (Sodas aren't the only place you'll find phosphorus in your diet, but we focus on them here because they contain no other nutrients, are consumed in large quantities, and may have plenty of empty calories—and caffeinated sodas pack a double-whammy.) This may be the easiest of all the things I recommend doing on behalf of your bones.

Phosphorus also binds with magnesium, manganese, zinc, and copper, interfering with the ability of those nutrients to do their work and so creating further problems for your valiant bones.

> **BONE BOOSTERS**
>
> Good news for those who like their drinks bubbly: seltzer
> still gets the thumbs-up, as it does not have phosphorus.
> Fruit juice spritzer, anyone? I like mine with a slice of lemon.

Before Diet Coke became something seemingly every other person drinks with breakfast, we got less than half the phosphorus we do now. Keep in mind that we get significantly *less* of most nutrients now than we did in the past. Not only does that make the increase in phosphorus seem more remarkable, but it also means we're getting ever more out of balance. Draw your line in the sand, and leave sodas with phosphorus on the other side (regular, diet, caffeine-free, even club soda).

PROTEIN

Generally speaking, the more protein you eat, the more calcium you excrete. When protein is digested, the parts it is broken down into are very acidic, and your body uses calcium to buffer them. That means whatever calcium you take in will be diverted to this task from building bone. And if there's not enough on hand, your body draws calcium out of your bones to do the job. It then passes out of the body altogether in the urine. For every gram of meat protein you take in, count on an average of one milligram of calcium going out. So for a 4-ounce portion of chicken, say, you're losing *nearly 100 milligrams* of calcium.

Protein also throws off the balance between calcium and phosphorus, which is crucial for healthy bones (see above). Without the proper levels of phosphorus, your body can't efficiently use whatever calcium it has.

Meat protein is more acidic during digestion than protein from fish, dairy products, beans, nuts, and seeds. They are made up of different amino acids (the "building blocks of protein," in case your high school biology isn't that fresh in your mind) with different levels and kinds of fatty acids. Not all fatty acids are bad: those in fish and nuts and seeds are the ones known as omega-3's and omega-6's, which have been proven to provide protection against heart disease.

So the quality of the protein you take in makes all the difference because we all need protein. Exactly how much protein a body needs depends on age, size, and overall diet and health, but for the average woman, 3 or 4 ounces a day is healthy (men usually need a little more). But almost all Americans consume more than twice that. Halfway through a quarter-pounder—or a can of tuna, for that matter—you'll have already met your protein requirements for the day. And for each ounce of protein that goes in, another 30 or 40 mg of calcium go out. Again, since you probably don't get enough calcium anyway, you can see that's a problem.

"BUT MY OFFICEMATE LOST 20 POUNDS ON 'THE ZONE,' AND SHE SAYS SHE FEELS AS GOOD AS SHE LOOKS!"

The Bone Density Diet is obviously different from and much more straightforward than The Zone and other very high protein weight-loss diets. But I don't want you to misunderstand me, because the underlying logic about blood sugar levels featured in those plans is essentially correct— and not unlike what I lay out in Chapter 8. You *can* focus your diet on protein and slim down, and stay healthy, *if* (and this is a big if) you eat it in the proper combinations with specific carbohydrates and fats. Even when done with exacting precision, a very high protein diet won't agree with everyone. For simplicity's sake, and for the benefits of the wealth of micronutrients and fiber in a plant-based diet, I take a low-protein approach I think is even better for overall health—and weight control.

That's one reason I recommend a diet—really a permanent way of eating—that leans toward the vegetarian. The less meat you eat, the less protein your body has to process. I replaced much of the meat I used to eat with a variety of beans, because beans not only have a lot of protein (and you do need some protein and trace minerals) but also require less calcium than meat as they are broken down. Soybeans also contain a plant estrogen called genistein, which is a great bone builder for women, so you get a double bonus there (see Chapter 11).

So forget very high protein diets if you want any chance of keeping your bones on your side for the long run. Limit the amount of meat you eat to 4 ounces a day or less (a piece the size of a deck of cards).

ALCOHOL

Too much alcohol interferes with the absorption of calcium, and thus with bone growth. Alcohol also seems to damage bone directly, and autopsies of alcoholics have shown skeletons that look as if they were 40 years older than they actually are. Heavier drinkers also suffer more fractures, which is partly explained by a higher rate of falls and other accidents while under the influence (even mildly). Yet people who have a few drinks a week have actually been shown to have higher bone density than nondrinkers. One reason is that moderate alcohol intake boosts estrogen, which in turn helps build bone.

Similarly, higher alcohol intake has been associated with increased cancer risk, while moderate drinking is protective of the heart. So this is a balancing act. When it comes to your bones, the benefits of alcohol are real but limited, and the potential for harm is serious. If you never or rarely drink, there is certainly no health reason compelling enough that you should start doing so now. But if you do drink, walk the line. Keeping it to no more than three alcoholic drinks a week would be ideal.

CAFFEINE

Caffeine, a diuretic, increases the amount of calcium you excrete in urine. (Urine also takes other minerals out of the body, including magnesium, another key nutrient for bones, as you'll see in Chapter 10.) To make up for the calcium lost thanks to the caffeine in one 6-ounce cup of regular American coffee (less than your average mug holds), you'd have to get at least an additional

SAFETY PROOFING

For those who already have bone density low enough to increase their fracture risk, there's another important level of risk reduction: safety-proofing your home to reduce the risk of falls or other accidents that might provoke a fracture. If these steps don't concern you directly, they may still be valuable advice for a friend or loved one. The following list will get you started:

- Avoid clutter on the floor, and especially on steps, so you won't trip or slip.
- Carpet slippery floors. Avoid cleansers, waxes, or polishes that make floors slippery. Wipe up spills as soon as they occur. Use rubber nonskid mats under area rugs.
- Install handrails in the shower and bathtub, and use rubber decals on the floor to keep you from slipping.
- Replace tables or other furniture low enough to be out of your normal line of vision that you might trip over.
- Keep phone and electrical cords short, off the floor, and properly affixed against walls or baseboards so you won't trip over them.
- Make sure hallways, closets, and especially stairs are well lit—bright enough, but without glare.
- Install handrails on both sides of all staircases.
- Keep flashlights handy, and put in night-lights anywhere you might be walking during the night. Don't walk around your house in the dark.

Some additional safety strategies:

- Choose supportive shoes without slippery soles, but also avoid those with such heavy rubber soles that they might actually trip you up.
- Avoid clothes long enough to get caught under your foot, particularly on stairs.
- Be aware of medication side effects or interactions that affect your balance or coordination, and ask your doctor or pharmacist about alternatives.

- Keep your blood pressure within the normal range.
- Exercise to build strength, flexibility, balance, and coordination, all of which help prevent falls.
- Have your hearing and vision tested and corrected as well as possible, and be rescreened regularly.
- Keep phones in as many rooms as possible in case you do fall and need to call for help.
- Use the appropriate assistance for walking: cane, walking stick, or walker. It won't do you any good to have one you don't use.
- If you fall and think you've broken something, don't move—or let anyone else move you—until you get professional assistance. In general, after a fall, don't put weight on an injury, and move slowly. See your doctor.
- If you have a pet, keep careful track of its whereabouts— and the whereabouts of its balls and toys—so you don't trip over a snoozing animal companion.
- Organize your things so you don't have to bend over or reach overhead for things you use frequently. Don't climb on chairs to reach what is up too high. Use a sturdy stepping stool designed for the purpose if you must, but you'd be better off asking for help.
- Get help with heavy lifting, or opening stubborn doors or windows.
- To pick up something from the floor, bend at the knees, not the waist.

As the old joke goes, the falling isn't so bad. It's hitting the ground that really gets you. Take the time to protect yourself so you don't have to find out for yourself.

40 mg of calcium. That's not much of a hurdle at one cup a day, but it quickly adds up for most coffee drinkers (that means you there, with your second latte grande of the morning). And chances are you don't get enough calcium to begin with, so you can't afford even small losses.

BONE BOOSTERS

The older you get, the more calcium each cup of coffee leaches out of your bones.

Studies have linked drinking two or more cups of coffee a day with significant increase in risk of breaking a hip compared to those who don't get as much caffeine. Tea has never proved to be a problem, as the caffeine amount in a cup of tea is usually much lower than in a cup of coffee, but the levels are certainly still significant if you're drinking it throughout the day. Chocolate, too, contains caffeine, in amounts that should catch the attention of serious chocoholics. Many medicines, including aspirin and other pain relievers, diet aids and diuretics, and cold and allergy pills,

---

HOW MUCH CAFFEINE AM I GETTING?

Note that the serving sizes listed here, though considered average, are certainly smaller than what you'll find in, say, a latte grande or a Big Gulp, or even a regular-size bottle of iced tea.

Food	Serving Size	Caffeine (in mg)
Coffee	6 oz.	103
Espresso	3 oz.	189
Instant coffee	6 oz.	57
Cola	12 oz.	37
Diet cola	12 oz.	50
Tea	6 oz.	36
Tea, instant	12 oz.	48
Chocolate candy	1 oz.	19
Baking chocolate (unsweetened)	1 oz.	58
Chocolate ice cream	½ cup	41

BONE BOOSTERS

Diet sodas have even more caffeine than regular—and plenty of sodas other than colas have caffeine in large amounts. We've noted that you should be steering clear of sodas because of their phosphorus contents, anyway, but if you are indulging, always check the label if you want to avoid the double whammy.

---

have caffeine as an ingredient, so read the labels carefully to be aware of exactly what you're taking. *To protect your bones, drink no more than one cup of caffeinated coffee a day.*

SMOKING

Smoking interferes with the maintenance of bone density. It also decreases the oxygen available to your cells (in a form of carbon monoxide poisoning) and creates damaging free radicals. Some of the damage to bones may be because smoking partially blocks estrogen, which is an important bone booster. Smokers go through menopause on average one to two years earlier than nonsmokers, giving them a couple bonus years in which to rack up bone loss.

DID YOU KNOW?

Smokers have almost double the risk of hip fractures of non-smokers.

Smokers also tend to drink more coffee and alcohol and have less well-rounded diets than nonsmokers, which adds another layer of risk. Smokers' bone density averages 15 to 30 percent lower than nonsmokers'.

Because of the many well-known disastrous health effects smoking causes, there is no good middle ground here: if you smoke, stop! If that is really beyond you, you can reduce your risks somewhat by at least cutting back. Your lungs can heal completely once enough time has passed without a cigarette, but a history of smoking, particularly in childhood, adolescence, and young adulthood, when your body is building bone at its fastest pace, will always carry some increase in risk to your bones. But the shorter the time

DID YOU KNOW?

Up to 20 percent of all hip fractures are attributed to cigarette smoking.

you smoke, the fewer cigarettes you smoke, and the longer ago you quit, the better off you'll be.

In the unlikely event you needed another reason to avoid secondhand smoke (or to not inflict it on others), add bone health to the list. There are many good strategies for stopping smoking, so seek advice on the many ways available to you to reach that goal.

SALT

Salt, too, increases the amount of calcium excreted from your body, which ultimately lowers bone density. Again, that's a small difference, but one that adds up. And—I've said it before, I'll say it again—most people don't have a high enough balance in their calcium accounts to be making constant withdrawals, even small ones. You lose a little here (salt) and a little there (caffeine, etc.), and next thing you know your checks are bouncing.

BONE BOOSTERS

Every 500 additional milligrams of salt (about what you get in a serving of canned soup) takes another 10 milligrams of calcium out of your bones.

As with high blood pressure, some people seem to be more sensitive to the effects of salt than others. But the group of sensitive people is large enough that everyone would be wise to use discretion when it comes to salt, since you don't automatically know whether you are sensitive. The more other risk factors you have, the more important the potential effect of salt will be. Stay within the American Heart Association's guidelines (2,000 mg a day or less) to be safe. (Most Americans come close to doubling that every day.)

SUGAR

Sugar intervenes in the absorption of calcium and increases the amount of calcium excreted, leaving bones without enough of a crucial ingredient. It lowers phosphorus, throwing the delicate calcium-phosphorus balance out of whack, and increases the output of your natural cortisol (a corticosteroid with its own detrimental potential). For these as well as many other reasons (see Chapter 8), we'd all do well to cut back on sugar.

HEAVY METAL POLLUTION

Polluted environments and food expose us to toxic heavy metals that can contribute to bone loss because the body draws calcium out of your bones to try to buffer them. Other chemicals in the air and water and additives in food also put you at risk. Alan Gaby, M.D., writes a lot about this, and I think his warnings are well taken. You can't always completely control what you are exposed to (for example, you can't stop breathing to avoid dirty air, and you can't necessarily relocate your home for fear of nearby pollution). But if you reduce your exposure as much as you can on your own, chances are that will be enough to keep you out of the danger zone.

High levels of lead in your body can cause bone abnormalities and interfere with progesterone, which in turn means bone formation is hampered. Low levels of nutrients, particularly calcium, boost the toxic effects of lead, but the good news is that addressing the deficiencies will lessen those effects. Some canned foods are contaminated with lead, and tens of millions of Americans drink water with lead levels above federal standards (15 parts per billion). Everyone should get his or her tap water analyzed and, if need be, switch to bottled water. Before using water from the tap, let it run for one minute to get rid of water that's been sitting in pipes long enough to potentially absorb lead from your pipes (even nonlead pipes may be joined with leaded components). Choose organic and fresh foods, or at least foods packaged in glass, over canned goods as much as possible.

Cadmium, too, causes mischief. It increases the rate of excretion of calcium and can ultimately cause osteomalacia, bone pain, and higher fracture risk. There's a lot of cadmium in cigarette smoke, which may explain the link between smoking and osteoporosis, and surely gives you another reason not to smoke and to avoid secondhand smoke.

Tin gets into food packed in cans containing tin, with acidic foods like pineapple and citrus juices being particularly likely to absorb it. Foods stored in open cans, or exposed to a lot of heat in closed cans, absorb even more. Once you ingest it, tin is deposited into the bone, in all likelihood interfering with normal remodeling processes there. The more tin you're exposed to, the more copper and zinc you'll need. Tin also restricts the making of stomach acid, which means the nutrients you do take in have a lesser chance of being absorbed and put to use.

Aluminum is stored in various tissues, including your bones. Once there, it interferes with creation of new bone cells and speeds up the breakdown of bone cells.

Don't allow yourself to be overwhelmed by the multitude of your bones' demands. Be smart! By identifying your individual concerns—and seeing their relative importance to your body— you'll be able to narrow your focus and concentrate on just what you need.

Chapter 7

What Tests Are Available . . . and Which Ones You Need

There are several types of tests available to gauge your current bone density, give you an idea of your future risk, and monitor related health concerns. Because developments in this field are so recent, and have advanced so quickly over the last few years, many people—and even some doctors—aren't fully educated about bone density screening and other tests. They may hesitate to take them, fearing exposure to radiation (in the case of density screening) and thinking that the results don't provide sufficient information anyway.

The good news is that the newest tests give a detailed and accurate picture of the state of your bones. You do need to know which tests to have and how to interpret them to make them useful, however. This chapter describes the available options and what you can learn from each test, and also guides you as to which ones you should consider having. As always, you should talk with your doctor about your concerns. My goal in this chapter is to help you make that a fully informed conversation.

Though the tests are expensive if you have to pay for them on your own, as bone density screening becomes more routine, more insurance companies, HMOs, and managed care plans are covering them. In most cases, the tests are now covered by Medicare.

> **TALK TO YOUR DOCTOR**
>
> Low bone density test results are a lot better predictors of fracture risk than high cholesterol levels are of heart disease, and at least as good a predictor as high blood pressure is of strokes. Screening for bone health should be at least as common as getting your cholesterol and blood pressure checked! But nearly three quarters of women with dangerously low bone density don't know they have it; only about 15 percent of women with it are currently being treated.

Knowing your bone density—so you can take appropriate action—is so crucial to your health and longevity that I'd recommend screening for most people even if you have to pay out-of-pocket, if there is any way possible to afford it.

Let me put the expense in perspective: bone fractures resulting from osteoporosis generate over $10 billion in health care costs each year in this country. No matter how much the tests cost, preventive efforts could save huge amounts of money on the societal level. And imagine the personal cost: hospital bills, doctor bills, lab bills, lost income from being out of work for an extended time, to say nothing of loss of quality of life.

WHO NEEDS BONE DENSITY SCREENING?

The questionnaire in the previous chapter gives you a good starting point. The greater the number of risk factors you have (the higher your points), the more concerned you should be about the state of your bones. The idea of low bone density, and how to prevent it, detect it, and treat it, is just sinking in with the general public (not to mention health professionals), so odds are you haven't led a perfect life as far as bone health goes. For anyone with red flags raised in the questionnaire, the first stop should be a thorough general health checkup, and then a discussion with your health care professional about screening for bone density.

In this chapter, you'll see three "Decade Planners" about working with your doctor depending on how old you are. Find the one for your age group (in your 30s, on page 93; in your 40s, on page 97; in your 50s and after menopause, on page 102) for specifics on the tests you should make sure your doctor performs and interprets for you.

Peak bone density is reached from age 30 to 40, and bone loss decreases measurably within ten years after hitting the high point. Every healthy woman should be initially screened for bone density during *perimenopause*, the period of time about one to two years before you stop having periods, when your hormones are downshifting and your periods become irregular or you start having menopausal symptoms. This is especially important if you are struggling with whether to take HRT.

If you have already gone through *menopause* but have never been screened, there is no time like the present. Make an appointment for a checkup and discussion about bone density between the ages of 30 and 35 if you have a lifelong pattern of poor diet and little exercise, or have had an eating disorder. Make the appointment as soon as you have a hysterectomy (or if you've had one in the past and have never been screened), or a fracture from minor trauma, or before you start any medical treatment that could affect your bones (like chemotherapy, thyroid treatment, or corticosteroids).

Otherwise, women should be making an appointment for that checkup-and-discussion by the *age of 40* if your risk factors are high, particularly if you:

- Have a family history (grandmother, mother, sister, brother, or father) of osteoporosis, or of losing height, developing dowager's hump or hunchback, or frequent fractures.
- Are slender and light boned.
- Are or have been a smoker.
- Have decreased sex hormones for any reason.
- Have spine abnormalities, like scoliosis.
- Have an endocrine or metabolic disorder.

- Have been treated for long-term gastrointestinal problems.
- Take thyroid medications, corticosteroids, or anticonvulsants, or have taken them over the long term some time in the past.

The more risk factors are present, and the longer they last, the greater the danger. Any one of them makes early screening worthwhile.

Men should be screened around the *age of 70*, or earlier if they:

- Have had a fracture from minor trauma.
- Have any of the medical conditions described that put them at increased risk.
- Use, or have used, any of the medical therapies that can affect bone density.

Just as with the "Rate Your Risk" questionnaire in Chapter 4, the more risk factors you have, the higher your cumulative risk, the more concerned you should be and the more aggressive action you should take. When it comes to screening tests, that means that the more risks you have, the earlier and/or more extensively you should be screened.

BONE DENSITY TESTS

DUAL-ENERGY X-RAY ABSORPTIOMETRY—DEXA to its friends—provides the most detailed information about the health of your bones, especially in the spine and hip, of any test currently available. This painless procedure takes only ten to twenty minutes, and exposes you to less radiation than a chest x-ray or a full set of dental x-rays or a year of just living in the world. Your only job is to lie on a table as a special x-ray machine passes over you, projecting energy at your bones and measuring how much of the energy passes through. The denser the bone, the less energy goes through. The resulting image has very high resolution, and so is very precise. The margin of error is just 1 percent. But the test is expensive, costing up to $300.

Case in Point: Ruth

I *have one patient who had a bone density scan just after her fortieth birthday, a time when many doctors are still reluctant to send a patient for the test. Ruth had a lifetime of excellent diet and exercise habits, but was concerned because her mother had osteoporosis. Since she felt strongly about it, I wrote the referral. The scan revealed that she already had low bone density. And her real danger zone—menopause—was still years away!*

With this knowledge, she stepped up her efforts to prevent further bone loss. She increased the amount of time she spent exercising, and began taking calcium and vitamin D supplements, along with a multivitamin-and-trace-minerals supplement, aiming to get herself back to the density of a healthy 30-year-old with peak bone mass.

Although encroaching osteoporosis in such a young woman is alarming, to me the truly scary part of this story is thinking about what would have happened if Ruth hadn't had the bone scan. Without knowing she needed to take positive steps now, and staying on top of her progress, I fear she would have ended up with a fracture before long, possibly before menopause. She would have lost a great deal of height, found an ever-increasing forward curve in her upper back, perhaps suffered bone pain, and maybe would have had to curtail her many and varied activities. Not only did the bone density scan perhaps save Ruth's life, it surely saved her lifestyle.

The machine takes measurements of your wrist, vertebrae, and hip, checking both trabecular (spongy) and cortical (rigid) bone. Trabecular bone turns over faster than cortical, so changes will show up there sooner. Results are expressed as a "T-score" comparing you to a healthy 30-year-old at peak bone density, and a "Z-score" comparing you to the average for your age, sex, and race. That gives you some perspective on how dense your bones really are. The hip measurement correlates well with your risk of hip fracture—the most deadly complication of osteoporosis.

For the record, DEXA, like all the bone scans described in

this section, measures only bone density, not *quality* of bone. Just having dense bones offers no guarantees on your skeletal health (strength, for example, is also crucial, but less measurable)—but it is by far the best insurance policy you can have.

DEXA is sometimes known as DXA, or dual-x-ray absorptiometry.

DUAL-PHOTON ABSORPTIOMETRY (DPA) is an older version of DEXA you might still run across. It checks the spine and hip. Compared to DEXA, it takes longer (20–40 minutes) but costs less ($75–$200). The image isn't as clear (the error rate is 8 percent), and the longer time period means you are exposed to more radiation. But the dose is still low, so if this test is cheaper or much more convenient, it will provide enough information for most people.

> ## THINGS TO THINK ABOUT
>
> Bone density screening tests are so low in radiation that the technician (unlike, say, your dental hygienist) will most likely stay in the room with you during the scan.

SINGLE-PHOTON ABSORPTIOMETRY (SPA) OR SINGLE-ENERGY ABSORPTIOMETRY (SXA) checks bone density at the heel or wrist. These machines are less expensive and portable, so you may be able to get the bone density of your wrist screened at a pharmacy, grocery store, or health club. It will involve nothing more than sitting

> ## TALK TO YOUR DOCTOR
>
> Osteoarthritis can make bone density scan results less accurate, so if you suffer from that you should be sure to get your NTX levels (see page 99) to have a second way to figure out your current situation and monitor your progress. A good technician will figure out which hip or wrist is better to scan (choosing one without arthritis where possible), and can see on the scan if the numbers and visual damage don't seem to match.

> ### TALK TO YOUR DOCTOR
>
> DEXA may result in mistakenly high bone densities in people with arthritis. Studies suggest that ultrasound, typically done of the heel, can predict fracture risk accurately. That method hasn't been in use long enough to feel 100 percent confident in those results either, and there is controversy over whether heel measurements (like wrist measurements) give you an accurate picture of other parts of the body. But if you have arthritis it may be a useful way to get a good picture of the state of your bones. There are ways to manipulate DEXA machines so a skilled technician can reduce the chances of an inaccurate reading, and as the machines improve over time, arthritis should become a nonissue in measuring bone density.

with your forearm under the x-ray for 10 to 15 minutes. It'll be considerably cheaper (as low as $35), but also will give a less complete picture since it measures only one site. Although you can project risk of hip and spine fracture from wrist measurements, obviously measurements at those sites give you the most accurate picture of your situation. But for many people without serious risk factors, this inexpensive testing is sufficient. If it reveals serious loss of density, further investigation may be required.

COMPUTER TOMOGRAPHY OR QUANTITATIVE COMPUTED TOMOGRAPHY (CT OR CAT SCAN OR QCT) is more expensive (up to $400) and exposes you to more radiation, so it isn't customarily used for bone density screening. But if you are having one for another reason, ask for a bone density measurement at the same time. The time required is comparable to that for DEXA (10–20 minutes), but there can be a higher margin of error. This is the only test that truly measures density (by volume), and the results you'll get are very detailed: a 3-D image showing both cortical and trabecular bone.

My Story: Marsha

I got my original baseline bone scan four years ago, right after I started taking hormone replacement therapy, and it showed my bones were normal density for my age. The nurse there specializing in bone health educated me about how much calcium I needed to take (1,200–1,500 mg a day, plus vitamin D), and about the different types of calcium and how to decide which one to pick off the health food store shelf.

A year later, I had a second scan to see how my bones were doing through my transition into menopause. I'd cut back on my usual daily exercise routine—aerobic walking or aerobics class—because of nagging shin splints, and at the same time hadn't been careful about the calcium I got in my food. I paid the price in my bones, which were still within the normal range, but less dense than they had been the year before. On top of that, an official doctor's office height measurement showed me I had lost almost an inch of my height.

The additional loss of density—even while I was on estrogen—combined with visions of my shrunken mother in tremendous pain from cracking a rib for no discernible reason, got me back on track. Fear is a big motivator! I'd been taking 1,200 mg of calcium every day, but now I've switched to up to 1,500. I eat yogurt and drink milk every day, and have found a way to work out without aggravating the pain in my legs.

It was an eye-opener for me to see that, at least for me, HRT wasn't a simple solution for protecting bones. All this has convinced me that exercising is important for more than just controlling my weight or protecting my heart, and that I'll need to make a bone scan a periodic part of my health care. I've also realized that there is no one answer that lasts forever, and that I'll have to adjust what I do over the years to stay as healthy as I can.

RADIOGRAPHIC ABSORPTIOMETRY (RA) is a regular x-ray of the hand analyzed by a computer as to density. This test takes just a few minutes and does not require a specialist to administer it, but the film must be analyzed at a special lab. The results, when you

> **TALK TO YOUR DOCTOR**
>
> Ultrasound techniques—using sound waves to measure bone density—are in development, and may provide an even easier screening option in the future.

get them, are as accurate as those from DEXA, and the cost is lower (about $120). Despite that, this test isn't used often.

X-RAYS can spot fractures, and they can tell you if your bones have low density, but they can't quantify the loss at all. But x-rays aren't sensitive enough to identify lost bone mass until 30 to 40 percent is already gone. So they may be able to tell you if you already have a serious problem, but by then you're pretty late in the game. X-rays also sometimes show what looks like osteoporosis, but isn't.

Right now we are limited to testing for bone density and fracture risk, but the missing piece I'd love to be able to fit in would be bone quality. How sturdily your bones are put together will turn out to be equally important to their density. Poorly built dense bones will still break easily, while strong but thin bones can have a lot of resistance. When the day comes that a company announces it has a test to evaluate the "microarchitecture" of your bones, your doctor will alert you to such an advance. The rate of change in this field is so rapid now, I hope we won't have to wait long for that day.

You may not need the most expensive or sophisticated tests right away. Together with your doctor, you should consider your risks—heredity, history, medications, lifestyle, diet, exercise—and decide which tests you need when. Even though the radiation involved is minimal, and even if the most expensive tests are covered under your health plan, you might as well not get something you don't need.

WORKING WITH YOUR DOCTOR

In Your 30s . . .

- Assume you are at peak bone mass until proven otherwise.
- Assess any risk factors (from the questionnaire in Chapter 4) and discuss with your doctor.
- If you are at elevated risk, get an NTX measurement (see page 99), followed by a bone density screening.
- Unless you have severe loss (unusual at younger ages), you have time to work with lifestyle changes before trying potent prescription drugs.
- Have your thyroid function checked.
- If you have irregular menstrual cycles, pinpoint the cause. In particular, you want to make sure that if it is due to "ovarian failure" you take steps to balance your hormones so your bones get what they need.
- Ask your doctor if you should rule out or modify any types of exercise, given your medical history (an old knee injury might mean you should swim crawl rather than breaststroke, or do less jogging and more weight lifting).
- If you have any questions about the content raised in this book, direct them to your health care provider.
- Otherwise, prevention is the name of the game, and the program in this book will give you all you need.

FOLLOW-UP TESTING

Everyone should be retested periodically to check on the rate of bone loss and the effectiveness of preventive measures or of treatments. To get the clearest comparisons, have your tests on the same machine, with the same technician, if possible. Each computer may be calibrated slightly differently, and you want your numbers to be consistent with each other. Switching machines may make it look as if you've gained or lost density when really

THINGS TO THINK ABOUT

Federal law now requires Medicare to cover bone scans in certain cases, including postmenopausal women— or any woman deficient in estrogen—at risk for osteoporosis (a judgment the law leaves to your doctor) and anyone taking a drug approved by the FDA for osteoporosis treatment (which would include Fosamax, Miacalcin, and Evista and traditional HRT), as well as people using steroid medications, with vertebral fractures and some other spine abnormalities (including osteopenia) or with hyperparathyroidism. The conservative guidelines call for covering one test every two years.

This law took effect only in 1998, and while it is better than nothing, it sets up an adversarial relationship among patients, doctors, and insurance companies when it comes to access to bone density screening. Why legislate who *can't* have such a procedure covered, rather than that everyone should, when prevention is so much cheaper than treatment, in dollars and in quality of life?

you've stayed the same or experienced just the opposite of what your results say—just the way different scales will tell you that you weigh a little more or a little less on the same day in the same clothes.

How often you should be tested depends in large part on the rate of change expected in your situation. People using drug therapy should have yearly scans until stable (spine measurements are most reliable for this purpose). Otherwise, you should get a scan every two or three years, unless there's reason to suspect an accelerated rate of loss. If subsequent tests show a decrease in bone mass, or no increase, you will need to alter your approach to making your bones healthy.

The bottom line is, you should be screened for bone density anytime the results will make a difference in deciding on whether to be treated, how seriously you need to pursue preventive strategies, which treatment is right for you, or how effective treatment is.

FRACTURE RISK

In addition to the density of your bones, a host of other factors contribute to your risk of fractures—the most serious concern related to having low bone density. So no matter what your bone scan shows, be aware of—and control to the extent possible—the other risk factors for fracture (some of which overlap with the risks of low bone density we've already discussed):

- Your mother broke a hip before she was 80.
- You had any fracture after the age of 50.
- You are taller than average (or were when you were 25).
- You rate your own health to be fair or poor.
- You can't get up from a chair without using your arms.
- You have poor perception of depth and/or contrast.
- You have a fast resting heart rate (over 80 beats per minute).
- You weigh less now than you did at 25.
- You have, or have had, hyperthyroidism, or are being (or have been) treated for hypothyroidism with thyroid supplements.
- You use, or have used over the long term, tranquilizers or anticonvulsants.
- You spend less than four hours a day on your feet.
- You have lots of caffeine in your diet.

With no more than two of these risk factors and low bone density, or more than two and normal bone density, your risk of fracture is reasonably low—about the same as that of someone without any of these risk factors. With five or more factors, combined with low bone density, your risk escalates to more than 25 times that of someone without risk factors.

WHAT DO MY RESULTS MEAN?

Whichever of these tests you have, the data you get may appear to be hard to understand. With the exception of CT scans and ultra-

---

TALK TO YOUR DOCTOR

"Does it matter what part of my body is checked for bone density?"

Whichever part of your body is checked for bone density will tell you mostly about fractures to that area of bone. Results at your spine or wrist, for example, don't tell you as much about your risk of hip fracture as you'd like, although the numbers can be extrapolated to predict bone loss in other areas. If different sites give you different levels of readings, use the lowest (worst) number as your guide, to be safe.

---

sound, you will get straightforward measurements of total bone weight (in grams) and weight per unit of area (in grams per centimeter squared). Just so you know, measurements of volume, not area, would show true density, but the results you get are good enough. (CT does measure volume, and so gives you true density.) Bone density predicts your risk of fracture eight to ten years into the future.

Anyway, the raw numbers alone do not tell you much, so your results will also be given in standard deviations (SD) from the mean (average). Don't be frightened off by the statistical jargon; a standard deviation is just a device to let you know where you stand compared to the rest of the population. One standard deviation equals roughly 10 percent. If your score is −1, then, that means your bone density is about 10 percent lower than the average; +2 means about 20 percent higher, and so on.

You'll get standard deviations for both your T-score (compared to young bones) and your Z-score (compared to the average for your age). So when you're 60 you might have a Z-score that is +2, putting you ahead of the pack of 60-year-olds. But your T-score would then be −1—cause for concern, but not alarm (see below). I use the Z-score only to give my patients a little perspective, and focus on the T-score instead. *There is no reason you can't aim for the bones of a 30-year-old. Why settle for anything less?*

WORKING WITH YOUR DOCTOR

In Your 40s . . .

- Assume you've started to lose bone until proven otherwise.

- Assess any additional risk factors with your doctor.

- Have your NTX levels (see page 99) checked to evaluate how serious (or minor) your loss is, and how aggressive you need to be.

- Get a bone density screening when you become perimenopausal (irregular periods, or night sweats, or mood changes), or sooner if you have significant risk factors found in the questionnaire in Chapter 4.

- Have all your major hormone levels checked, including estrogen, progesterone, FSH (follicle stimulating hormone), LH (leutinizing hormone), testosterone, and DHEA. The tests of levels in saliva are cheaper and easier to do than levels in the blood. More important, because they are done every few days over a month's time, in order to see the overall pattern, the results are far more useful than a blood test that just gives you information about a single point in time in a system we well know is cyclic.

- Have your vitamin D level checked.

- Have your thyroid function checked.

- Ask your doctor if you should rule out or modify any types of exercise, given your medical history (an old knee injury might mean you should swim crawl rather than breaststroke, or do less jogging and more weight lifting).

- If you have any questions about the content raised in this book, direct them to your health care provider.

- Unless you have severe loss or rapid progression, give lifestyle changes a fair try before using potent prescription drugs.

- Otherwise, prevention is the name of the game, and the program in this book will give you all you need.

The World Health Organization (WHO) provides a conservative framework for evaluating your bone density. To WHO, an SD of −1 to −2.5 compared to peak bone mass (T-score) means osteopenia, or bone loss, and below −2.5 means osteoporosis. It may be more helpful to realize that for each decrease in standard deviation—or for approximately every one-tenth decrease in bone mass—your risk of hip fracture doubles or triples. That is, −1 means you have twice the risk as you would for a score of 0 (being average), −2 means four times the risk, −3 means eight times— and so on. Unless your bones are at peak mass, I recommend taking action to address any loss at all. Even if you are at peak right now, you won't stay there unless you take some precautions.

OTHER TESTS

As I've said, I think the average woman should be screened for bone density before menopause, and the average man should be screened by around age 70. But before you get expensive scans, consider cheaper, simpler, noninvasive tests, at least for baseline measurements. Certain chemicals in your blood and urine are markers of bone formation and loss. Checking their levels can help predict your fracture risk, estimate the quality of your bone, and evaluate effectiveness of treatment. In terms of follow-up care, these tests allow monitoring of progress and they are simpler and cheaper than bone density scans.

Just what levels are normal in the following tests depends on the person, so your results are relative, not absolute. Every lab will print out the normal range *for that lab* in addition to your results, to give you a general idea of where you fall. You want to be as far on the positive side of that range as possible. You should repeat the tests periodically to see if the levels are changing, and if so, in positive or negative directions.

The levels of markers of bone formation and destruction found in blood vary about 10 percent in an individual, and markers in the urine range over about 30 percent, even on the same day. Time of day and season may affect the results. Bone breakdown may naturally speed up in the winter and slow down in the summer. Have your tests at the same time of day each time, and be aware if you are comparing numbers from the same or different times of year. Have the tests processed by the same lab each time. The best way to keep variation to a minimum is to have blood drawn first thing in the morning or collect a urine specimen the second time in the day you urinate, as excretion of these substances generally peaks early in the day.

Home versions of these tests are in the works; these would allow you to monitor your progress more closely, or at least independently, as easily as you can do a pregnancy test. In any event, all these tests could stand further study in the interests of making them more precise.

Presently, the single most important test outside of bone density scans is the one that measures *N-telopeptide of cross-lined type I collagen*. For simplicity's sake, I use the medical shorthand "NTX." This simple, fast, and reliable urine test measures the rate of one kind of bone metabolism. N-telopeptides are molecules used in forming collagen (a major component of bone), and are the first things broken down when bone is destroyed. So high levels mean a rapid rate of bone destruction—in all likelihood outpacing formation of new bone. This test can indicate your risk of fracture and the rate of progression of bone loss, both of which can be high even with reasonably dense bones in some cases. That is, with DEXA you may discover you have density that is on the low side but pretty close to what is expected, but then your NTX might reveal rapid progression and a high risk of fractures. In that case, you'd want to take aggressive preventative action.

Studies show that NTX levels predict changes in the density of your spine, and that women with the highest rates of bone turnover measured this way also had the biggest response—in terms of improved bone density—to HRT. All of which is exactly why this test is so important.

The normal NTX range is from zero to 40 or 50, and the lower it is, the better. You should have your NTX levels checked twice, about six months apart, to give you the best idea of how you are progressing.

The newest tests I've found to be useful, released in the year after this book was first published, are for prydidoline and deoxy-prydidoline. Like NTX these are cross-linked collagens which can be identified in the urine. Prydidoline levels measure collagen loss from any and every source, including rheumatoid arthritis and joint destruction, as well as bone destruction. Deoxy-prydidoline, on the other hand, is very specific for bone. Particularly in patients with arthritis, these results are useful because they help sort out the source of bone loss of osteoporosis and distinguish it from other collagen breakdowns in the body.

A DEXA scan will tell you the current density of your bones. The lab tests help reveal whether you are not building bone or losing it—or both. After you have this information, the next level of tests can help you find out why these things are happening—all of which you need to know in order to make the best individualized plan of attack in order to regain strong bones.

In addition to basic health screening, think about having the following:

- A blood test to measure *calcium*. High levels of calcium in your blood indicate either that bone is being broken down or that calcium is getting into the body but not into the bone (and so is still floating around in the blood). If you are not efficiently absorbing your calcium supplement, you will see high calcium levels in your blood. Checking your NTX and parathyroid hormone (see below) can tell you if bone turnover is causing high calcium levels. Otherwise, your body's absorption and use of calcium is at issue.
- A blood test to check *serum bone-specific alkaline phosphatase*, an enzyme produced by the osteoblasts in building bone. In the blood, it indicates bone formation is taking place—always a good sign. The same substance (alkaline phosphate) is produced at other places in the body, too, so this measurement became useful only with the recent development of a test that distinguishes the source of the chemical.

HOW TALL ARE YOU?

If you do nothing else, at least measure your height scrupulously and regularly. Even a half-inch decrease from your lifelong normal height is a matter of serious concern. The best thing I can say about this test and the protection it offers is that it is absolutely free. But obviously, by the time you begin shrinking, your bone density loss is advanced. When symptoms begin appearing, you have already lost about 30 percent of your bone mass (30 percent below peak density is considered the threshold for being at risk for fractures). By tracking your height, you can find out about bone loss before complications set in, but not before symptoms appear. So although this doesn't give you enough advance warning to work seriously with preventive measures, it is better than nothing.

THINGS TO THINK ABOUT

The average American woman loses an inch and a half of height every ten years after menopause.

The problem with both of the above tests is that sometimes the levels in the blood are normal even when you have osteoporosis. Abnormal levels might indicate bone loss, but might also reveal other metabolic disorders, like hyperparathyroidism, that may or may not be connected to bone loss.

- A blood test to check your *vitamin D* (as "25-hydroxy-vitamin D") levels. If they are too low (under 9 nanograms per milliliter), your body won't be able to use the calcium you ingest. Low levels may indicate that you should have a bone scan.
- A blood test to measure *procollagen I extension peptides*, which results from the making of collagen, a crucial ingredient in bone structure. This is a new test not commonly in use yet, but may well prove to be very valuable in the future.

WORKING WITH YOUR DOCTOR

In Your 50s . . . (and every decade after menopause)

- Assume you have osteoporosis until proven otherwise.
- The tests you need are the same in your postmenopause 50s, 60s, 70s, 80s, and beyond, and you should have everything rechecked at least every ten years.
- Assess your risk factors with your doctor.
- Get a bone density screening.
- Get your NTX levels measured.
- Have your vitamin D levels checked.
- Check levels of DHEA and testosterone. If you're taking estrogen and progesterone, you need to have those levels checked, too, in order to monitor their relationship to each other and to make sure you're taking the correct amount for you.
- Have your levels of thyroid stimulating hormone checked.
- Get a parathyroid evaluation.
- Get a serious diet review by a nutritionist (if your doctor isn't up to it). Look for someone who can talk to you about health on a biochemical level who will deal with you as a specific individual with specific individual needs. You're looking for a lifelong way of eating optimally, not a time-limited, calorie-restricted diet or a "good enough" approach.
- Get a knowledgeable assessment of your current fitness, and your exercise strategies. Work with a physical therapist or licensed, trusted personal trainer. Find out if you have any limitations on the kinds of movement you should do, given your medical history, and discover ways to use exercise to help your body. If you have some arthritis, for example, just resting the joint would be shortsighted, and what you really need is something to support the joint and moderate the

pain. Whatever your regimen, it should make you feel better, not add stress to your already busy life. Have a complete and thorough physical, including colonoscopy and a stress test.

- Don't wait for symptoms. Get all the information you need to make a plan now, so you know what to do for the rest of your life to stay healthy. This isn't about finding out if there is anything wrong right now, but it is an opportunity to create wonderful quality of life for the many years to come.

- If you have any questions about the topics in this book, direct them to your health care provider.

- Otherwise, prevention is the name of the game, and the program in this book will give you all you need.

- A blood test to check *osteocalcin* levels. Osteocalcin is a protein in bone matrix involved with bone formation, and levels in the blood can indicate the pace of bone building. One study showed that, as with NTX levels, women with the fastest turnover of bone had the biggest gains in bone density when taking HRT. Osteocalcin levels are the best way to monitor women taking calcitonin (see Chapter 20), and are a good way to assess bone formation.

Many new screening tests are being developed out of cutting-edge research about bone metabolism, so in the future we will be able to get better and better pictures of just what is going on, and figure out what to do about it. Eventually, we will be able to cure the aging of bone, not just monitor it.

TESTS FOR MONITORING TREATMENT

There are other, less commonly available tests for markers that can be useful in monitoring the effect of drug treatments. Once you've started on a prescription, these markers could change by

50 percent or more in the first few months, letting you know what kind of progress (or lack thereof) you are making. Your doctor may order the following:

- A urine test to check the rate of bone breakdown by measuring levels of hydroxyproline, hydroxylysine, pyridinoline, and deoxypyridinoline. All four are used in creating collagen, and one is also used in elastin. These substances are crucial for forming bone, so their presence in the urine means that bone is being broken down.
- A blood test to measure plasma tartrate-resistant acid phosphatase (TRAP), another indicator of bone destruction.

In the future, these and other tests will be very useful and important.

TESTS FOR GENERAL GOOD HEALTH

I mentioned that you should have an overall health checkup as the first stage in evaluating your level of risk regarding bone density. That should include:

- A mammogram, especially in considering HRT
- A cholesterol check, also helpful in deciding about HRT
- A check of your thyroid, since abnormal levels of thyroid hormone can lead to bone loss
- A check of your parathyroid (if your calcium levels are abnormal)
- Liver function
- Kidney function
- Urine analysis
- Sex hormone levels

NOW WHAT DO I DO?

So you've had whatever screening tests were appropriate. Now what do you do?

Gather all your test results. Start with your bone density—T-score and Z-score—and compare your most recent results with any previous scans you may have had. How do you compare to others your age (Z-score) and to peak bone mass of an average healthy young person (T-score)? If you have NTX results, is the number high enough to indicate a higher than expected risk of fracture or a faster than expected rate of bone loss? Do any other tests show results that affect bone health?

If your bone density is at peak levels and all your other tests are normal, good for you! But don't celebrate so long that you forget to work on keeping your bones that way. Check out how diet, exercise, and supplements can be your strongest allies, and look into "alternative" approaches. Unless your last period was more than five years ago, you should also consider HRT (see Chapter 18) if you have not already.

> **THINGS TO THIINK ABOUT**
>
> Your goal should be not to keep your bone density where it is, but to return it to a level that would make any 30-year-old proud.

Odds are, however, that you will have some risks you want to tame. Learn how to use diet, exercise, and supplements to build and maintain bone strength (see Parts II and III), and launch a preventive attack. Consider HRT if you are in or beyond perimenopause, balancing your risk of bone loss with your risk of breast cancer, heart disease, Alzheimer's, and other major health concerns (see Chapter 18). If your results show you need to take immediate strong action, consider prescriptions that can slow and/or reverse bone loss (see Chapter 20). Investigate "alternative" health approaches to keeping your bones healthy (Chapter 19).

Good bone density means something drastic has to happen to break one of your bones—the kind of car accident, falling from a ladder, or skiing accident trauma we think of as leading to broken bones. But the lower the bone density, the less is required to produce a fracture. The danger zone is generally considered to be when you reach levels that put you in the lowest 20 to 25 percent of people, but *most* people who get fractures from minor trauma (tripping, twisting, etc.) have denser bones than that. It is much easier to prevent bone loss than it is to replace lost bone, so you should start preventive efforts well before you reach the danger zone—just what the remaining weeks of this program are designed to help you do.

❋ ❋

WEEK 1 FOCUS

- Evaluate your risk factors for bone loss and fractures, and pinpoint where you could make improvements.
- Get a thorough physical.
- Get a bone density screening (if indicated) and any other relevant tests to evaluate where you stand.
- Establish your health care team.

WEEK 1 ACTION PLAN

1. If you haven't already started a "bone density" notebook to keep track of your plans and your progress, please do so know, such as how many milligrams of calcium you should be getting each day or the name of a hormone you want to ask your doctor about. Use it to record answers to questions in the Action Plans. Use it for the specific journaling projects described in later Action Plans. Your notebook will be a great reference for you as you design your bone density strategies, tailoring my suggestions to your actual life.

2. What is your overall health like? Think about your energy levels, sleep habits, general diet, exercise routines, family medical history, digestion, bowel habits, chronic complaints, relationships with your health care provider, support network, psychological issues, stress levels, friendships, love relationship, family, knowledge about health, skin condition, and general appearance. What is serving you well? What isn't currently contributing to your overall wellness?

3. What is your mental image of old age in general? Yourself in old age? Are these the images you want?

4. What phase of bone growth pattern are you in (see page 26)?
   —Phase one (bone building, up to peak mass by mid-20s)
   —Phase two (stable peak bone mass, mid-20s to mid-30s)
   —Phase three (bone loss because of increased bone break-down, mid-30s to late 50s or mid-60s)
   —Phase three acceleration (first five to ten years after menopause)
   —Phase four (bone loss because of decreased bone formation as well as increased bone breakdown, mid-60s on)

5. Take the "Rate Your Risk" quiz (page 46), and calculate your score.
   • What is your score?
   • Are you at increased risk (score 50 or more)?
   • Note the areas you're strong in (negative scores, or zeros).
   • Note the areas where you need improvement (highest scores).
   • What puts you at the most serious risk?
   • Which things will be easy to change?
   • Based on your score, do you feel you should have a bone density screening?

6. Do you have five or more of the conditions that give you an increased fracture risk independent of your bone density?

7. Establish your needs and goals. For now this is general, along the lines of "drink more milk," "cut out that second cup of coffee," "start exercising," and "ask my mom about her bone density." Later in the program, you'll get more detailed. Right now write the whole list in your notebook. Then choose your top three priorities. Commit to working on those first, and then continue on to improve your health.

8. Get a thorough physical.
   • Get a bone density scan and your NTX levels checked if indicated. Call your health insurance carrier or HMO and find out if bone density screening (particularly DEXA) is covered for you. If it is not, call your doctor and find out how much it costs.
   • Anyone who gets a scan should also get an NTX test. If

the more involved test is not yet indicated for you, or you are not sure if you need it, a simple NTX result can be a guide. What is your NTX level?

- If you are perimenopausal, arrange to have a bone density screening. If you are menopausal, and have never had a screening, arrange to have one now.
- From the Decade Planners for age-specific issues to take up with your doctor, note in your journal what tests to talk with your doctor about.
- Adjust medications and management of medical conditions to the extent that you can to protect your bones. As you put the lifestyle changes described in this book into place, you may be able to reduce the medications you take (in consultation with your doctor).

9. If you've had a bone density screening—or when you get tested—what are your results? If your doctor just told you generally ("nothing to worry about" or "good for your age" or "a little loss"), ask for a copy of the results and ask him or her to go over them with you thoroughly if you can't decipher it yourself. Your doctor may think being close to the average for your age is OK, but you may be worried about any loss compared to a young adult, so you want to have all the information in hand in order to make your own decisions.

- What is your T-score (compared to average peak bone density)?
- What is your Z-score (compared to women your age)?
- Get both scores in percentage of loss as well as standard deviations, so you can use the figure that's most meaningful to you.
- If you've had more than one test, what has changed? Why?

10. Check with your health care professional to get a clean bill of health for undertaking a new exercise program. If you have any injuries or physical limitations, discuss what movements will protect or improve weak spots, and what you should avoid for safety's safe.

11. Bring all the health care practitioners you work with up to date on what you're doing with their colleagues.

12. Do you have the right health care team for you in place? Have you evaluated your physician's attitude toward and knowledge level about nutrition and exercise and other lifestyle health habits? Nutritional supplements? Alternative health care traditions? If you work with any other health professionals, ask yourself the same questions about them. If you work with anyone in a complementary or integrative field, what is his or her attitude toward high-tech Western medicine? Are you getting all the information, options, and support you need overall?

❋ ❋ ❋ ❋ ❋ ❋ ❋ ❋ ❋ ❋ ❋ ❋ ❋ ❋ ❋ ❋ ❋ ❋

EVALUATE YOUR DIET AND CHOOSE YOUR SUPPLEMENTS

The second step on your journey to a lifetime of healthy bones is to give your diet as thorough a checkup as you just did for yourself. The first chapter in this section is an overview of the principles of a healthy diet. Eating a wide variety of nutritious foods is the best way to get your body what it needs, and a diet that is low in meat, moderate in protein, low in saturated fat, but which includes healthy fats (the omega 3, 6, and 9 oils from fish, nuts and seeds, and whole grains), is low in simple carbohydrates and sugars, is high in complex carbohydrates and whole grains, and is rich with fruits and vegetables and nuts and seeds, is good for you, in general, and also good for your bones in particular. And while this program's recommendations are aimed primarily at keeping your bones strong, following the diet will also help you shed unwanted pounds or maintain a healthy weight.

Because even the most carefully planned diets aren't always perfect—and since a few nutrients are hard to come by in the food chain—I recommend supplements as a kind of inexpensive insurance plan. The second chapter in this section focuses on calcium, the most crucial of all the nutrients for bone health. After looking at how to get as much of it as possible from the foods you eat (dairy and nondairy), the chapter gets into all the technical details you need to know in order to find a supplement that's right for you (without spending any more than you have to) and how to take it for maximum effectiveness.

The following chapter does the same for each of the other nutrients also necessary for bone health. Calcium is the most famous for its role, but you also need vitamin D and magnesium and others to allow calcium to do its work, and this chapter covers where to find them in food and how much you need every day. A list of additional nutrients with key parts to play in bone remodeling completes the picture.

This week is devoted to assessing where you stand in regard to diet, setting goals for where you want to be, and planning for which supplements you will use to fill in any remaining gaps.

Chapter 8

Eat Your Way to Healthy Bones

Food is the fuel for the human machine. If you want the machine to hold up, you've got to give it enough fuel to keep it going. That's the minimum, and if you don't care about the inconvenience and expense—not to mention the heartache—of frequent trips to the mechanic, that'll about cover it. Maybe you're just leasing. But if you've bought and intend to be in it for the long haul, you'll have to do some thinking about the type and quality of the fuel you use.

Before I stretch that analogy to the breaking point, I'll come right to the point: what you eat has an enormous effect on how—and how long—you live. Proper diet lowers our risk of cancer, heart disease, and diabetes, keeps us slim or helps us lose unwanted weight, and even lets us think more clearly. Shelves are full of books that have been written on each of those topics, so you can look up the information if you don't want to simply take it from me. Less well known is the fact that your bones, too, thrive when you eat right and weaken without enough nutritious foods. When your bones weaken, *you* weaken. Your skeleton is the foundation on which your body depends, and without a solid underlying structure, the house cannot stand.

The basic principles of healthy eating still apply when you shift your primary focus to your bones: low saturated fat, high fiber, moderate protein, vegetables and whole grains. But just when you think you learned everything you need to know from the famous "Food Pyramid," you find that your bones have special requirements the builders of the pyramid never mention. In this and the next three chapters, you'll get a generally healthful way of eating designed to build and preserve bone strength. Another chapter shows you how to ensure your body is prepared to make good use of all the nutrients it takes in. Then we'll go one step further and pull all this together into a specific, delicious, easy-to-follow diet, including recipes to get you started.

The proper supplements can fill in the gaps of an imperfect diet (and aren't they all) and push overall health further toward its highest potential, and the next two chapters detail all the specific nutrients that are crucial to your bones and how to take them as supplements. Still, the best option will always be getting the nutrients you need in your food. Your body may or may not be the perfect temple of life, but still it is your body—the only one you've got. Be good to it.

THINGS TO THINK ABOUT

The right fuel for the body depends on the specific body. You wouldn't put water in the gas tank of your car or gasoline on your flower beds. But whatever fuels you, you want it to be of the highest quality possible.

THINGS TO THINK ABOUT

Food is information for the body. It tells it how to react, organize itself, and set itself up to reach the dynamic balance of overall good health called homeostasis. So the same principle that computer programmers cite applies to your body and how you fuel it: garbage in, garbage out.

EAT RIGHT FOR LIFE

No diet will work if you think of it as something you do for a limited time, before going back to business as usual. That's certainly true for weight loss, and it is equally true for building and maintaining bone density. In next week's section, you'll get to our 21-day eating plan, but that is intended just to get you started. By the time you've been eating this way for three weeks, new habits should be taking hold, and you'll be able to venture forward on your own, incorporating the principles you've learned from this book into your everyday life. Eventually, you won't be conscious of being on a diet; you'll just automatically choose the foods you need and avoid the ones that aren't contributing anything to the bottom line: good health and a body that functions smoothly and efficiently.

Before you get to the chapters on specific nutrients and the menu plans, there are a few general guidelines you should follow:

- Educate yourself about nutrition, cooking strategies, and exercise.
- Make it a habit to read food labels, so you know exactly what you're getting (and not getting).
- If your family's favorites don't meet bone density diet standards, don't just forget about them—look for ways to alter them to make them healthier but still delicious.
- Adjust the other seasonings in your food so they won't require as much salt and/or sugar.
- Buy organic whenever that's an option.
- Choose whole grains over refined, and fresh foods over canned, frozen, or packaged, because any kind of packaging destroys nutrients.
- Recognize that as you get older you need even more nutrients, although most people take in even fewer as they age.

Experiment with using less meat. Pick dishes more like stews or stir-fries, where a small amount of cut-up chicken, mixed with a variety of vegetables, goes a long way, rather than roasted chicken or whole chicken breasts. Everyone needs a certain

PRINCIPLES OF A BONE-HEALTHY DIET

- Maintain a diet low in saturated fat.
- Cut back on animal protein. Aim for no more than 4 ounces of meat a day (a piece about the size of a deck of cards).
- Focus your menus on vegetables, fruits, beans and legumes, and whole grains.
- Get at least five servings a day of a variety of vegetables and fruits.
- Eat at least one green leafy vegetable every day.
- Have at least one serving of beans or legumes each day.
- Learn which foods are high in calcium, and include several servings every day.
- Add soy products and other sources of phytoestrogens into your diet.
- Limit the amount of soda you drink to no more than one a day.
- Limit caffeine to no more than one cup of coffee a day.
- Keep salt within the guidelines set out by the AHA: 2,000 mg a day or less.
- Drink no more than one alcoholic beverage a day.

amount of protein in his or her diet for good health, but Americans generally get too much of it. Protein, especially meat protein, draws calcium out of your bones during the digestion process. Meat, the usual source of protein in the typical American diet, also tends to be full of saturated fat, and eating a lot of it (as most of us do, without even thinking of it as a lot) puts you at increased risk of many diseases, including heart disease, and breast and colon cancer. Vegetarians also lose less bone as they age, so I recommend leaning as much toward a vegetarian way of eating as you are comfortable with. You do not have to forswear steak forever (though there's certainly no harm in doing so), but you can't dine on it nightly and expect to keep your bones and heart happy. The more you cut back, the better.

EAT YOUR VEGETABLES

I've got a decided bias in favor of an *almost* vegetarian way of eating. Fish is such a healthy food that I wouldn't advise you to give it up for anything other than philosophical reasons. I see nothing wrong with eating chicken and poultry as a part of your diet, and even (gasp!) red meat on occasion. I would advise, however, always choosing free-range meat and chicken, eating lean cuts with skin and visible fat removed, eating much smaller portions than we usually put on our plates, and limiting yourself to one meat entrée each day. Better still, don't think of meat as an entrée, but as a condiment or side dish. That will keep your animal protein intake to safe levels (too much protein draws calcium out of the bones, you'll remember). It will also leave you with an appetite for all the other foods that are rich in the nutrients your bones need, most of which are not found in meat.

> ### BONE BOOSTERS
>
> Just 1 ounce of meat requires 24 mg of calcium as a buffer during digestion.

Vegetarians and vegans (strict vegetarians who eschew eggs and dairy products) have significantly lower risk of osteoporosis (not to mention a range of other diseases) than carnivores. Total bone mass is not much different, but once bone loss begins, vegetarians have the advantage because their rate of loss is much slower. They aren't building more bone, they're just hanging on to more of it for longer, which is the name of the game for anyone playing in the second half. The benefit comes as a result of taking in less protein and less phosphorus (made in the process of digesting meat), both of which can increase the amount of calcium excreted from your bones. Your bones can't afford to let their calcium go! (See Chapter 9.) Doubling the amount of protein coming in can double the amount of calcium going out. Levels that high are not at all uncommon in the United States.

To protect your bones, your low-fat, limited-protein, quasi-vegetarian diet must be rich in calcium, vitamin D, magnesium, and soy products (see Chapters 9, 10, and 11). It also must be reasonably low in salt, sugar, caffeine, alcohol, and phosphorus (which comes primarily from sodas; see Chapter 6). It should also

THINGS TO THINK ABOUT

When it comes to getting a good balance of nutrients, try a "traffic light diet." Eating a variety of green, yellow, and red* fruits and vegetables every day is the best way to get what you need.

*And orange (what you get when you combine yellow and red!).

incorporate nutritional supplements as an insurance policy, if nothing else (see Chapter 10). All this is aimed at building up the densest possible bones in the first place, and losing as little of them as possible thereafter.

Good nutrition is also a boon to those who already have low bone density. Improving the diet, or adding supplements, decreases the rate of fracture and reduces the rate of death following a fracture. It also saves money. It has been a while since I mentioned it, so let me take this opportunity to remind you: it is never too late.

IS IT HEALTHY TO BE A VEGETARIAN?

Your grandmother might worry you won't get enough protein, but as we've seen, the reality is that just about every American gets *too much* protein, and vegetarians certainly don't lack for it, either. A vegetarian diet is richer in nutrients than the average American diet and may be lower in fat. Vegetarians have lower rates of many common health concerns, including:

- Osteoporosis
- Heart disease
- Cancer, particularly breast and colon cancer
- High blood pressure
- High cholesterol levels
- Stroke
- Arthritis
- Macular degeneration
- Type II diabetes

If that's not enough to make you look twice at how much meat you eat, and how much you can cut out of your diet, try this on for size: vegetarians are much closer to ideal weight than the average American.

My Story: Julie

When I went to have my bone density checked, I figured the results would come back telling me I was "at risk"—isn't every woman over 60? But I was very surprised when it turned out I already had osteoporosis. I've always had a pretty balanced diet, and been a generally active person. I'm no athlete, but I am a half-decent weekend skier.

I am small-boned and thin, like my mom, who was very bent over by the time she died, well into her 80s. As I've read about the things that have an impact on your bones, I've learned more about my risks. I never have soda, but do usually drink a cup or two of coffee each day. I smoked for more than ten years when I was very young, but I stopped as soon as the Surgeon General's report about the cancer dangers came out. I didn't have any menopausal symptoms, so I never even really considered hormone replacement therapy. My doctor brought it up again after my scan, but I cut her off immediately. I'm about to be 65, and have no intention of starting that now, if I haven't needed it otherwise.

When I found out how much bone I had lost, I started taking Fosamax. After two years on it, a second DEXA scan showed I had increased density by 7 percentage points. That puts me on the borderline between osteopenia and osteoporosis, but definitely on the denser side and out of immediate danger. Though I never had any side effects from it, Fosamax is a difficult medication to take because you have to wait a half hour after you take it before you eat, and you have to stay upright during that time, so you can't exactly crawl back in bed with the New York Times. Besides, I don't want to be on this or any drug forever. And in fact, I'm not at all certain just what caused the improvement, since I started a strength training program, became a vegetarian, and began taking vitamin and calcium supplements on the same day I started Fosamax!

That's why I've decided to stop taking the drug and rely on diet and exercise. I'm now a vegetarian, but not vegan—I do eat eggs and dairy. I always say, "I don't eat anything that had a heartbeat." That was an enormous change for me, because before that I ate meat at least once a day. I certainly always had meat at dinner, and sometimes it seemed like

I was the last woman alive who would admit to regularly enjoying a steak. It's funny, though, because giving up meat hasn't really bothered me. Once I got on a roll with it, it just became second nature.

Regular exercise was also a major lifestyle change for me. I've never been a couch potato, but I never followed any particular routine before. Now I exercise daily. I do half an hour of aerobic exercise seven days a week—a cross-country skiing machine, though I don't use the arm part (I read). Plus, twice a week I work out with weights.

My doctor recommended taking a calcium supplement and a multivitamin, so now every day I get 1,000 milligrams of calcium in pills that also contain vitamin D, magnesium, and trace minerals. I also take a common multivitamin to make sure I cover everything.

I've been off Fosamax for six weeks now. This is an experiment on my part, to see if I can maintain the changes I've made, without the medication. I'll get another DEXA scan in a year and then reevaluate my situation. If I lose bone, I suppose I'll go back to the Fosamax, but I believe the healthy changes I've made in my life will give me the strong bones I need.

THE INSULIN RESPONSE

Our ancestors were hunter-gatherers who ate only what they could catch or pick—meat, fish, berries, nuts, and some fruits and vegetables. Agriculture is only about 10,000 years old, so, in the grand scheme of things, humans haven't been consuming wheat and other grains, especially those milled into flour, or dairy products, for very long. Our digestive and immune systems still haven't completely evolved to deal with them. That's part of the reason our bodies so often react negatively to the way we eat in the United States today. The meat our ancestors ate was game—not factory farmed or even "free range"—and rich in nutrients, low in fat, and without chemical exposure. Their vegetables and fruits were also truly organic, grown in soil that hadn't been depleted of nutrients by decades of industrial farming, and so containing a full complement of nutrients without any chemical contamination.

INSULIN RESISTANCE

Insulin resistance causes excess adrenaline and cortisol to be released in the body, and those hormones can accelerate bone loss. On top of that, insulin resistance is often a red flag that you're on the road to diabetes and/or obesity. So it pays to know the warning signs of insulin resistance. *Type 2 diabetes* is the most dramatic manifestation, but a host of other findings can warn you to get your insulin levels checked. "Normal" insulin levels are generally considered to be anything up to 20, but I think you hit the danger zone between 9 and 12 and should take action at that early stage, cutting back on sugars and simple carbs. Two or more of the following in combination should be enough to get yourself checked out:

- Gestational diabetes
- Triglycerides above 150
- HDL cholesterol under 35
- Blood pressure above 140/90. Your risk actually starts to increase at 125/85.
- Polycystic ovaries
- Heart disease before age 60
- Uric acid over 8 mg/dl
- Family history of type 2 diabetes, high blood pressure or heart disease before age 60, or high triglycerides
- Low birth weight
- Lack of exercise
- Gaining more than 15 pounds after age 18, having a BMI over 25, or being an "apple" shape
- Being African American, Japanese American, Latino, Melanesian, Polynesian, Indian, Australian aboriginal, Micronesian, or Native American

Subsisting largely on meat, at least the meat widely available today, isn't ideal, either, so I don't recommend a "caveman diet" for everyone. In terms of our general health, the other big problem with the American diet—along with fat and protein overload—is

Case in Point: Grace

*G*race smoked her last cigarette just weeks before her first bone scan. The smoking, a history of heavy drinking (though it ended thirty years ago), chronic digestive problems requiring various medications, and an extremely stressful job from which she recently retired had taken their toll: she had osteoporosis in both her hip and spine, falling more than three standard deviations below normal bone density. Grace had never taken hormones and wasn't about to start now, nor did she want any prescription medications, despite the severity of her loss.

Instead, she began exercising—walking and doing yoga on alternate days—started taking supplements of calcium, vitamin D, and trace minerals, and changed her diet to lower simple carbohydrate intake, increase protein, and generally improve the nutritional quality of the food she ate. On top of that solid foundation she added a regimen of herbs to help her balance her hormones and handle stress, including red clover, black current seed oil, omega-3 oils, and amino acids. She also used natural digestive enzymes to control her troublesome digestive symptoms and improve her absorption of nutrients.

Although I usually recommend waiting at least a year for a follow-up to allow plenty of time for improvements to take full effect, Grace had a second bone scan six months later and her progress was already apparent. While her spine showed very minor increases in density, her hip went from −3.62 SD to −2.94. She obviously still had a way to go to eliminate her risk of fractures, but felt confident that her "all natural" approach was serving her well.

that simple carbohydrates (starches and sugars) have such a central place in our diets.

Complex carbohydrates are the good stuff, but we eat much more white flour, pasta, white bread, white rice, cakes, cookies, bagels . . . you get the picture. All those simple carbohydrates are quickly broken down into sugar once they are in your body. All that sugar—together with the sugar we take in directly—makes your body release insulin to process it. (That's just where diabetics get into trouble: their bodies aren't making the insulin they need.) The insulin does its job, and your sugar levels retreat. But the insulin response lags behind the sugar's demand for it. As the sugar is being used up, the insulin levels are still rising, and remain elevated after the sugar is depleted. That lowers sugar levels below normal, making you crave more, and eating it makes the whole cycle begin anew.

Each new burst of sugar, then, puts your insulin level higher still, while your sugar levels drop far enough to make you crave more carbohydrates and sweets to raise them again. This vicious cycle triggers the release of stressor hormones in an attempt to quell the insulin-sugar response. This is a constant general stress on your body and leads to weight gain, poor sleep, loss of concentration, tiredness, and lack of energy. If you can no longer hold your head up at about 2:30 in the afternoon, when you had a full night's sleep the previous night, I bet you had a plate of pasta for lunch or a sugary dessert after, or a carbohydrate breakfast. And for our purposes here, those extra hormones, in addition to corralling the insulin, also can wreak havoc with your bones.

I'll give you an example of how this cycle works. Say you eat a bagel for breakfast and accompany it with a large glass of OJ. You used jam instead of fatty cream cheese, and chose calcium-enriched juice, so you're pretty proud of yourself for starting your day out right. But your body's just been dosed with sugar, sugar, and more sugar, and your insulin level rapidly rises—then stays high even after the sugar has gone. For lunch, then, you have a sandwich and potato chips, and another glass of juice. Your sugar and insulin levels soar again. By dinner, you are ravenous and craving still more carbs—your body's way of trying to equalize the high insulin and low blood sugar levels. So you eat—and eat, and eat—and whether you eat healthfully or not, overnight as insulin levels normalize, your sugar level drops very low. The brain requires sugar, and low levels deprive it of an easy energy source, giving you less than optimal functioning. And you wake up craving . . . sugar. Each quick fix of pasta or a cookie makes you feel better, but only temporarily, and crashing can make you feel worse than you did to start out. It becomes a constant game of catch-up. Sugar raises insulin, which decreases sugar, which makes you crave more sugar . . . it is an endless cycle.

To avoid that insulin response, choose complex carbohydrates. The best grains are the ones closest to how nature intended them: whole, *chunky* grains. Think oatmeal, barley, wheat berries, quinoa, millet, and bulgur wheat. Brown rice is better than white, but still relatively quickly converted to sugar. Vegetables are almost all excellent choices, though potatoes and corn are also quickly made into sugar (they do come with fiber, however, which puts them a notch above, say, macaroni). You wouldn't guess it, but sweet potatoes are actually a better choice than white potatoes. Fruits will deliver fiber, and some complex carbohydrates, but their sweetness comes from sugar, so you have to be careful to eat them in combination with a small amount of protein or healthy fat. (Beans and legumes are good choices, as are nuts and seeds, cheese, and yogurt.) Whole-grain flour is better than refined, but simply by being ground into flour, they are no longer technically whole grains. So oatmeal you have to cook for five minutes is better than the one-minute, or quick variety, which is better than instant, which is better than oat flour. You'll have to read bread labels carefully, as almost everything sold in your grocery store is made primarily with white flour, even rye, whole wheat, and multigrain loaves. Don't be fooled by the listing "wheat flour"—unless it says "whole wheat flour," it isn't. High-fiber foods are usually complex carbohydrates.

BONE BOOSTERS

Breakfast is a common simple-carbohydrate pitfall, getting your whole day off to a bad start. Here's one simple solution: cook a large batch of the best oatmeal over the weekend, then refrigerate it and reheat one serving at a time in the microwave. Add fruit to it for extra benefit and flavor.

The idea is not to subsist solely on barley and broccoli, but to moderate the overall amount of sugars your body has to contend

POOR CARB METABOLISM

Watch out for signs your body is having real trouble with carbohydrate metabolism: craving carbohydrates and sweets, feeling tired after meals, being irritable, having poor concentration or low energy. Red clover herb and omega oils are very helpful (used according to package instructions), along with substances like coenzyme Q10, B-complex vitamins, chromium, L-carnitine and acetyl L-carnitine, and other supplements that help regulate sugar and insulin levels. These work best in conjunction with a diet that is protein rich but low in meat, low in simple carbohydrates, and high in fruits and vegetables.

with so you eliminate the haywire insulin response. As with so many things, balance is the key. If you can't do without pasta, use whole wheat or vegetable pasta, at least, and choose more vegetables than fruits. If you snack on fruit three times a day, switch one serving for a handful of nuts, or go with oatmeal in the morning instead of a bagel.

RECOMMENDED DAILY DOSES

CoQ10	100–300 mg
B-complex vitamins	50–100 mg
Chromium	200 mcg
L-carnitine	1,500–2,000 mg
Acetyl L-carnitine	500–1,000 mg

QUALITY COUNTS

Whether you are out to lose weight or to maintain your current healthy weight, don't be fooled into thinking that just counting calories will get you there. Before we get into all the specific reasons why, and explain what else you have to consider, I want to give you an example to bring this point home: if you are eating all healthy foods, how many calories you take in, exactly, will be

Myth: The development of "nonfat" products has been a positive development for health-conscious people.

Fact: While low- and nonfat dairy products have been a boon to those seeking calcium and protein without eating too much fat or meat, most of the new products are loaded with sugar and artificial ingredients found nowhere in nature, are very high in calories, and create the illusion you can eat a lot with impunity.

irrelevant, and if you are eating all junk foods, you'll put on or be unable to lose weight no matter how low you keep your calorie counts.

Imagine this: You start your day with a large bowl of oatmeal with sliced fruit, cinnamon, and nonfat milk or soymilk. Your midmorning snack is a handful of nuts. For lunch you eat an enormous green salad with a variety of vegetables, topped with feta cheese, sunflower seeds, and olives, and a cup of lentil soup. You have a snack of no-sugar-added yogurt and an orange. For dinner you have a small piece of chicken, barley pilaf, greens sautéed with garlic, and sliced tomatoes with basil. You eat some sugar-free frozen yogurt with homemade granola during the evening.

You are on a diet.

Now imagine the next day you stop by the drive-through window on your way to work to pick up sausage, eggs, and cheese sandwiched in a buttered biscuit, and a cup of coffee. Before you've even reached the office, you've probably eaten about half as many calories and two-thirds of the fat you did the day before. (And it'll be days before you need any more salt.) Your schedule is crazy right through lunch, and you're feeling a bit guilty about breakfast anyway, so between phone calls you down a pickle left over from your officemate's lunch and keep on working. But you're starving by the time the snack cart rolls by, so you buy a jelly donut. Or you pass up the snack cart, but then can't stay away from the candy jar on the desk down the hall. By dinnertime, you're too tired to fix anything, but you know you really have to eat better. So you microwave a "lite" entrée you have in your freezer for just such occasions: fettuccine Alfredo. The portion doesn't really fill you up, but at least, at only 6 grams of fat, you know it is good for you. Plus, it had a few peas in it, so that gives you a serving of vegetables, right? And you already had that pickle at lunch.

Both days you probably had about the same number of calories. But the first day you were never hungry (in fact, you couldn't even finish that salad), and ate a lot of the foods you love. You also got a wide range of the nutrients your body needs for overall health and for healthy bones. The second day, after the unsettled feeling of having a lump of sausage sitting in your stomach passed, you never felt like you really ate. And your body certainly didn't get much of what it needs.

I'll give you one guess which way of eating would make you feel better over the long term. On top of that, making consistently smart choices will allow you to lose inches, and probably pounds, too—on the same level of calories that would keep you puffy and fat if it mostly came from junk food. If you eat too many calories, even if they all come from carrot and celery sticks, you will gain weight. But even on a reasonable number of calories, you won't get or stay slim if the foods aren't nutritious. You should also keep in mind that however poor the effect is on your outsides, it is even worse for you on the inside.

WEIGHT CONTROL

The bone density diet is aimed primarily at giving you healthy bones. But it also supports (as would any nutritious, well-rounded, low-fat, high-fiber diet) overall good health and weight control. Being 20 percent over your optimal weight puts you at increased risk for high blood pressure, heart disease, and diabetes, just to name the most common of the chronic diseases caused or exacerbated by excess weight.

The best way to simply evaluate your weight, and keep it within an appropriate range, is to calculate your body mass index (BMI), or your height divided by weight. Unfortunately, the people who made this up thought in metrics, so you have to do a little

FUN WITH COMPUTERS

To have a computer do the work for you, you can get your BMI calculated at the "OnHealth" website. Go to *http://onhealth. com/ch1/index.asp,* and click on the Interactive Tools link. You'll see a list of "interactives" that includes a BMI calculator. Or put "Body Mass Index Calculator" into your favorite search engine, and you can pick from a number of places that will do the number crunching so you don't have to! Some will do it for you in kilograms and centimeters, or stones, if you prefer that to pounds and inches.

extra math to account for the conversion. Ready? Multiply your weight, in pounds, by 703. Square your height, in inches (multiply it by itself). Divide the weight answer by the height answer, and that gives you your BMI. If you don't have a calculator handy just now, you can get an estimate of your BMI from the chart on page 128. Short of getting tested by full immersion in water (which could set you back $200), BMI is the easiest way to estimate your lean body mass, as opposed to body fat.

HOW MANY CALORIES SHOULD I GET?

To maintain your healthy weight, figure out roughly how many calories you should take in each day by multiplying your target weight by 14 if you are moderately active, 13 if you are sedentary, and 15 if you are extremely active. Don't forget that calories come from food—and are burned off by exercise. No matter how many calories you do or don't swallow each day, you'll never completely control your weight or be as healthy as you can be without incorporating regular exercise into your life (see Week 4).

Here's the best news you've heard about your weight: bone density is higher the higher your BMI. But a BMI above 26 has other health risks attached—heart disease, cancer, and diabetes, to name a few—so whatever further gains you might get in bone

HOW AM I GOING TO KEEP TRACK OF ALL THIS STUFF?

It may seem overwhelming to keeping running tallies of so many things, but once you increase your awareness by noting them specifically for a couple weeks, you'll begin to approximate the appropriate levels automatically, and you'll no longer need consciously to measure and add up every morsel that passes your lips. If you don't want to take on all of these new goals at once, choose one and concentrate on that for two weeks, and as you get on autopilot on that one, start with another. It will take longer to get yourself on track, but since we are talking about a lifetime plan, the investment of a few extra weeks now will have plenty of time to pay off. The most important thing to remember is that it is not so much the calories or fat grams or cholesterol counts that matter, but the actual foods you choose. If you choose all wholesome, nutritious foods and eat a variety of them, you'll get all the nutrients you need, won't take in too many of the no-nos that are so hard on your body, and will stay within a healthy range of weight.

density are outweighed by the additional risks. But BMI below 21 puts you at increased risk of fractures (and losing the ability to live independently after a fracture), which just goes to show you: you *can* be too thin. The bottom line: you want to maintain a weight that puts your BMI between 21 and 26, and not to worry a bit if you are at the upper end of that range.

Calories are not the only game in town. Keep an eye on your fat and fiber grams each day. Make sure you get at least 25 grams a day of fiber. And you should get no more than 30 percent of your calories from fat, including 10 percent of calories from saturated fat. One gram of fat has 9 calories, which means, for example, no more than 50 grams of fat a day on a 1,500-calorie diet (with no more than 17 of those grams from saturated fat). Going as low as 20 percent of your diet from fat would be even better, and some experts recommend as low as 10 percent. Remember, however,

Body Mass Index
Height (in feet and inches)

Weight (in pounds)	5'	5'1"	5'2"	5'3"	5'4"	5'5"	5'6"	5'7"	5'8"	5'9"	5'10"	5'11"	6'	6'1"	6'2"
100	20	19	18	18	17	17	16	16	15	15	14	14	14	13	13
105	21	20	19	19	18	17	17	16	16	16	15	15	14	14	13
110	21	21	20	19	19	18	17	17	16	16	16	15	15	15	14
115	22	22	21	20	20	19	19	18	17	17	17	16	16	15	15
120	23	23	22	21	21	20	19	19	18	18	17	17	16	16	15
125	24	24	23	22	21	21	20	20	19	18	18	17	17	16	16
130	25	25	24	23	22	22	21	20	20	19	19	18	18	17	17
135	26	26	25	24	23	22	22	21	21	20	19	19	18	18	17
140	27	26	26	25	24	23	23	22	21	21	20	20	19	18	18
145	28	27	27	26	25	24	23	23	22	21	21	20	20	19	19
150	29	28	27	27	26	25	24	23	23	22	22	21	20	20	19
155	30	29	28	27	27	26	25	24	24	23	22	22	21	20	20
160	31	30	29	28	27	27	26	25	24	24	23	22	22	21	21
165	32	31	30	29	28	27	27	26	25	24	24	23	22	22	21
170	33	32	31	30	29	28	27	27	26	25	24	24	23	22	22
175	34	33	32	31	30	29	28	27	27	26	25	24	24	23	22
180	35	34	33	32	31	30	29	28	27	27	26	25	24	24	23
185	36	35	34	33	32	31	30	29	28	27	27	26	25	24	24
190	37	36	35	34	33	32	31	30	29	28	27	26	26	25	24
195	38	37	36	35	33	32	31	31	30	29	28	27	26	26	25
200	39	38	37	35	34	33	32	31	30	30	29	28	27	26	26
205	40	39	37	36	35	34	33	32	31	30	29	29	28	27	26
210	41	40	38	37	36	35	34	33	32	31	30	29	28	28	27
215	42	41	39	38	37	36	35	34	33	32	31	30	29	28	28
220	43	42	40	39	38	37	36	34	33	32	32	31	30	29	28
225	44	43	41	40	39	37	36	35	34	33	32	31	31	30	29
230	45	43	42	41	39	38	37	36	35	34	33	32	31	30	30
235	46	44	43	42	40	39	38	37	36	35	34	33	32	31	30
240	47	45	44	43	41	40	39	38	36	35	34	33	33	32	31

that no one can thrive, or even survive, on a *no*-fat diet. Fat is good—provided you get the healthy kinds—and necessary for smooth functioning of the body. You need essential fats, like the omega-3s in fish and soybeans, and fatty acids. The omega-6 oils in nuts and seeds are also beneficial, so the only reason to watch your intake may be *calories*, not fat. "Bad" fats, which do nothing for you but block your arteries and strain your immune system, hurt the body's ability to use the good ones, another reason to maintain a positive balance.

If you need to lose weight to reach your target BMI, cutting your calories by 500 a day will allow you to lose about a pound a week. Be sure to cut empty calories, not nutritious ones. Remember that exercise is the best way to eliminate calories, particularly when you're eating mostly wholesome, healthy foods. Weight loss from diet alone—without benefit of exercise—is unlikely to last. Slow and steady weight loss is the best way to lose weight and keep it off. The faster you lose weight, the more likely you are to simply regain it. No matter what your current or target weight, you should always get a *minimum* of 1,200–1,500 calories a day. (That's a generally good level for most women, unless you are still growing, or very athletic, in which case you'll need more calories to fuel your body. Men generally need more calories each day because they have a larger body mass, on average.) Lower calorie intake makes you likely to miss out on sufficient levels of a variety of nutrients, especially (but certainly not only) calcium. And your metabolism will eventually adjust to whatever level of caloric intake it usually gets, and providing fewer calories will mean your body gets used to using less. Restricting calories in the short term may help you lose weight initially, but it will eventually lose its effectiveness. Most people experience this as a plateau—they'll stop losing weight, even though they are still eating less. What's more, to keep off the weight you have lost, you have to stay at that same low level. As soon as you add anything else, you begin to gain back whatever you lost—and probably more.

The caloric goal you set for yourself when you are trying to lose weight should be the same as what you plan to continue eating ever after. If that number of calories is not allowing you to lose weight, your best bet is to step up the type, amount, or frequency of exercise you're getting. When you reach your desired weight, you could cut back on exercise *gradually* if you don't want to continue losing weight. You have to do it slowly to avoid gaining weight by quickly reducing the number of calories you're using, and allow your body to gradually adjust and find a new "homeostasis" or

LOSING WEIGHT THE WRITE WAY

Try writing down every single thing you put in your mouth for a week, including portion size: "6 M&Ms" or "huge plate of spaghetti" or "a handful of grapes and a slice of cheese." Weigh yourself every day you're doing this. Most of my patients, even the ones who come to me complaining they can't lose weight no matter what they do, usually begin to see the weight coming off that very first week—without following any plan aside from committing what they eat to paper. After the initial shock of seeing exactly how much they do take in, they automatically begin to modify what they eat. It goes something like this: "If I eat that cookie, I'm going to have to write it down! And then I have to show my list to Dr. Kessler! I think I'd rather not eat it today." Even just one week of this is enough to make those forced healthy choices into habits—and the pact is sealed as you see the first pound come off.

steady state at your desired weight. Of course, you might just enjoy exercise and all its attendant benefits enough that you won't want to cut back. Then you'll have no choice but to increase the number of calories you take in, if you want to maintain your weight! The idea is to change your "set point" to your desired weight. Whatever you do, since exercise is good for you for many reasons beyond weight control, you'll want to keep exercise a part of your life forever, even if you find four days a week is more to your liking than five or six over the long run.

If you have specific health concerns, like diabetes or high blood pressure, you should also design your diet with your doctor to make sure it meets all your needs.

The recipes and menus in Chapters 13 and 14 are designed to be flexible according to your caloric requirements and personal preferences. The keys to weight loss are already well known to you. No book, including this one, can tell you more about generally how to do it than you already well know: eat moderate, well-balanced meals and snacks, and exercise. There are no quick fixes—and in fact, the quicker the fix, the faster and higher the rebound.

ARE YOU AN APPLE OR A PEAR?

A pear-shaped figure (hips wider than waist) offers health benefits compared to an apple shape (waist greater than hips), which has been associated with higher rates of high blood pressure, heart disease, stroke, and type II diabetes. Abdominal fat usually indicates more fat around the internal organs, which is part of the problem. There's also apparently a connection to higher insulin levels and poor carbohydrate metabolism (due at least in part to too many simple carbohydrates in the diet). The increase in cortisol and other stress hormones that results is what leads to the chronic health problems mentioned above—and, in all likelihood, to low bone density as well.

Beyond glancing in the mirror to see your general shape, the best guide to where you fall is your waist-to-hip ratio, which you find by dividing your waist measurement by your hip measurement. (Take the measurements a few times, and average them, to ensure accuracy—tape measures are very fickle.) To be a "pear," the number should be .8 or less for women and up to .9 or 1.0 for men. Anything higher makes you an apple.

If you find you have an apple shape, you should cut back on sugar and carbohydrates to protect your health. When you do, you'll also probably lose weight and move closer to being a pear. If you need more motivation to make the change, get a fasting blood sugar level and a fasting insulin level, then a "two-hour postprandial" sugar and insulin test—your numbers after drinking a sugary drink your doctor prescribes—to see how your body handles sugar (a simple carbohydrate). Anything up to 22 is considered normal according to conventional wisdom, but issues surrounding carbohydrate metabolism are generally underrecognized, and I think you should be concerned about anything over 14 (or even a 9 or 10 fasting). Higher numbers are considered prediabetic.

The pear shape is more common in women, thanks to the wider hips childbearing requires. A pear can have just as much body fat as an apple, but the distribution lower on the body is not as dangerous as right around the middle (the spare-tire look).

Some women don't fall clearly into one category or the other—big thighs, big tush, big stomach. If that's you, I'd recommend playing it safe, and considering yourself open to the hazards of the apple shape and taking action accordingly.

The specifics are simple to learn (and truthfully not all that hard to stick to, once you get used to a new way of eating). As mentioned earlier, select your foods to get less than 30 percent of your calories from fat, with less than 10 percent being saturated fat. Less than 15 percent should come from protein, which, like carbohydrates, has 4 calories per gram. Everything else should be mainly complex carbohydrates, vegetables, and fruits. That catchall category would also include any sugar and white flour, but you obviously don't want to trade in too much in the way of nutritious foods for those empty calories. You want about half of your calories to come from complex carbohydrates. Just don't expect to add everything up to an even 100 percent, since almost all foods have various kinds of nutrients. Foods with fat may also have protein or carbs, or vice versa. Eating a pork chop or a tofu burger gets you both protein and fat, for example, though you'd tally one under saturated fat

FUN WITH COMPUTERS

If you want to know if you are an apple or a pear, but you never liked division and percentages, all you have to do is take your measurements (in inches) to have your waist-to-hip ratio calculated via computer. Go to *http://onhealth.com/ ch1/index.asp*, and click on the Interactive Tools link, and then on All Calculators. You'll see a list of "interactives" that includes a waist-to-hip ratio calculator.

and animal protein and the other not. This point bears repeating: it isn't just the calories or fat grams that count, but the overall nutritional quality of the food containing them. That is, choose the tofu more often than the chop.

Regular exercise of the proper sort is indispensable when it comes to living at a healthy weight, and is described in more detail in Week 4. It is the only way to increase your metabolic rate, the surest way to lose weight or maintain a healthy weight.

AM I WELL NOURISHED?

If you generally feel you are in optimal health, you'll do just fine following the bone density diet. Actually, if you are in optimal health, I bet you adhere to many of these principles already, and will just be fine-tuning for the specifics of bone health.

If you have any chronic health concerns, you should always consult with your health care professional before embarking on any new health plan, and taking up a new way of eating is no exception. And, if you have a reason to suspect a particular deficiency, you may need a formal nutrition evaluation. A good nutrition assessment should include a thorough medical history and physical examination. A blood cell count gives you an indirect indication if

THINGS TO THINK ABOUT

One good study showed that in young women in generally good health, a low-protein diet led to *decreased* calcium absorption. Similar women on a high-protein diet absorbed significantly more calcium. So is a high-protein diet therefore good for everyone? Myopic studies can easily miss the big picture.

The study did not distinguish between meat and nonmeat sources of protein. But since we know much acid is produced when meat (and most grains!) are digested—and that the body draws calcium out of the bones, if necessary, to neutralize it—the key is to include a wide variety of fruits and vegetables in your diet to counteract the acidity before your bones are affected. And the more of your protein that comes from nonanimal sources, the better, since nonanimal proteins become less acidic during digestion.

there is a deficiency in iron, B_{12}, or folate, and calcium and phosphate levels are good to know for anyone concerned about low bone density. Your health care provider may recommend some other tests that can point up nutritional deficiencies if they exist. Discuss the medications and supplements you take, and how you take them, with your physician to make sure they don't interfere with one another or with absorbing nutrients from what you eat. Knowing your weight, blood pressure, sugar and cholesterol levels, and thyroid and kidney function (though they don't measure nutrients directly) can, among other things, give you a sense of how healthy you and your diet are, and where you can make improvements.

A health professional can help you tell how well you digest, absorb, and metabolize nutrients. But all of that is secondary to getting the nutrients in your body in the first place. If you do have a formal workup with a nutritionist, you may be asked to keep a written log of everything you eat for three days or more—which will be no problem if you've already started following the guidelines in this book, as you'll already have a food journal going. On the assumption that that gives an accurate reflection of your usual diet—and that you've been completely honest—your nutritionist would then do a specific evaluation of the amount of all the nutrients you're getting, along with cholesterol, fat, and calories. You should ask for an assessment of the nutrients specifically related to bone health (see Chapters 10 and 11) as well.

BONE BOOSTERS

Oranges are a good source of calcium, particularly for fruit. Nature often packages necessary nutrients together, which is why food beats supplements as a quality source of a nutrient every time. But fortified orange juice is one of the best ways to get supplemental calcium—since along with the added calcium, you'll get a pinch of naturally occurring calcium— and all the complementary nutrients Mother Nature intended. That is, you're getting what makes your body make the best use of calcium at the same time you get the calcium, naturally.

Case in Point: Maggie

My favorite patient story is a really short one. Maggie is in her mid-40s, but already menopausal—which puts her at higher risk for bone loss. She's a serious hiker and devoted student of yoga, and she takes a calcium supplement. Her diet is excellent, mostly vegetarian, though she eats fish, with loads of soy and whole grains and organic vegetables.

And she's got the bone density of a 35-year-old. Her bones are still at their peak, even years into menopause with no additional hormones, no prescriptions, not even any nutritional supplements beyond calcium. Nothing but good nutrition and regular exercise.

You may not have the fancy software, or the detailed knowledge, to do precisely the same scientific thing as a professional nutritionist or dietitian. But you can learn a lot by keeping your own written list. Seeing exactly how you eat has a way of bringing a little bit of reality home to you, particularly if you are forthcoming about the leftover half of your kid's peanut butter and jelly sandwich you scarfed down rather than throwing out, and the six Hershey's Kisses you swiped from the jar on your officemate's desk. You'll easily be able to check on some basics, such as whether you even eat three recognizable meals each day, and if

CHECK INCHES AS WELL AS POUNDS

I tell all my patients to measure their chest, waist, hips, arms, and thighs at the start of any changes to their usual diet, so they can track the loss of inches as well as pounds (especially since a lot of people decrease the first without a change in the second). Muscle weighs more than fat and burns many more calories, so a healthy combination of diet and exercise may well keep you at the same weight— or even (don't panic!) increase it—at the same time as your measurements decrease and you look trimmer.

they are made up of reasonably nutritious foods. Breakfast bars eaten in the car don't count.

With your current diet laid out for you in black and white, it should be easy to tell how often you eat something high in calcium, or how much you get in the way of vegetables, or if you eat soy foods regularly. Even if you *think* you get a glass of milk and a cup of yogurt every day, a test like this is bound to point up how often the best-laid plans go wrong. You might get sidetracked by a meeting that lasts all afternoon, or a trip away from home, or a weekend full of social plans that involve eating out. Or you simply run out of your supplies and don't get to the grocery store for a few days.

Remember to count up how many sodas or caffeinated or alcoholic beverages you take in. Even without calculating exact salt intake, you can see how many prepared or packaged foods you rely on, any one of which can easily put you halfway to your daily limit. You run into a similar situation with sugar. You don't have to add up micrograms and milligrams to see whether you get a variety of fruits, vegetables, grains, and beans. If you do, you can feel reasonably sure you're getting most or all of what you need in the way of vitamins and minerals. If you don't get some at every meal, or eat the same few types over and over—if you're "an-apple-a-day" type and not much more—you're depriving your body of what it needs to serve you well indefinitely.

A BRIEF DETOUR THROUGH YOUR PSYCHE

Finally, step back and take a look at your behavior patterns surrounding food. Though we may not be able to quote chapter and verse, most of us know the basics of healthy eating. Yet we continue to eat as we do—which has little in common with ideal nutrition. Ask yourself why. Do you stand in front of the refrigerator every time you get nervous? Gorge yourself when you are angry with someone—or with yourself? Fall back on old habits when you are upset? Know good ways to celebrate that don't involve food? Center every social occasion on eating?

I'm not a psychologist, so I'm not able to give you the secret to eliminating any or all of this type of thing. There is no one easy answer for everyone. But I think becoming aware of your tendencies is the most important first step. Just recognizing your habitual responses will start you down the path to changing them, if necessary. As long as you keep eating out of habit or as an unconscious response to stresses in your life, you won't have the first clue how to change your approach. However, once you realize, for example, that you eat to entertain yourself when you are bored, you can make alternate plans to prevent or cure boredom, cutting yourself off at the pass by substituting a healthy behavior for an unhealthy one.

Food *is* a pleasure and a comfort, and there's nothing wrong with enjoying what you eat, and eating what you enjoy. The problem is when you don't know any other ways to find pleasure and comfort, and so rely solely on food to evoke positive feelings for you. You also do yourself no favors if you find only unhealthy foods pleasurable. While I'm not immune to the appeal of a chocolate truffle, I'd rate a fresh, ripe mango right up there with it. Some people just can't get enough of Japanese-style boiled soybeans, or would trade their own mothers for a plate of brie and apple slices. Find ways to hit the pleasure centers in your brain and nourish your body at the same time. Then, while you work at expanding your repertoire of ways to manage stress, at least if you choose to soothe yourself with food, you'll do it consciously and healthfully.

Most Americans could stand to improve their diets, and will have to if they want long, full, and healthy lives. You may not notice the effects of a poor diet in your younger days, but I guarantee they'll catch up to you (probably before you turn 40). Your bones are definitely noticing the effects all the time, and registering them in their very cell tissue, whether you are or not.

Just following the advice in this chapter will put you on the path to a healthier you in general. All the major health organizations, whether their rallying cry is cancer or heart disease prevention, or diabetes awareness, recommend the same diet: low fat, high fiber, moderate protein. That's not a coincidence: no matter what your particular health challenge, the components of a healthy diet are the same. Building bone density is no exception, though as you'll see there are specific additional ways to help bone health in particular. You don't have to be 100 percent perfect in meeting all the nutritional requirements this book lays out every day. A missed magnesium supplement here or an extra slice of pizza there isn't going to make or break you, or prevent you from enjoying the benefits of good nutrition. But you do need an overall healthy lifestyle, including good nutrition, to be generally healthy. When you make smart choices *most* of the time, then you don't need to worry about eating that birthday cake.

Good nutrition is not just vitamins and minerals and fats and proteins. It is getting your body the materials it needs so that your cells have the best chance to work and interact correctly. The program in this book, when you make it your own, facilitates that.

Chapter 9

The Three Secrets of Healthy Bones: Calcium, Calcium, Calcium

Cement is made from sand, gravel, water, and a mixture of minerals, including iron, lime, and silica. Mixed in a certain combination and a certain way, you get solid, strong cement. If you use the wrong substances, or the wrong proportions, or low-quality ingredients, you get bubbly, brittle cement. Variations of good mixing technique and top-quality components will get you different grades in between: cement capable of absorbing great impacts, cement that withstands wide fluctuations in temperature, cement that stays flat come wind or rain or sleet or snow.

Think of creating healthy bones as mixing good cement. You need just the right balance of a variety of things—nutrition, exercise, genetics, dietary supplements—to get the end product you want. In this case, we're going for the densest cement. No holes. No cracks. Built to last. Your success depends on the quality of your ingredients, and the one thing you absolutely must have plenty of on hand at all times is calcium.

In addition to its job of building and strengthening bones (and teeth), calcium helps muscles contract and relax (including the heart muscle) and assists nerves in transmitting impulses. It helps manage cell membranes—and the chemicals, hormones, nutrients, and pathogens they let through and keep out—and

> **DID YOU KNOW?**
>
> Calcium is the mineral found in the largest amounts within the body, and 98 percent of it is located in the bones. The other 2 percent is evenly split between the teeth and various soft tissues. In 160 pounds of human, you'd find 3 pounds of calcium. A fifth of total bone mass is calcium.

helps bind cells together. It is necessary for proper secretion from many glands, and plays a role in dilating veins and arteries. It works as a messenger for certain hormones, aids in blood clotting, assists some enzymes in completing various chemical transactions throughout the body, and is necessary for regulating blood pressure. The hormones and enzymes influenced by calcium help control the digestive process, including the metabolism of fat and the production of saliva.

> **DID YOU KNOW?**
>
> Three-quarters of Americans are deficient in calcium. Women over 50 years old get, on average, less than half of what they need. Elderly women get an average of about 500 mg a day, and younger women about 600 or more.

The body places a premium on keeping calcium in the blood at optimal levels in order to keep all these things running smoothly, and "optimal" is a very narrow range. The body regulates the levels by storing any extra in the bones, and by releasing calcium from the bones anytime blood levels drop too low. Don't make your body steal from your bones: make sure you take in enough calcium.

WHAT IS IT GOOD FOR?

Because calcium plays many roles in your body, getting the recommended amounts brings a wide variety of health benefits. Correct levels of calcium cut the risk of angina, heart disease, and heart attacks by up to two-thirds, and reduce the risk of strokes caused by blood clots in the brain (80 percent of strokes are this ischemic kind). It protects against colon cancer and may slow growth of cancer cells in general, offering protection against breast and prostate cancer, among others. Some evidence connects calcium to protection against endometrial cancer, underlining the argument for taking calcium in conjunction with HRT (or any other treatment for bone density). Calcium helps lower blood pressure, making it a possible first strike in treating high blood pressure that isn't in the critical realm, and a useful adjunct to any other treatment. It can reduce cholesterol levels, help heal periodontal disease and prevent loss of permanent teeth, and mitigate allergies and allergic symptoms. It evens out mood swings connected to the menstrual cycle, as well as other PMS complaints. Any one of those benefits could help your quality of life, and perhaps even save your life.

> **THINGS TO THINK ABOUT**
>
> Some researchers speculate that PMS symptoms are a warning sign that you are not getting enough calcium. Others have connected the intensity of PMS symptoms with the intensity of menopausal symptoms. Either way, PMS might be a big warning sign that you are at particular risk of bone loss—so the earlier you take action, the better. Just getting more calcium may make you feel better right now, too.

TAKING CALCIUM PROTECTS YOUR BONES

Studies have demonstrated many kinds of bone benefit from getting enough calcium. High calcium intake has been proved to reduce postmenopausal bone loss and to reduce the risk of fractures, even in those who had previous fractures. Even before menopause (and in men), calcium supplements have been shown to increase peak bone density and to slow bone loss after age 30 from as high as 1 percent a year to close to nothing. Childhood diets richer in milk—and therefore calcium—have been connected to denser bones at menopause, and so to less risk of osteoporosis. Sufficient calcium before adolescence provides a large lifetime reduction in fracture risk.

After 35 or so years of age, we may not need calcium to build bone, but we do need it to slow or stop bone loss. Some evidence points to greater effectiveness perimenopausally than post-menopausally in reducing bone loss. It slows the pace of bone turnover, particularly in cortical bone (at the hip, among many other places). Supplements may be more beneficial for women well past menopause than in women currently going through menopause. Women taking HRT with calcium may get better results from calcium than women using calcium alone.

The lower your usual intake, the more benefit you'll see from getting higher amounts of calcium. Supplements of calcium and vitamin D alone have been shown to decrease the risk of fracture by 40 percent (and the risk of dying after a fracture by 16 percent), *even when bone density doesn't change.* Calcium supplements prevent and slow bone loss. With sufficient calcium, bone quality and strength improve even if density stays the same. Calcium taken with a multivitamin and mineral supplement worked better than calcium alone. Calcium taken with prescription treatments for low bone density provided better results than the prescriptions alone.

Taking into account all the variables you'll see examined in this chapter, the bottom line is that using calcium supplements over the long haul benefits bones, and particularly women's bones, no matter what stage of life you are in.

HOW MUCH CALCIUM DO YOU NEED?

The RDA underestimates what you need for developing and maintaining peak bone mass. The National Institutes of Health more recently set higher goals that I think are more appropriate: 1,200 to 1,500 mg daily up to age 24, and for pregnant and breast-feeding women; 1,000 mg a day for men under 65, for women before menopause, and for women after menopause taking estrogen. For women not on estrogen after menopause, and men and

---

THE U.S. RDA

The official government Recommended Daily Allowance (RDA) for calcium is 1,200 mg a day for everyone under 25 and 800 mg for everyone 25 and older. This is an important number to know, because it is the basis for food labeling. A yogurt label saying it contains 25 percent of your calcium needs actually has about 200 mg, or only 20 percent of what a premenopausal woman needs and 13 percent of what a menopausal woman not taking HRT needs.

---

women over 65, 1,500 mg a day is the recommendation. Most women get less than that—and many get less than half what they ideally should. Lower levels of calcium have been shown to provide benefits, so every little bit helps. But if you want to build peak bone mass, you'll have to get more than the RDA.

All the numbers about how much calcium you need are based on the amount of calcium you take in, and the recommendations assume you'll absorb a normal amount of it. This is an important distinction because, as you'll see, you absorb only a small portion of the calcium you eat in even the best of circumstances. If for any reason your digestion or absorption is off, you might need to take in even more. The signs of inefficient digestion are belching, gas, irregular bowel movements, indigestion, and bloating. Poor absorption is harder to detect, but it can cause hair loss, brittle nails, and dry skin, among other things.

Even higher levels of calcium may not make any difference if your body can't use what you take in, so it pays to develop excellent digestion (see Chapter 12), generally, and to make sure you have all the other nutrients your body needs in order to make use of calcium (see Chapter 10).

EAT YOUR CALCIUM

The best way to get enough calcium in your diet is, without question, to eat foods rich in it. Getting calcium as part of foods—as

HOW MUCH CALCIUM DO YOU NEED?

Infants up to 6 months	400 mg a day
Infants 6 months–1 year	600 mg a day
Children 1–5	800 mg a day
Children 6–10	800–1,200 mg a day
Teenagers and young adults (11–24)	1,200–1,500 mg a day
Women over 25 but not menopausal	1,000 mg a day
Pregnant and breast-feeding women	1,200–1,500 mg a day
Women after menopause, taking estrogen	1,000 mg a day
Women after menopause *not* taking estrogen	1,500 mg a day
Men 25–65	1,000 mg a day
Men over 65	1,500 mg a day

part of meals—means taking in a range of other nutrients at the same time. That gives your body the best preparation for making the most of what it gets.

The easiest way for most people to get calcium is to include more low-fat dairy products in their daily diets. The "low-fat" part is important for everyone over the age of 2, since whole milk and cheeses are creamy because they contain so much fat, which isn't good for your heart, your cancer risk, your waistline, or your health in general. (Up to age 2, children need fat and should get whole milk.) Luckily, when the fat is removed, the calcium sticks around. Actually, skim milk has a bit *more* calcium than whole

BONE BOOSTERS

Yogurt is the single best source of calcium for those who eat dairy, with more calcium than even the tall, cold glass of skim milk leaving mustaches on all those famous faces. Just one cup of yogurt gets most women a third of the way to their daily requirement.

milk. Plain nonfat yogurt has more calcium than milk, but no vitamin D. Milk on your cereal in the morning, a yogurt snack, and some cheese in your dinner entrée will get you much of the way to your goal.

If you are *lactose intolerant* (and over half of older Americans are), you don't digest milk sugar, so dairy products give you diarrhea, gas, or cramps. But you have options when it comes to calcium in dairy products (on top of all your nondairy options, described below). You can buy milk with lactase enzymes added that break down the lactose that causes your body problems. Or you can buy those enzymes separately to add to or take along with any dairy product. Yogurt and acidophilus milk (fortified with "good" bacteria like those found in yogurt) are sometimes not a problem to people who don't tolerate other dairy products well. If you want to experiment for yourself, read the labels to make sure you get brands with live cultures of (naturally occurring) bacteria, as those bacteria break down the lactose for you. Not every kind of yogurt has them—and frozen yogurt almost never does. Goat and sheep's milk and cheese are worth a try (check the labels to make sure they aren't blended with cow's milk). Try hard, aged cheeses, since most are low in lactose. Finally, try eating small portions, spread out. Many people who are lactose intolerant get by with no symptoms as long as they don't eat too much of what bothers them at once.

THINGS TO THINK ABOUT

The average American gets between 200 and 600 mg of calcium a day—far below anyone's minimum requirement for good health. To make matters worse, diets without enough calcium tend not to have sufficient levels of a host of other nutrients, either. On the flip side, increasing the calcium in your diet usually means raising the level of nutrients across the board, including other nutrients crucial for healthy bones.

BONE BOOSTERS

Cottage cheese, unlike most low-fat dairy products, is not a particularly good source of calcium unless you choose a brand that has been enriched.

CALCIUM CONTENT OF DAIRY FOODS

Choosing a variety of foods from this table (and the following one on nondairy sources of calcium) will help you provide plenty of this most important mineral for your bones. You do have to watch out for the fat content of dairy foods, but the good news is that low- or nonfat products actually have *more* calcium than their more full-fat counterparts. The calcium counts here are approximate, and you should always check the nutritional information on food labels for more precise numbers when possible. Remember that most labels give nutritional values as a percentage of the RDA, which in the case of calcium is just 800 mg a day, much less than I recommend to ensure healthy bones.

Food	Serving size	Calcium, in mg
Milk		
Nonfat (skim) milk	1 cup	300
Whole milk	1 cup	290
Evaporated milk	½ cup	320
Powdered, nonfat milk	¼ cup	380
Buttermilk	1 cup	285
Dairy Foods		
Cottage cheese, low-fat	1 cup	150
Cottage cheese, low-fat, enriched	1 cup	320
Cream cheese, regular	2 tablespoons	25
Cream cheese, light	2 tablespoons	40
Yogurt, plain, low- or nonfat	1 cup	480
Yogurt, flavored, low- or nonfat	1 cup	330
Cheese		
Hard cheese (average)	1 oz.	210
Soft cheese (average)	1 oz.	130
American	1 oz.	195
Blue cheese	1 oz.	90

Cheddar	1 oz.	205
Feta	1 oz.	140
Goat cheese	1 oz.	85
Mozzarella (part skim)	1 oz.	200
Muenster	1 oz.	200
Parmesan or Romano, grated (fresh has more calcium than dried)	1 oz.	335
Ricotta (part skim)	½ cup	335
Ricotta (whole milk)	½ cup	255
Swiss	1 oz.	250

Desserts

Boston cream pie	Average serving	80
Custard, baked	½ cup	145
Cream pie	Average serving	120
Cheesecake	Average serving	80
Pudding	½ cup	140
Rice pudding	½ cup	140
Tapioca	½ cup	150
Frozen yogurt, low- or nonfat	½ cup	150
Ice cream	½ cup	95
Soft-serve ice cream	½ cup	130
Ice milk	½ cup	125
Sherbet	½ cup	50

Combination Foods

Bean burrito	Average	208
Beef taco	Average	175
Cheese enchilada	Average	320
Cheese lasagna	Average serving	350
Cheese manicotti	Average serving	250
Cheeseburger	Average	170
Chili with meat and beans	1 cup	80
Cream of . . . soups	1 cup	180
Macaroni and cheese (homemade)	1 cup	360
Pizza	1 slice	165
Quiche	Average wedge	300

My Story: Cecelia

I started taking calcium supplements fifteen years ago, when my aunts started breaking bones. My mother, too, was shrinking dramatically, and I'm lactose intolerant and so I get very little dairy calcium in my diet. Let's just say I saw the writing on the wall. Along with 1,200 mg of calcium every day, I take a multivitamin that contains vitamin D and magnesium (among other things), as well as a supplement of several B vitamins.

I had a bone scan when I was just past 60 that showed that the calcium—and ten years of hormone replacement therapy—had done its job. My bones were of average density and well out of the danger zone. Walking two to three miles a day surely hadn't hurt, either. I'm doubly glad my bones are strong because one of the inert ingredients in Fosamax is lactose, so I wouldn't be able to take it!

I also had to stop taking HRT when I had breast cancer a few years ago. Now I take Tamoxifen to help prevent a recurrence, and I'm counting on some bone protection from that, although I know there haven't been studies on that aspect of it. I've also started using 100 percent lactose-free milk, and I can tolerate cheddar cheese and yogurt with live cultures. I eat beans a few times a week, but I don't get nearly enough dark green leafy vegetables. I'm working on that. But for now I'm glad to know supplements can make up for the times I can't get calcium in my diet.

Dairy products provide most of the calcium in the American diet, but they are also one of the top two types of food that cause allergic reactions (wheat is the other contender). As you'll see below, there are many nondairy options when it comes to calcium. Even if you are allergic to milk—usually a sensitivity rather than technically an allergy—you may be able to tolerate some kinds of dairy. Try cheese and cooked foods with dairy in them, since heat breaks down the protein that affects you. Goat and sheep's milk also probably won't bother you.

Goat's milk has more calcium than cow's milk, so everyone ought to at least try it.

TOP 5 CALCIUM SNACKS (DAIRY)

Pick any of these quick snacks for a big boost in your daily calcium intake:

1 cup plain low- or nonfat yogurt (480 mg)
½ cup part-skim ricotta (335 mg)
1 cup flavored, low- or nonfat yogurt (330 mg)
1 cup cottage cheese, low-fat, enriched (320 mg)
1 cup nonfat milk (300 mg)

YES, VIRGINIA, THERE IS CALCIUM WITHOUT MILK

I've said that eating more dairy food is the *easiest* way to get enough calcium in your diet. But it is not necessarily the ideal way, and it certainly isn't necessary. Osteoporosis is very rare in Asia, and Asians consume very little dairy. They get their calcium from leafy greens and soybeans. They also have diets much lower in protein than Americans do, so they don't need to take in as much calcium in the first place. Sea vegetables are high in calcium—and just about all the minerals important for healthy bones—and a diet rich in them may be another part of the secret. (They also help lower blood pressure and cholesterol, and provide antioxidant protection against heart disease and cancer, which I think gives you more than enough reason to experiment with different types, as vegetables or as condiments, to discover which you like best.)

Three-quarters of all the calcium in all the foods we eat in this country is in dairy food. On average, just under 10 percent comes from fruits and vegetables, and about the same amount from meat; another 4 percent from grains, and 2 percent from other foods. I'm all for shifting that balance in favor of the fruits, vegetables, and grains, because the more animal protein you take in, the more calcium you need. So milk and dairy products ironically increase your need for calcium at the same time as they boost your calcium levels, making it hard to stay ahead of the game. Studies have linked high milk consumption with denser bones and lower risk of osteoporosis—probably because of the calcium content. But in

CALCIUM IN NONDAIRY FOODS

These approximate values will help you choose a variety of foods richest in calcium. Always check the labels for nutritional information when available. I've included a few calcium-fortified foods here, but don't rely on just a banner touting "Now! With Calcium!" or some such claim without checking to see just how much calcium that means. Amounts can also vary widely by brand.

Food	Serving size	Calcium, in mg
Fish, Seafood, and Eggs		
Gefilte fish	1 cup	65
Mackerel, canned (w/bones)	3 oz.	260
Perch	3 oz.	115
Salmon, canned (w/bones)	3 oz.	200
Salmon, cooked	3 oz.	130
Sardines, canned (w/bones)	3 oz.	340
Shrimp, canned	3 oz.	95
Oysters	3 oz.	80
Clams	3 oz.	60
Lobster, cooked	3 oz.	55
Egg	1 extra-large	30
Soy		
Soymilk, fortified	1 cup	160
Tempeh	4 oz.	170
Tofu	4 oz.	130
Tofu, processed with calcium sulfate or calcium chloride (firm tofu has more calcium than softer varieties)	4 oz.	400
Beans and Legumes		
Dried beans, cooked	1 cup	90
Black beans, cooked	1 cup	135

Food	Serving size	Calcium, in mg
Black-eyed peas, cooked	1 cup	210
Chick peas, cooked	1 cup	135
Great northern beans, cooked	1 cup	130
Lima beans, cooked	1 cup	160
Navy beans, cooked	1 cup	120
Pinto beans, cooked	1 cup	130
Soybeans, cooked	1 cup	200
White beans, cooked	1 cup	160
Vegetables		
Bok choy (cooked)	1 cup	230
Collard greens (cooked)	1 cup	350
Kale (cooked)	1 cup	180
Mustard greens (cooked)	1 cup	160
Turnip greens (cooked)	1 cup	230
Broccoli (cooked)	1 cup	160
Brussels sprouts	1 cup	55
Cabbage	1 cup	50
Okra (cooked)	1 cup	220
Rutabaga (cooked)	1 cup	100
Sea Vegetables		
Nori	¼ cup	300
Hijiki (cooked)	¼ cup	150
Wakame (cooked)	¼ cup	130
Agar-agar	2 tablespoons	120
Kombu (kelp)(cooked)	¼ cup	75
Fruit		
Blackberries	1 cup	45
Kumquats	6 medium	65
Orange	1 medium	55
Dates, dried, pitted	½ cup	50
Figs, dried	5 medium	135
Raisins	½ cup	50

Food	Serving size	Calcium, in mg
Nuts and Seeds		
Almonds (shelled)	½ cup	190
Brazil nuts (shelled)	½ cup	130
Hazelnuts	½ cup	140
Walnuts	½ cup	140
Soy nuts (dry roasted soybeans)	½ cup	185
Poppy seeds	1 tablespoon	125
Sesame seeds	1 oz.	280
Tahini (sesame seed paste)	¼ cup	135
Sunflower seeds (hulled)	2 oz.	65
Baked Goods, Cereals, and Grains		
Biscuit	Average	90
Bran muffin	Average	115
Corn bread	2½-inch square	115
Pancake (homemade, enriched)	2–4-inch diameter	115
Waffle (homemade, enriched)	7-inch diameter	180
Corn tortilla	Average	60
Cold cereal (fortified) (check the label, as values vary widely by brand)	1 cup	250
Oatmeal	1 cup	20
Instant oatmeal (fortified)	1 packet	100
Amaranth (cooked)	1 cup	275
Quinoa (cooked)	1 cup	80
Beverages		
Grapefruit juice, fortified	1 cup	280
Orange juice, fortified	1 cup	300
Mineral water	1 liter	200
Rice milk, fortified	1 cup	240
Other		
Blackstrap molasses	1 tablespoon	135

THAT'S WHY THEY CALL IT MINERAL WATER

Mineral water can be a good source of minerals you need, but check the labels to find out what you're getting, as they vary widely in their calcium content. For example, Perrier has 140 mg per liter and San Pellegrino has 200 mg per liter, to name two common brands, and some go as high as 450 mg per liter.

some countries where dairy is not a usual part of the diet, osteoporosis occurs much less commonly than it does here. Generally speaking, the countries with the highest rate of dairy consumption also have the highest rate of low bone density—probably because of the animal protein. If yogurt and milk are the only ways you're likely to get calcium, stick with that. But seek out nondairy options to both expand your range of choices and lower the amount of animal protein in your diet.

If you're already committed to avoiding animal products for philosophical or health reasons, add the bone benefits of lower protein intake to your list of good reasons why. Rest assured that you, too, can have the healthiest possible bones. Vegetarians and vegans (strict vegetarians) have a lower risk of osteoporosis. Their bones have about the same density as nonvegetarians' up to the age of 50 or so, and they do lose bone mass as they age, but the loss seems to be slower. If you've considered going vegetarian or relying less on dairy products for whatever reason, I encourage you to go ahead. There are a wide range of health benefits to cutting animal products out of your diet; you will not harm your bones, and you will probably help them. Even if you have no intention of swearing off the milk mustache, the more calcium you get from other lower-protein sources, the better off you'll be.

BONE BOOSTERS

Read labels carefully on all calcium-fortified juices to find out exactly what you're getting. Calcium amounts vary widely in general, and you also have to watch out for concoctions that are all corn syrup and artificial flavorings, usually sold as "fruit drink."

FOODS TO WATCH OUT FOR

You do have to watch out for a couple foods that are high in calcium but are not actually good sources of calcium. For starters, oxalates in food interfere with calcium absorption. You can absorb only 5 percent of all the calcium in spinach, for example, because it also contains oxalic acid. Kale, on the other hand, has little oxalic acid, so you can absorb 40 percent of all the calcium in kale. To give you a little perspective, you absorb 20 to 25 percent of the calcium in milk. From that we can learn two things: (1) kale and similar vegetables are not only good sources of calcium, the calcium they do have is more available to your body than the old standby, dairy products; and (2) whatever you eat, you absorb only a portion of all the calcium. The recommended doses in this book (as elsewhere) take that into account, and tell you how much you should take in to get what you need once it is absorbed. But this situation underlines why good digestion (and so good absorption of nutrients, including calcium) is so important (see Chapter 12).

TOP 5 WAYS TO DRINK YOUR CALCIUM

1 cup fortified orange juice (300 mg)
1 cup nonfat milk (300 mg)
1 cup fortified grapefruit juice (280 mg)
1 cup fortified rice milk (240 mg)
1 cup fortified soymilk (160 mg)

TOP 5 NONDAIRY SOURCES OF CALCIUM

Fish and shellfish
Soy products
Beans and legumes
Dark green leafy vegetables
   (especially sea vegetables)
Nuts and seeds

Oxalates are also a major component of kidney stones, another reason to limit the amount you take in.

Spinach, asparagus, parsley, chives, green beans, sorrel, rhubarb, Swiss chard, beets and beet greens, dandelion greens, and summer squash all have oxalates (along with calcium). You can also find it in cocoa (and so chocolate), peanuts, cashews, almonds, and tea. The oxalic acid in one food does not affect any other foods eaten at the same time, so this dilemma has a simple solution: go easy on foods with oxalic acid (though there's no need to avoid them altogether); don't count all the calcium in them in your daily total; and when you eat greens high in calcium and oxalic acid, sprinkle them with lemon juice or vinegar to break down the oxalic acid.

BONE BOOSTERS

Calcium is better absorbed from ground sesame seeds (tahini) than whole seeds.

Other substances called phytates (they are related to phosphorus) also bind with calcium and prevent it from being absorbed. The effect is less pronounced than with oxalates, but you have to watch out for high-calcium foods that also contain it. That includes some whole grains, especially oats and wheat bran, and some legumes, like some dried beans and peas. There's no need to avoid them, since they are generally healthy foods and don't seem to interfere with anything else eaten at the same time. Just don't count them in your tally for how much calcium you've taken in on any given day.

Fiber, like bran, can cause another complication. It speeds foods through the digestion process, and as a result there may not be time for all the calcium to be absorbed. Wheat bran in particular may also bind with calcium and keep it from being absorbed. You need a lot of fiber in your diet for overall good health, and most Americans don't get enough as it is. I am not telling you to cut back. But be aware that when you combine, say, raisin bran cereal and milk, you shouldn't count on getting all the calcium you'd get if you drank the same amount of milk on its own. There is no official formula for figuring how much you do get, but at least some of your high-calcium foods should be eaten at different times from very high-fiber foods. And don't take a calcium supplement at the same time as very high fiber food (one reason to take your calcium at bedtime). You probably do want to keep your intake to 35 grams of fiber a day, or calcium and other minerals may not be properly digested and absorbed. It is very hard for most people to reach that level, so don't lose a lot of sleep over it. Just read the labels to make sure you are not going overboard. You may well find that label reading opens your eyes to how little you're getting, so while you're at it, keep in mind that you *should* be getting at least 20 grams a day, and see how you measure up. Eating a variety of whole grains, vegetables, and fruits along the lines of the Bone Density Diet should provide you with plenty of fiber.

High levels of fructose can interfere with calcium absorption. Check the labels on sodas, juices, "fruit juice sweetened" products, and other drinks and foods for "high fructose corn syrup" and avoid those that have it. Sodas also have a high phosphorus content, so skip them.

CHOOSE THE RIGHT SUPPLEMENT

Getting enough calcium in your daily diet is eminently doable, as you'll see in the menus provided for the Bone Density Diet in Chapter 14. But since you don't always eat as you should, on many days you don't get all the calcium you need, particularly if you have higher requirements or if you don't eat dairy. So I recommend an insurance policy against a diet that isn't always up to snuff: a calcium supplement.

Standing in front of the supplements shelves in the drug or health food store, you'll be confronted by a choice among many kinds of calcium. *Calcium carbonate* is the most common, and also usually the least expensive. It has the most pure calcium by weight, so you will need the fewest pills to get enough calcium with this form. It can be difficult to digest, however, and constipates some people or causes gas or other bowel symptoms. Taking calcium with magnesium (see next chapter) can prevent constipation, as magnesium has laxative properties. (The calcium-magnesium combination also works as a mild muscle relaxant, so it is good for insomnia and nighttime leg cramps— more reasons to take at least some of your calcium at bedtime). Another way to prevent getting constipated from calcium is to get plenty of liquid and plenty of exercise. Drinking plenty of fluids also helps increase absorption, no matter what kind of calcium you take.

One newly popular form of calcium carbonate is antacid tablets like Tums or Rolaids. You have to read the labels carefully to make sure there is no sodium or aluminum in any antacid you buy as a calcium supplement. The ones to look for are nothing but calcium and sugar (and artificial flavor and color, just for fun). Many people like the fact that these tablets are chewable, since most of the calcium pills you swallow are rather large. Any chewable, liquid, or effervescing form eliminates concerns about whether the calcium dissolves in your stomach. Capsules, as opposed to tablets, accomplish the same thing.

Calcium citrate is also well absorbed, easier to digest, even with low stomach acid, and is less likely to constipate or cause gas. It has a lower risk of contributing to kidney stones, which is an important consideration for men (who have a higher rate, generally, of kidney stones) and anyone prone to stones. It has less elemental calcium than calcium carbonate, meaning you have to take more pills to meet your needs. It is more expensive, but for anyone who has gastrointestinal trouble with calcium carbonate, or who believes the carbonate is not being well absorbed, calcium citrate is a good choice. This is the form most commonly used to fortify juices and cereals.

Another option is *calcium lactate*, which is also more easily digested than calcium carbonate. Anyone wanting to use it will have to cough up more money than for carbonate. *Calcium aspartate* has a similar plus/minus rating: easy to digest, costly to buy. *Chelated calcium* is marketed as being better absorbed and more "bioavailable," but I've seen no proof that it is different enough to justify the much higher price tag. *Calcium phosphate* costs more than carbonate but less than citrate, is well absorbed, and is less likely to cause gas or constipation. You'll also see *calcium gluconate*, *calcium malate*, and *microcystalline hydroxyapatite*, or MH. Despite the manufacturers' various claims, some studies show that your body absorbs just over a quarter of the calcium it takes in as a supplement—and sometimes up to 40 percent— regardless of the form. Other studies support a particular form or combination of forms. The bottom line is: get your calcium. The word after "calcium" on the front of the label matters less than the number after "elemental calcium" on the back, which tells you how much calcium you're actually getting. But if one kind of calcium disagrees with you, you'll have plenty of others to choose from.

Bone meal or dolomite is sold as a calcium supplement as well, and sometimes touted as "natural." Calcium from oyster shells is another "natural" option, and is sometimes sold as simply "natural calcium carbonate," with no mention of oysters. (If it doesn't say "natural" or "oyster," it is made in a lab, out of limestone.) But I'd steer clear of these because they can have a higher rate of contamination with lead or other toxic metals. Many of the other types of supplements are also sometimes contaminated with lead, particularly MH, but it is most likely in the "natural" forms. Check the labels on any supplement to find the ones that have been screened for lead content and found to have less than 2 parts per million.

Several brands offer combinations of two or three different forms of calcium in one pill. You might be able to get the best of both worlds by using a carbonate-citrate combination. It should be easier on your digestion and your wallet than just carbonate or citrate, respectively.

Whatever calcium supplement you take (including antacids), read the label to check how much *elemental calcium* it contains, so you can figure how many pills you'll need each day. (See "How Much Calcium Do You Need?" chart on page 145 for the total amount of calcium that's right for you.) If the label doesn't say "elemental calcium," look for a listing of just plain "calcium"—making sure not to confuse it with "calcium carbonate" or "calcium citrate" or any of the other specific names. Take note of how many pills are required to get the amount of elemental calcium listed on the label; some brands make it look as if they have more calcium by listing the amount in more than one pill, complicating the comparison shopper's burden.

Finally, check for calcium brands with labels saying they've met USP (United States Pharmacopoeia) standards. The USP is a nongovernment organization that sets standards for supplement manufacturing (including how well a calcium supplement should dissolve). If you choose one not approved by USP, or you want to double-check despite the "seal of approval," you can perform this simple home test: drop one pill into half a cup of vinegar. It should be dissolved within half an hour. If it isn't, try different brands until you find one that is. If calcium doesn't dissolve quickly in vinegar, it won't dissolve in the stomach, either. It won't do you any good to have simply swallowed the pill if it isn't available to be put to use. Don't waste money and effort on pills you can't absorb.

Every time you've seen calcium touted in a magazine or doctor's office pamphlet, I bet you've read contradictory instructions on how best to take supplements. "Take calcium separately from other foods," some say, to avoid conflicts with other nutrients that can interfere with absorption. "Take calcium with a small snack to ease digestion," others will tell you. Or maybe, "Don't take calcium pills too close to eating high-calcium foods like yogurt or tofu, since your body can handle only so much of it at one time." Of course, with the bone density diet, you'll be including those foods throughout the day, so avoiding them could get to be quite a trick. All this conflicting advice is almost enough to make you want to forget the whole thing.

Let me try to make it clearer. I think there's some wisdom in each of these paths of reasoning, but I realize you can't simultaneously follow all of them strictly. So what I recommend is dividing your doses of calcium and spreading them out through the day to give your body the best chance to digest and absorb all it can. Take no more than 500 mg at a time; anything more than that will just go to waste. Take one dose before bedtime to give your body all night to make use of it without competition from other foods. But since some foods actually improve absorption (just as some others impede it), I advise my patients to then take one or two more doses (depending on the total level they need) with snacks or small meals. Doing it at consistent times improves the chances of your remembering to do it, but the specific times don't matter. You might like to take one with breakfast and one with your afternoon snack—in addition to the one at bedtime—or just one more at lunch. Whichever you choose, you should keep it separate from foods high in wheat bran or calcium.

By taking one dose at bedtime and one or two more at different times during the day with food, you can cover all the bases, letting your body work both ways (with food that may help absorption, and without to ensure no interference).

Calcium can interfere with iron absorption, so if you take iron supplements, including a multivitamin with iron, make sure to take calcium and iron at separate times. When taking calcium with a snack, make sure the snack is not high in iron. Anemic individuals should be particularly aware of how much of each mineral they take in, and when, in relation to each other. No one should stop taking iron prescribed or recommended by a doctor. But if you are dosing yourself, consider if you really need iron. Most Americans get enough. Particularly if you're using a multivitamin with iron, you may be able simply to switch to one without iron without adversely affecting your health. You may want to get a blood test (while you are *not* taking a supplement) to measure your iron levels in order to determine if you actually need a supplement.

CHECK YOUR MULTIVITAMIN

If you take one, don't forget to check your multivitamin to see how much, if any, calcium it contains, and factor that in when you're counting how much you get in a day. It is unlikely you will get enough calcium in your multivitamin alone, as most usually contain only around 100 mg (if any).

Calcium can interfere with thyroid medications, and some antibiotics (like tetracycline), anticonvulsants, and corticosteroids, so don't take supplements within two hours of those medications, and talk with your doctor before you begin calcium supplements. Ask your pharmacist whether calcium affects your medication whenever you fill a prescription. Potential interactions like these are another reason it is important for you to tell your doctor everything you take, including supplements.

When it comes to calcium, more is not always better. Too much calcium (just about impossible to achieve without supplements), or too much unabsorbed calcium, can upset your body chemistry just as too little can, so you don't want to go over 2,000 mg a day from all sources, including foods. Above that level, your risk of kidney stones increases. Other problematic health effects have been linked to excessive calcium, including arteriosclerosis, arthritis, and glaucoma. Too much calcium can interfere with nerve function, and cause sleepiness and lack of energy. Very high levels of calcium also hamper the absorption of other crucial trace minerals, like iron and zinc.

To get 2,000 mg would require a gallon of milk a day, or its equivalent, so you can see too much calcium is not really a problem unless you take supplements. Used judiciously, calcium supplements are a great boon to bone density. Get as much calcium as you possibly can from food sources, but don't let a less-than-perfect diet deprive you of the benefits of calcium and other vital nutrients.

CALCIUM AND THE ELDERLY

Metabolism slows with age, and as a consequence, so does food intake in general—and calcium intake in particular. This is one reason weight gain becomes a concern for women around menopause, and that effect increases with age. In addition, low calcium intake is a common problem in elderly people when dental problems discourage eating vegetables or other foods that are challenging to chew, or when getting to the store regularly becomes more difficult, making it harder to keep fresh fruit and vegetables—and healthy, perishable foods in general—on hand. If any of these situations crops up for a loved one, help the individual focus ever more vigilantly on choosing healthy foods, and talk to them about the increased need for the "insurance" of a supplement.

FORTIFIED FOODS

Lately, Madison Avenue seems to be touting a new calcium-fortified food every time you turn around. You can now get "enriched" fruit punch, and along with the stingy amount of calcium it includes, you get the bonus of a sugar shot and a palette of artificial colors. But other products are more promising. Calcium-fortified orange juice delivers calcium that is already dissolved, together with natural sugars that (although still sugars) aid in digesting it further, as well as other naturally occurring nutrients your body needs. The acid in orange juice also helps boost calcium absorption, especially in people with low stomach acid (see Chapter 12). Fortified soymilk allows you to avoid dairy for health or philosophical reasons—or add soy for health reasons (see Chapter 11) without missing out on the calcium that comes with cow's milk. Some cold cereals, breads, breakfast bars, and other processed foods have calcium added, offering another convenient way to increase your intake. Reading nutritional labels is a good habit anyway, so you always know just what you are eating. Certainly you should check to see which products you use are (or could be) boosting your calcium intake.

No research indicates if the calcium in fortified foods is as beneficial as naturally occurring calcium, or if its effects are equivalent to those from taking supplements. No doubt the truth lies somewhere in between the two. Personally, I'm in favor of using whatever healthy means get calcium into the body. I wouldn't be a big advocate for "New! Improved! Candy Bars PLUS Calcium!" as a regular part of your diet. But if you are not going to eat enough tofu and kale to get your 1,200 mg, by all means drink a cup of calcium-fortified orange juice as part of your bone density diet.

Do be sure to read the labels to see how much you're actually getting, both to make sure you get enough all together, but also (now that at least one cereal claims to provide 100% of the RDA of calcium) to make sure you don't get *too* much, particularly if you are also taking supplements. If you have to choose between food and supplements (and calcium-added foods count as supplements), it is always better to have natural food (not fortified) as the source.

KIDNEY STONES

People with kidney stones are often advised to cut down on how much calcium they eat because kidney stones are largely made up of calcium. But the more natural calcium you get from the foods in your diet, the *less* likely you are to develop kidney stones. You should be careful with supplements, however. Protein and oxalates in the body have more to do with causing kidney stones than calcium does. Keeping them low is key.

The recommended levels of calcium from foods and supplements shouldn't be a problem for anyone who has never had a kidney stone.

CALCIUM BALANCE

Your body performs some elaborate choreography to maintain appropriate levels of calcium in the blood. Levels change according to how much bone is being formed, how much bone is being broken down, how much calcium is being absorbed in the intestine, and how much calcium is being excreted in urine. Vitamin D, parathyroid hormone, and your body's calcitonin, along with other hormones, all perform in that dance. When blood calcium levels are low, more parathyroid hormone is released, which stimulates greater absorption of calcium and also stimulates bone breakdown as a way to increase available calcium. When blood levels are high, parathyroid hormone isn't released at the same rate, and calcitonin, which stimulates bone-building osteoblasts, is released. Parathyroid hormone also controls the making of the active form of vitamin D, which in turn boosts absorption. Calcium absorption is hampered by lack of vitamin D. Calcium and vitamin D deficiencies become more common as people age, and can cause constantly high levels of parathyroid hormone. That in turn causes bone loss.

Protein and phosphorus both affect the amount of calcium in the blood. In digesting animal protein—including dairy products—your body uses calcium to reduce the acidity of the process. The more animal protein you take in, the more calcium you need and the more your body will pull from your bones if adequate amounts aren't otherwise available. This is why a vegetarian diet is protective of your bones, and why people who eat diets low in protein and calcium still have strong bones. The body strictly maintains phosphorus (which Americans overdose on daily in the form of sodas) in a particular ratio with calcium. When phosphorus levels soar—as with a multi-soda-a-day habit—calcium is drawn from the bones in an attempt to maintain that ratio.

WHEN ENOUGH CALCIUM ISN'T ENOUGH

Several factors in your diet can interfere with the absorption or action of calcium, as we saw in Chapter 6, on risks you can control. Keep salt, alcohol, and caffeine to a minimum so they don't impede your body's use of calcium. Americans get way more animal protein than they need for good health, and the more protein you take in, the more calcium gets rerouted from rebuilding your bones to buffering the acid created by the digestion process. Keep your meat to one or two small servings—the size of a deck of cards or smaller—a day. (If you don't eat meat, you probably have an appropriate amount of protein in your diet.) Smoking, too, raises your risk of low bone density, regardless of how much calcium you get.

Just as the star of any show is made to shine more brightly by an excellent supporting cast, calcium needs the company of other nutrients to do its best for your bones. *Not everyone with low bone density has insufficient calcium.* Some people lack magnesium, or vitamin D, or have insufficient digestion, or don't get enough exercise. The next chapter looks at the other foods and supplements you need to maximize the benefits your bones get from calcium. Taking a calcium supplement may be the simplest thing you can do to ensure the health of your bones. So start there. Just remember that you may need to do even more.

As a society we are not so much calcium deficient as we are overloaded with things that cause us to lose calcium (and magnesium and other nutrients). Protein is the biggest culprit. So even though we start by stressing calcium, calcium alone is not the answer.

Chapter 10

In the Mix: Key Nutrients for Bone Health

Because the bone-making process is so complex, many other nutrients besides calcium are necessary for a lifetime of strong bones. One study showed that calcium supplements taken together with a complete multi–vitamin and mineral slowed bone loss much more than calcium alone, so don't stop being open to making changes after the last chapter! Going back to the cement analogy, strong, solid concrete depends on having quality ingredients mixed in careful proportions. All cement might be made of the same basic ingredients, but cement can be made fine and smooth, coarse and granular, or dense and shock-absorbing, depending upon its components. We want strong bones that aren't hard and fragile or soft and nonsupportive, so we need a host of other nutrients along with our calcium.

This chapter reviews the other vitamins and minerals your skeleton will thank you for, explains their part in protecting your bones, tells you what foods are good sources of them, and shows you how much you should get every day. Vitamin D and magnesium are particularly crucial, so I'll focus on them first. After that I've listed the nutrients in alphabetical order. Other nutrients, like the antioxidants beta-carotene and vitamin E, are well known to benefit your overall health, but here I'm including only the ones with direct bearing on your bones.

Once again, you need to try to get as much of what is good for you from food sources as you can, since foods already contain a variety of naturally balanced nutrients. But even with an excellent diet, some nutrients are hard to come by in sufficient quantities. And since few of us maintain an excellent diet all the time, I advocate supplements as an inexpensive insurance policy. High levels of some nutrients affect the levels of others, and most are interdependent for their effectiveness. Just as too much calcium can cause an imbalance of other nutrients, nutritional supplements can cause similar problems. In general, I recommend taking a multi-vitamin-and-mineral supplement to try to keep things reasonably proportional. You can probably find one that gives you most of what you need to take in addition to calcium. I tell my patients to look at Osteologic brand by Physiologics, since it contains good levels of all the nutrients that are important for healthy bones. Any number of other brands would do just as well, and if the one you like leaves something out, you can always add an individual supplement. Some calcium supplements come with magnesium or vitamin D included, and those may be a good option for you as long as the calcium is of high quality (as described in the last chapter) and the total amounts you take don't exceed recommendations.

Anyone with kidney problems and anyone taking medication for a chronic illness must be sure to check with his or her health professional before using supplements.

VITAMIN D AND MAGNESIUM
Vitamin D
After calcium, this is the most important substance to have for bone health. Without vitamin D, the body cannot adequately absorb calcium or put it into bones. Vitamin D also promotes phosphorus absorption (preserving the crucial calcium-phosphorus balance) and protects against bone loss by lowering excessive

BONE BOOSTERS

Even though just 20 minutes in the sun gives you enough vitamin D for the day, most people don't get enough. On average, we meet the RDA only halfway, and, as with so many nutrients, the RDA amount alone isn't enough to protect your bones.

levels of parathyroid hormone. It may have a role in bone formation and may also help to decrease the risk of fracture overall.

DID YOU KNOW?

While milk is fortified with vitamin D, most milk made into dairy products is not, so you can't count on cheese or any other dairy source of calcium as having vitamin D.

You do get some vitamin D in a generally healthy diet, but vitamin D is unique in that most of what you get in your body comes from what your body makes when it is exposed to sunlight. Ultraviolet light (like the sun's rays) turns cholesterol in the skin into vitamin D.

Levels of vitamin D in the body fall in the winter, when we get less sun, so during that season, particularly in the North, we need to pay attention to getting sufficient vitamin D. Strict vegetarians, or anyone else who does not drink milk, will need to be diligent about getting out in the sun or taking a supplement. Absorption of the vitamin D you ingest decreases with age, and older people tend to spend less time in the sun and drink less milk, so vitamin D deficiency is common. There are no early symptoms of D deficiency, but lowered absorption of calcium will accelerate bone loss because bones will release calcium into the blood to keep levels normal. Deficiency can lead to osteomalacia (loss of calcium in the bones, which softens them), which can cause pain in the ribs, lower back, pelvis, and legs, or to osteoporosis. In children, vitamin D deficiency can lead to rickets, which involves bone abnormalities.

Vitamin D needs other nutrients, including fats, in order to be absorbed or to be created in your body. That's one reason a *no*-fat diet is unhealthy. You should have the level of vitamin D in your

> **Myth:** I get all the vitamin D I need in milk.
>
> **Fact:** Despite government regulations, the amount of vitamin D actually in each glass of milk varies widely.

blood checked (or rechecked) a few months after beginning supplementation to make sure you are in the normal range.

WHAT (ELSE) IS VITAMIN D GOOD FOR? Breast and colon cancer prevention; lowers blood pressure by increasing calcium absorption.

BONE BOOSTERS

Taking calcium supplements is fruitless if you don't also get 20 minutes a day in the sun (or a vitamin D supplement).

FOODS RICH IN VITAMIN D: Fortified milk and dairy products (though almost all milk is fortified, be aware that most milk products, like cheese and yogurt, are not), fortified breads and cereals, fish (especially salmon, herring, mackerel, sardines, and tuna), eel, fish-liver oils, egg yolks, organ meats, and avocado. Keep in mind that although milk is supposed to be fortified with 400 IU of vitamin D per quart, in reality the amount you get in a glass of milk varies widely.

RECOMMENDED DAILY DOSE: 400–800 IU. If you need only 1,000 mg or less of calcium a day, a lower dose (200–400 IU, the RDA) will be sufficient. Most multivitamins contain 400 mg, and you can also get a combination supplement of calcium and vitamin D. Twenty minutes of noontime sun each day (no sunscreen, no hat, palms up) would give you all you need, though in the winter, or in northern or less sunny climates, you might still need a supplement, or plenty of fortified milk (100 IU per cup). I recommend supplements as a backup measure, even if you're getting good sun exposure. If you are often out in the sun, just take a dose at the lower end of the suggested range.

Too much vitamin D can contribute to kidney stones, so if you are at risk for them, you should carefully monitor your calcium levels while you take vitamin D to make sure you're not going overboard. Anticonvulsant medications can deplete levels of vitamin D, so if you take them check with your doctor about appropriate supplements. No one should take more than 1,000 IU a day.

Magnesium

Magnesium is the third most crucial nutrient for healthy bones, after calcium and vitamin D, but a Gallup survey showed that almost three-quarters of Americans are deficient in it. Most women over 40 have low levels of magnesium; by the time you are 70, you are absorbing only two-thirds of the magnesium you did in your younger days. Half of all magnesium in the body is found in the bones, and it is necessary for bone growth, as well as for muscles and connective tissues. Magnesium supports the underlying structure of bone that calcium crystallizes on; magnesium deficiency has been shown to cause abnormal crystals of calcium in bones, and crystals of calcium in abnormal locations. A strong structure helps even less dense bones be stronger. Stress spurs excretion of magnesium, as do alcohol and some prescription drugs (including diuretics, digoxin, and cisplatinum). Magnesium prevents calcium from being excreted, helping it to be used properly. Magnesium is required to activate vitamin D, and with low levels of magnesium, levels of vitamin D also decrease. That means the body will have difficulty absorbing calcium. Magnesium also has a role in controlling estrogen, parathyroid hormone, and calcitonin, all of which are important in bone formation. Magnesium deficiency can cause muscle weakness and nausea. Taking calcium and magnesium together at bedtime can put an end to night leg cramps.

THINGS TO THINK ABOUT

People with osteoporosis have lower levels of magnesium than people without osteoporosis. We don't need any more test cases to prove the point, so get your magnesium!

WHAT (ELSE) IS IT GOOD FOR? Because magnesium plays a role in all kinds of chemical reactions all over the body, it has been linked

BONE BOOSTERS

The balance between calcium and magnesium is crucial, and getting high levels of calcium but low levels of magnesium can actually contribute to bone loss. When you use supplements, keep the ratio of 2 to 1 calcium to magnesium

to many health benefits, including controlling high blood pressure; lowering high cholesterol levels; countering PMS; reducing likelihood of recurrent kidney stones (and perhaps preventing them in the first place); lowering risk of respiratory diseases like bronchitis and respiratory complaints like wheezing; decreasing the risk of asthma, chronic fatigue syndrome, gum disease and gingivitis, headaches, multiple sclerosis, bursitis, and tendonitis; and protecting against irregular heartbeats and angina, and irritable bowel syndrome. Low levels can make diabetes more severe, and have been linked to arteriosclerosis and heart attacks. A deficiency has been linked to mental illnesses, including depression, agitation, and hallucination, though it is not clear if supplements would be of any help. You get the idea: magnesium is a *really* important nutrient.

FOODS RICH IN MAGNESIUM: Milk, green vegetables (especially green beans and celery), green leafy vegetables (especially spinach and lettuce), fish and seafood, whole grains (especially oats and wheat germ), brown rice, seeds (especially sunflower seeds and poppy seeds), nuts (especially almonds and cashews), legumes (especially soybeans, cow peas, and dried beans and peas), molasses, dairy products, meat, and water, and the herbs purslane, stinging nettle, licorice root, coriander, and dandelion.

RECOMMENDED DAILY DOSE: 600 mg. Most of us get only about 250 mg. Most multis don't have enough, so you should consider a separate supplement, or buying a combination supplement of calcium and magnesium. (You'll see many, many varieties of magnesium on the shelves, but for the most part, magnesium is magnesium. If you consult a professional nutritionist, he or she may prefer a specific type, but I don't recommend a particular kind.) Too much magnesium could cause loose bowels—if that happens to you, just cut back on the dose until the symptom clears up. Don't take magnesium if you are in renal failure.

OTHER NUTRIENTS
Boron
The trace mineral boron is important in calcium metabolism, and lack of it can make your bones more brittle. It activates estrogen and other hormones important in bone health, and supports other substances in your body that slow or stop the loss of calcium and the breakdown of bone. Without enough boron, you lose magnesium and calcium, both of which are necessary for strong bones; sufficient boron reduces excretion of calcium and magnesium. A diet low in magnesium creates a higher demand for boron, so you can see it is a vicious cycle. Boron also helps activate vitamin D, which is key in absorbing and using calcium. Boron is also required by the endocrine system in its work maintaining bones and joints.

WHAT (ELSE) IS IT GOOD FOR? Boron is an enzyme that facilitates critical chemical reactions all over the body.

FOODS RICH IN BORON: Nuts and seeds (especially almonds, peanuts, and hazelnuts), noncitrus fruit (especially apples, pears, grapes, strawberries, cherries, apricots, peaches, dates, raisins, currants, and figs), legumes (beans and peas) (particularly soybeans and soybean products like tofu), vegetables (especially cabbage, tomatoes, asparagus, broccoli, beets, and green leafy vegetables), honey, and some herbs and seasonings (dandelion, poppy seeds, parsley, stinging nettle, dill, and cumin seeds).

RECOMMENDED DAILY DOSE: 3 mg. You should be able to get that in a diet that includes a variety of fruits, vegetables, and nuts. But the average American gets only half that amount, so you might

> **Myth:** Taking a calcium pill every day pretty much covers it.
> **Fact:** You need other nutrients to make the calcium useful in your body—the most crucial being vitamin D and magnesium—and if you don't get enough of those the calcium alone won't do you much good.

want to consider a supplement to be sure. Boron could theoretically be toxic, but it is not known to cause harm in doses less than 100 mg a day.

Copper

Copper slows bone breakdown and assists in repairs. Making collagen (the main component of bone matrix) requires it. Low levels of copper can negatively effect heart function.

WHAT (ELSE) IS IT GOOD FOR? Making red blood cells, heart muscle function.

FOODS RICH IN COPPER: Whole grains, nuts, organ meats (especially liver), shellfish, eggs, poultry, legumes (especially dried beans and peas), and green leafy vegetables.

RECOMMENDED DAILY DOSE: 2.5–10 mg a day. Copper and zinc need to be in careful balance with each other, so if you take a supplement of one, make sure you get enough of the other to keep them in a ratio somewhere between 1 to 10 and 1 to 20. Calcium can interfere with the absorption of copper, so you should take a copper supplement if you take a calcium supplement—but take them at separate times.

Folate (Folic Acid) (Vitamin B₉)

Folate—the naturally occurring form of the B vitamin folic acid—is not stored in the body, so you have to be sure to get enough every day. You may have deficiencies in particular parts of the body even if the levels in your blood are normal, so it is worthwhile paying attention to make sure you get sufficient amounts in your diet. The more protein you take in, the more folate you need, which is part of why a vegetarian diet helps protect against osteoporosis as well as heart disease. Folate helps break down homocysteine, which is formed from the breakdown of protein. Homocysteine levels rise after menopause, and play a role in promoting osteoporosis (by meddling in the making of bone matrix), as well as the formation of plaque in the arteries of your heart. Alcohol and birth control pills can interfere with absorption, so you may want to cut back on or eliminate them, or get more folate. Folate competes against zinc, so if you take a supplement of one, be sure to take one of the other as well to preserve a healthy balance.

WHAT (ELSE) IS IT GOOD FOR? Preventing spina bifida and neural tube defects (devastating birth defects). Preventing strokes and heart disease. Chronic fatigue syndrome, infertility, and depression. Fighting viruses. Helping form RNA and DNA, your genetic material, and influencing cell division. Forming and breaking down proteins. Forming red blood cells.

FOODS RICH IN FOLATE: Legumes (especially soybeans, pinto beans, navy beans, peas, chickpeas, white beans, kidney beans, lima beans, and lentils), rice, barley, asparagus, avocado, spinach, sprouts, sweet potatoes, cabbage, endive, beets, broccoli, okra, brussels sprouts, leafy green vegetables (especially kale and turnip and mustard greens), fruit (especially raspberries, oranges, and orange juice), whole grains, wheat and wheat germ (there is twice as much folate in whole wheat bread as in white bread), bulgur wheat, rye, brewer's yeast, nutritional yeast, sunflower seeds, fortified cereals, calf's liver, chicken liver, and the herbs jute and pigweed. Parsley is a good source of folate, but also contains a compound that is a uterine stimulant, so don't eat large amounts (as in tabouli) if you're pregnant unless you're about to deliver and not concerned about speeding things up.

RECOMMENDED DAILY DOSE: The official RDA is 400 micrograms (mcg)—(.4 mg)—though the average American gets only about half of that. Because lack of folic acid is a major contributing factor to

Case in Point: Charlotte

At 87 years old, Charlotte had lost 60 percent of her bone mass compared to the average young person at peak bone density, and a sky-high NTX score of 200 indicated rapid progression and very high risk of fracture. So she started taking Fosamax, and after a year, retesting showed good news and bad news. First, the good: she'd gained ten percentage points—excellent progress, but that still left her at 50 percent below ideal levels of bone mass. Then, the bad: her NTX level hadn't budged. So I recommended a supplement of trace minerals in addition to the calcium she'd started along with the Fosamax. Within a year, her NTX was just 13—the low end of normal!—and while she still had a way to go in building up her bone density, she no longer lived in fear of an immediate fracture. She felt able to be more active, which would in turn benefit her bones still more. Charlotte had always believed in eating well to get the nutrients you need, but she couldn't argue with these results: her usual diet, though generally healthy, still hadn't given her bones everything they needed to make the most of the drug therapy she was using. The supplement had made all the difference.

a certain kind of birth defect, more products are being fortified with it in an attempt to make sure everyone gets enough. Using a lot of aspirin and ibuprofen can lower your folate levels, so you should explore cutting down on the drugs or make sure to take a supplement. Very high doses of folic acid may interact with dilantin or other anticonvulsant drugs, so check with your doctor. Folic acid can also compromise some lab tests, so it is important for your doctor to know if you are taking supplements. No one should take more than 1 mg (1,000 mcg) a day without being closely followed by a medical professional, but megadoses like that are never really needed.

Manganese

Manganese, another trace mineral, is needed for the formation of cartilage and other components of bone. It stimulates the production of compounds that make up the matrix structure calcium attaches to. It is also necessary for the production of sex hormones, which are, in turn, necessary for proper bone formation and remodeling. Deficiency is common in women with osteoporosis, and deficiency in anyone can cause or exacerbate bone loss.

WHAT (ELSE) IS IT GOOD FOR? Activating enzymes that enable a wide variety of crucial chemical reactions throughout the body to take place.

FOODS RICH IN MANGANESE: Pineapple (fruit or juice), oatmeal, nuts and seeds, whole grains and cereals (especially brown rice, rice bran, oatmeal, and whole wheat), beans, green leafy vegetables (especially spinach), meat, and tea.

RECOMMENDED DAILY DOSE: 5–10 mg. Calcium and magnesium can interfere with manganese absorption, so it makes sense to take a supplement of manganese if you take the others (and you should definitely be taking calcium!). Check the label of your multivitamin; it should be easy to find one that has enough. It can theoretically be toxic, but the only time that's been known to happen is to miners and steel mill workers who inhale manganese dust, so people not falling into one of those categories don't have to worry about standard supplements.

Selenium
Selenium is a building block of bone matrix, and is another nutrient critical for a wide range of enzyme reactions in the body. Deficiency of selenium has been linked with heart abnormalities and heart failure.

WHAT (ELSE) IS IT GOOD FOR? Selenium is an antioxidant, so it protects cells and organs from damage. It works with vitamin E to prevent breast cancer, and is a good antiviral agent. It prevents— or slows down progress of—cataracts. It is also an antiviral agent.

FOODS RICH IN SELENIUM: Seafood (especially swordfish, clams, oysters, and canned tuna), chicken, meat, organ meats (especially chicken livers), egg yolks, milk, garlic, whole grains (especially whole wheat flour, wheat germ, puffed wheat, and oat bran), broccoli, cabbage, celery, cucumbers, mushrooms, onions, sunflower seeds, and nuts. One average Brazil nut gives you your RDA for selenium.

RECOMMENDED DAILY DOSE: 200 mcg.

Silicon (Monosilic Acid, Silicon Dioxide)

This mineral is needed for healthy connective tissue, which means bones as well as cartilage and tendons. It is important for the structures in the bone that support calcification. With age and declining hormones, levels of silicon in the blood and skin decrease (part of why arthritis so often comes with age), so supplementation may become more important as you get older.

WHAT (ELSE) IS IT GOOD FOR? Treating fractures; arthritis, bursitis, and tendonitis; balding; kidney stones and general urinary tract health (it increases excretion of urine).

FOODS RICH IN SILICON: Brown rice, rice bran (sometimes sold as "rice polish"), barley, cucumbers, walnuts, brazil nuts, cashews, pistachios, string beans, turnips, and the herbs parsley, stinging nettle, chickweed, and horsetail.

RECOMMENDED DAILY DOSE: 1–2 mg. There is no RDA for silicon, and we don't really know if we get enough of this mineral in our diets. At the very least, if you have osteoporosis, you should take a supplement. It may be included in your multivitamin.

Strontium

Strontium has a structure similar enough to calcium that it can work as a body double. When it does help out in your bones and teeth, it adds strength and helps stave off bone breakdown. It also draws extra calcium into the bones. It is attracted to bone remodeling sites, so it surely has some role in the process, though we don't yet understand exactly what it is. The human body contains about 320 mg of strontium, and almost all of it is found in the bones and connective tissue.

WHAT (ELSE) IS IT GOOD FOR? Osteoarthritis and bone pain

FOODS RICH IN STRONTIUM: A wide variety of foods, though levels vary greatly depending on the condition of the soil and water used in producing them. Water can be a good source, but, again, that would depend entirely on how much is in your particular water supply.

RECOMMENDED DAILY DOSE: .5–3 mg, which is the amount included in many multivitamins. Most people get that much in their diets anyway, and some experts recommend up to 10 mg a day, though it remains unclear whether higher doses make a difference. I think it is worth making sure it is in your multi.

Vitamin B₆ (Pyridoxine)

This B vitamin supports the protein structures in bone, as well as helping produce the bone-building hormone progesterone. People deficient in B₆ who get fractures heal more slowly. Like folate (folic acid), it metabolizes homocysteine, an action that protects the heart and bones, so more B₆ may be required after menopause, when women lose the protection of estrogen and progesterone on those systems. Deficiency is more and more common the older you get. Smokers are often deficient, and a high-protein diet also makes your body require more B₆ because the vitamin is important to protein metabolism.

WHAT (ELSE) IS IT GOOD FOR? Asthma, carpal tunnel syndrome, infertility, osteoarthritis. It influences the nervous system and helps red blood cells form.

FOODS RICH IN VITAMIN B₆: Cauliflower, watercress, spinach, garden cress, okra, onions, broccoli, squash, kale, kohlrabi, brussels sprouts, peas, radishes, avocados, carrots, tomatoes, lentils, soybeans, pinto beans, black-eyed peas, chickpeas, sunflower seeds,

Case in Point: Janet

*J*anet came into my office because of hip and low back pain she'd had for years. She'd had a hip fracture years before, followed by a hip replacement. A standard x-ray showed arthritis was at least part of the problem, then a bone density scan showed she was 34 percent below normal in the spine and 41 percent low at the hip. She got limited exercise because of chronic emphysema and joint pain. She'd been taking thyroid hormone for years, and went through menopause without taking any other hormones because she had had breast cancer. All of that should have been like big red flags warning about bone loss to Janet's doctors, but in all her 78 years no one had laid out a plan to slow or stop her bone loss or build her bone density. Despite the options available to her now (from which she chose to take Fosamax), the more helpful medical advice would have come years ago, so she could have maintained the bone mass she started out with.

Janet did eat a reasonably healthy diet, and took nutritional supplements as well. In fact, when she came in, she brought 13 bottles of vitamins and minerals to show me exactly what she was taking. One she started after she heard something on the news about it, another was something her neighbor takes, something else her daughter bought her . . . and on it went. She was using a lot of important nutrients, and even more that she didn't really need, and all of it was in a very piecemeal fashion, with no rhyme or reason behind the mixture.

Along with a prescription for Fosamax, I gave her a revamped list of vitamin and mineral supplements consisting of just four items: calcium with vitamin D and a comprehensive multivitamin with trace minerals, specifically for her bones, and a strong antioxidant combination and vitamin E for her overall health. The regimen would be both more efficient and more effective; not only did she need many fewer pills but also she saved a lot of money. She told me she noticed a difference within a few weeks. "I feel great," she said. "I'm so much better that my husband, who has always said he doesn't believe in vitamins, is taking them now, too."

Two years later, Janet had another bone density test and found she had gained four percentage points in her spine—and sixteen in her hip *(about twice what you'd expect, statistically speaking)! The gains were so great in her hip that she was no longer considered to have osteoporosis, but was now in the osteopenia range and out of immediate danger of a fracture. On the strength of these results, she started exercising without excessive fear of injury. I referred her to a pulmonary rehab center because of her emphysema, where she learned not just to exercise her muscles but also to improve her heart and lung function. Without the shortness of breath that had plagued her, she found she really enjoyed exercising. With newfound ease of movement and breath, Janet felt and acted years younger than when I first met her. I'm pleased to know that more vibrant person, and I'm also pleased to know her activity level will mean still more improvements for her bones.*

whole grains (especially rice, bran, buckwheat, whole wheat, and wheat germ), watermelon, bananas, fish (especially tuna and salmon) and shrimp, chicken, beef, pork, liver, eggs, brewer's yeast, and nuts (especially hazelnuts).

RECOMMENDED DAILY DOSE: 5–25 mg. The RDA is just 2 mg, and since B_6 is hard to get in even an immaculate diet, we usually get even less than that. Most B-complex pills have 50–100 mg, which is fine. But don't take more than that unless you're working closely with an expert: huge doses can cause nerve damage—one study suggests 500 mg might be enough to cause problems. If you do run into bad side effects at high doses, the conditions usually will be reversed, for the most part, by stopping taking the supplement, but some abnormalities may persist. Taking B_6 may increase your need for magnesium, so take a supplement of that, too, if you take one of B_6.

Vitamin B_{12}

Like B_6 and folate, vitamin B_{12} protects the bones against the effects of homocysteine. Levels in your body generally decrease with age, so as you get older you should pay more attention to this nutrient.

WHAT (ELSE) IS IT GOOD FOR? Forming red blood cells; protecting nerve fibers; forming DNA; cell division.

FOODS RICH IN VITAMIN B_{12}: Beef, liver (especially beef liver and liverwurst), fish (especially flounder, herring, mackerel, and sardines), seafood (especially clams), blue and Swiss cheese, cottage cheese, yogurt, milk, eggs, tempeh, miso, soy sauce, and nutritional yeast.

RECOMMENDED DAILY DOSE: 1,000 mcg (1 mg). Since in food it comes mainly from animal sources, strict vegetarians should take nutritional yeast. Absorbing vitamin B_{12} requires a special protein, which some people don't produce. (Consult with your doctor if you are experiencing signs of fatigue, tired or weak muscles, loss of concentration, and tingling of the feet.) In those cases, you may need periodic B_{12} injections, or a supplement that dissolves in the mouth, where absorption is easier than in the stomach.

FAT-SOLUBLE AND WATER-SOLUBLE VITAMINS

Vitamins A, D, E, and K are fat soluble and so can be stored by the body. That means you can take a supplement once a day, and your body will use it or store it, as appropriate. The rest of the vitamins are water soluble, and stay in the body only for about four hours after you take a supplement, so you should divide any large doses to allow your body the best chance to absorb what it needs before it passes through.

Vitamin C

Vitamin C is important for the formation and repair of cartilage, collagen, and other organic components of bone. It increases calcium absorption. Severe deficiency of vitamin C can result in scurvy, a disease that sometimes has bone abnormalities associated with it.

WHAT (ELSE) IS IT GOOD FOR? Boosting the immune system and fighting infections (the reason it is touted for colds); healing cuts, bruises, and other wounds; helping absorb iron and metabolize protein. Vitamin C is an antioxidant, so it protects all cells and organs from damage.

FOODS RICH IN VITAMIN C: Sweet red peppers, green bell peppers, guavas, cantaloupe, papaya, strawberries, brussels sprouts, citrus fruits and juices (especially pink or red grapefruit and oranges), sweet potatoes, potatoes, tomatoes, broccoli, cauliflower, peas, kale, and snow peas.

RECOMMENDED DAILY DOSE: 1,000 mg, preferably in divided doses. The RDA, at 60 mg, is just enough to stop you from getting scurvy, but it isn't enough for you to reap all the benefits. (The RDA generally is set at levels necessary to prevent deficiency diseases, which is much too narrow a view, given what we now understand about the complex roles nutrients play in every area of your body.) Too much vitamin C can cause upset stomach or diarrhea, and large doses can interfere with the anticoagulant Coumadin. Taking vitamin C with food (or lowering your dose) should clear up any gastrointestinal side effects, but you should talk with your doctor if you are using a blood thinner. Don't take vitamin C supplements if you have kidney failure.

TALK TO YOUR DOCTOR

Vitamin K helps blood clot, so if you are taking an anticoagulant (including a daily baby aspirin or a vitamin E supplement), discuss it with your doctor before you increase your intake of vitamin K, as the vitamin and the medicine could counteract each other. For the most part, you're fine unless you notice you start bruising easily.

TOP 5 SOURCES OF VITAMIN K

	Micrograms of vitamin K per ½ cup (cooked) serving
Collard greens	440
Spinach	360
Brussels sprouts	235
Scallions (raw)	150
Broccoli	113

Note: Cabbage, asparagus, Swiss chard, romaine lettuce, and kale are also good sources.

The presence of vitamin K in so many of the same foods that are a good source of calcium and other bone-healthy nutrients is another argument for concentrating on getting the nutrients you need from food rather than supplements. Nature prepackages complementary nutrients together.

Vitamin K

Vitamin K is going to be the "new" bone-building vitamin. The word is pretty much out about vitamin D and magnesium, so marketers are next turning their attention to this lesser-known vitamin, which attracts calcium to the bones and helps hold it in place there. It activates osteocalcin, a protein crucial in bone matrix (the second in command after collagen). Without enough high-quality bone matrix, your bones would be fragile even if they were dense (like chalk, which is mostly calcium). So vitamin K is good for both formation and maintenance of healthy bone, and studies suggest it also has a role in slowing or stopping bone loss. It can also speed healing of fractures. Deficiency is common in people with osteoporosis, though we don't know if that is a cause or an effect of the disease.

Vitamin K is manufactured by bacteria normally found in your intestines. When you take antibiotics for any reason, you also do away with these friendly bacteria, which may account, at least in part, for the link between antibiotic use and damage to bones.

> **DID YOU KNOW?**
>
> One of the largest studies ever done about women and nutrition found (among many other things) that women who got over 100 mcg of vitamin K a day were almost a third less likely to fracture a hip than women who took in less of the vitamin. Vitamin K was shown to be particularly helpful to women not using hormone replacement therapy.

When you take antibiotics, consider following your treatment with probiotics (see Chapter 12 on digestion) to limit the negative effects.

WHAT (ELSE) IS IT GOOD FOR? Clotting of blood, cell membrane maintenance, and fat synthesis.

FOODS RICH IN VITAMIN K: Dark green leafy vegetables (in case you didn't have enough reasons already to eat them!), and liver. You get small amounts in dairy products.

RECOMMENDED DAILY DOSE: 100–300 mcg, taken with a meal. Levels as low as 50 mg can be toxic, so don't overdo it. Don't take supplements of vitamin K if you are on a blood thinner like warfarin or Coumadin (though it won't interfere with heparin).

Zinc

Most of us get less than two-thirds of the RDA of zinc, and deficiency is even more common in elderly Americans. But it is necessary for bone formation; it is used in creating both osteoblasts and osteoclasts, and in making some of the proteins found in bone. It assists with repairs, and also helps vitamin D function. Stress greatly depletes zinc, so unless you've attained some kind of permanent Zen state, your body probably makes frequent high demands on your zinc supply.

WHAT (ELSE) IS IT GOOD FOR? PMS (it stimulates the release of hormones, including progesterone); shortening the duration

THINGS TO THINK ABOUT

Laboratory studies suggest that zinc improves some phytoestrogens' ability to boost bone metabolism (see Chapter 11)—another reason to make sure you get enough of the trace minerals.

of colds; protein metabolism; healthy hair; prostate health; coping with stress; and wound healing. Zinc is a catalyst for numerous vital chemical reactions throughout the body.

FOODS RICH IN ZINC: Meat (especially beef, calf's liver, pork, and lamb), poultry (especially chicken and dark meat turkey), egg yolks, fish, milk, oysters, crab, sesame seeds, sunflower seeds, pumpkin seeds, legumes (especially soybeans). Whole grains (especially wheat bran and wheat germ) contain significant levels of zinc, but also have phytates, which block absorption of zinc.

RECOMMENDED DAILY SUPPLEMENTS FOR BONE HEALTH

VITAMINS

Folate (folic acid) (B$_9$)	400 mcg
Vitamin B$_6$ (pyridoxine)	5–25 mg
Vitamin B$_{12}$	1,000 mcg
Vitamin C	1,000 mg, divided
Vitamin D	400–800 IU
Vitamin K	100–300 mcg

MINERALS

Boron	3 mg
Copper	2.5–10 mg
Magnesium	600 mg
Manganese	5–10 mg
Selenium	200 mcg
Silicon (monosilic acid) (silicon dioxide)	1–2 mg
Strontium	0.5–3 mg
Zinc	50–100 mg

TIMING WHAT YOU'RE TAKING

To help you sort out the timing for all the supplements you should consider taking to ensure healthy bones ("Don't take calcium and copper at the same time," "Don't take manganese at the same time you take calcium and/or magnesium," etc.), below is a schedule that will accommodate all the recommendations for dosing. This is just one possibility, and you'll be able to work out variations if something else works better for you.

Your total list of supplements will look something like this: calcium (or calcium/vitamin D or calcium/ magnesium combination), multi–vitamin and mineral, vitamin D (if not combined with calcium or the multi), magnesium (if not combined with calcium), vitamin C (in divided doses), and any vitamin, mineral, or trace element not found in your multi in sufficient amounts.

This schedule is one good way to work out the timing of the various nutrients:

- **With br eakfast:** Calcium, magnesium (if taking as a separate supplement), vitamin D (if taking as a separate supplement), vitamin C
- **With lunch:** Calcium (if you're taking more than 1,000 mg a day)
- **With dinner:** Multivitamin, vitamin C
- **At bedtime:** Calcium (and magnesium if taking as separate supplement)

If you're taking a separate supplement of manganese or copper (if they aren't in your multi, or there isn't enough in your multi), take with lunch or dinner to keep them separate from calcium. If you take iron (or if your multivitamin contains iron), make sure not to take it at the same time as calcium.

RECOMMENDED DAILY DOSE: 50–100 mg (the RDA is 15), which you can probably find in a multivitamin. Calcium can interfere with zinc absorption, so take supplements at different times. Even a well-balanced diet might be low in zinc. When you are looking for a supplement, look for zinc picolinate, zinc citrate, or chelated zinc. Zinc sulfate is not as well absorbed and may irritate the stomach. Zinc oxide is only for external use. Zinc depletes your copper stores, so you should take copper if you take zinc, getting ten to twenty times as much zinc as you do copper to keep both levels in the normal range. In some people, zinc causes nausea or a metallic taste in the mouth. If that happens to you, just decrease your dose until you find a comfortable dose. Zinc can be toxic, but not until you reach levels around 150 mg a day over the long term.

❁ ❁ ❁ ❁ ❁ ❁ ❁ ❁ ❁ ❁ ❁ ❁ ❁ ❁ ❁ ❁ ❁ ❁ ❁ ❁

WEEK 2 ACTION PLAN

1. In your bone density notebook, keep track of everything you eat this week, noting portion size, calories, fat grams, fiber, and calcium for each day. If you can afford it, a professional nutritionist can analyze your list of what you ate, saving you the research and addition. But you can certainly do it yourself, and at least be close enough to give yourself a general picture of how you're doing. If you're doing it yourself, and have Internet access, the "Kitchen Counter" Web site may be useful. If you can find all your foods in its extensive database, which includes many brand-name products, it will add up most of the important nutritional information for you. (Go to *http://homearts.com/helpers/calculators/caldocf1.htm*, or try typing "Kitchen Counter" into your favorite search engine.)

2. At the end of the week, look at the numbers you've come up with to see where you're already doing what's healthy and where you could use some improvement, and commit to a plan for making any necessary changes by writing it in your Bone Density notebook.

3. On one day this week, pay particular attention to how much saturated fat is in your usual diet. Read labels. Make note of foods high in saturated fats (generally speaking, animal products, particularly meats and cheeses and

other full-fat dairy products) you use regularly. How much saturated fat do you get on an average day?

4. Spend a day gaining the same kind of awareness of protein. Pay attention to how much animal protein you get, as opposed to vegetable-based protein, and how much of the animal protein is from meat.

5. Take another day to focus on simple carbohydrates (pasta, bread, rice, corn, potatoes, sugars). How much do you get in an average day?

> ### WEEK 2 FOCUS
>
> - Evaluate your current diet and your family's eating habits.
> - Choose appropriate supplements of calcium, vitamin D, and magnesium, and a good multivitamin that includes trace minerals.
> - Cut down on or eliminate the foods that leach calcium from your bones.

6. Take one more day to look at how much salt you have in your diet, and be particularly suspicious of all packaged foods. Do you automatically salt what's on your plate before you eat it? Do you rely on salt when you're cooking, or do you just use it to accent a variety of other flavors and spices?

7. In the four areas above, pinpoint your strengths and weaknesses, and make a plan for changing your habits where necessary.

8. At the end of the week, check to see if you made a minimum of five servings of vegetables and fruits each day. Do it without counting juice (since it has no fiber, one of the important nutritious components of fruits and vegetables). If you didn't make this minimum, brainstorm some easy ways to bring up your totals (snacking on precut baby carrots as you prepare dinner, or carrying a small bag of nuts in your briefcase, and so on).

9. Weigh yourself, and measure your chest, waist, hips, arms, and thighs, to give you a baseline to compare yourself against as you make changes in your lifestyle. Muscle

weighs more than fat, so don't focus only on the scale. You may stop losing pounds on the program in this book, but your shape may still change for the better.

10. What is your BMI? (see page 129)

11. Is your body apple or pear shaped? (see page 132)

12. How many calories do you need a day? (see page 127) (If your BMI is between 21 and 26, figure what you need to maintain your current weight. If your BMI is above 26, figure out a target weight that would put you in the healthiest range of BMIs, and calculate the number of calories necessary to maintain that weight.)

13. If you want to lose weight to put your BMI into the healthiest range, make a plan for eliminating up to 500 calories a day. (Don't go under the number of calories necessary to maintain your target weight.) How many will be from cutting out "empty" calories from your diet, and how much will come from increasing exercise?

14. In your journal, write down your behavior patterns when it comes to food that you want to change.

15. How much calcium do you need each day? (see page 145) How much calcium do you generally get? If your daily diet falls short, make a list of ways you can add in more calcium. How much calcium do you want to get from a supplement?

16. Try three new calcium-rich foods this week (or three new ways to serve familiar favorites).

17. Cut back on coffee, sodas, and alcohol—drinks that leach calcium from your bones.

18. If you have children, how much calcium should they be getting? (Go to page 32 for recommendations by age for the under-25 crowd.) Work on ways to get more calcium into your whole family's diet—you'll all benefit—and think about a supplement for your kids.

19. Which calcium supplement sounds right for you? Buy some, and do the vinegar test (see page 160) to make sure the calcium will be available to your body. If it doesn't agree with you, or something keeps you from taking it regularly, keep trying different types and brands until you find one you like.

20. How much sunlight do you get each day? Look at your journal to see how many foods rich in vitamin D you got this week. If you get less than 20 minutes of sun, and aren't a regular drinker of vitamin D–fortified milk, take a vitamin D supplement. Check how much you might get in your multi, or try one of the calcium–vitamin D combinations.

21. Check your food journal against the list of foods containing magnesium to see if you're likely to be getting enough in your diet. Is your calcium supplement combined with magnesium? Or does your multi have sufficient levels? If not, get a separate supplement, or try the calcium/magnesium combination.

22. Food is the best source of nutrients, but good-quality supplements are also an excellent source. So check your food journal against the list of foods containing each of the nutrients your bones rely on to discover where you may have gaps. Choose supplements carefully to cover those gaps.

23. Find (and buy) a multi–vitamin and mineral that will meet your bones' needs, checking trace minerals in particular. If you already take a multivitamin, check the label to see if you're getting the appropriate amounts of nutrients for your bones. If not, find a new one that covers all the bases, or buy single supplements to fill in any gaps.

24. Use supplements from a company with high standards for the raw nutrients used, and strict standardization of production. The nutritionist I work with gets samples from every conceivable company and runs his own tests on them to see what meets with his standards. I use his choices in my office. The list is ever changing, but right now includes Biotics Research, Thorne Research, Ecological Formulas, Designs for Health, Physiologics, and Tieraon's Herbals, among others.

25. Buy at least a six-week supply of the supplements you need. Throw out any you already have that are expired or don't have the right levels of nutrients.

26. Make a schedule for when you will take your supplements.

❖ ❖ ❖ ❖ ❖ ❖ ❖ ❖ ❖ ❖ ❖ ❖ ❖ ❖ ❖ ❖ ❖ ❖ ❖ ❖

EAT RIGHT FOR
HEALTHY BONES

After last week's focus on what you eat right now, you're ready to move on to planning how you *will* eat for the rest of your life. You probably have some good habits in place by this time, but you'll be learning new strategies here that will increase your level of bone strength for years to come.

The first chapter this week covers the health benefits of soy foods and other phytoestrogens, plant hormones that mimic some of the beneficial properties of estrogens in your body. For anyone not familiar with the wide variety of healthful soy products available, the chapter includes an introduction to the most important ones, with plenty of tips on how to use them that are simple enough for even an inexperienced cook to put into practice right away.

A second chapter, on digestion, emphasizes that no matter how many nutrients you put into your mouth, without a healthy and efficient digestive process, much of the valuable stuff will never become active in your body. The market is flooded with all kinds of remedies, and now even preventive drugs, but they all just disguise symptoms rather than get to the root of the problem—and won't help your body absorb crucial nutrients properly. But a healthy diet often clears up bothersome symptoms, and if that isn't enough—or isn't quick enough—there are a variety of gentle, natural strategies explained here that can help.

With all that background, you'll be ready for the low-saturated-fat, moderate meat, whole-grain, vegetable-centered—and delicious and easy to prepare—recipes in Chapter 13, and the three weeks' worth of menus incorporating these recipes that follow. Eating this way will help you achieve or maintain your ideal weight, but in addition the Bone Density Diet is the heart and soul of the 6-Week Bone Density Program. The Action Plan at the end of this section will get you started on it so that you can build new habits gradually, allowing them to become a permanent part of your life. When you are ready for the diet, the three weeks of menus will give you lots of ideas and inspiration for continuing on your own. By the end of that time you'll already be seeing positive changes in your body and your energy levels, and will be well on your way to building strong bones that last—and you'll be slimmer, leaner, and stronger, too.

Chapter 11

The Phytoestrogen Promise

Most health claims on food labels tell you what's been left out, claiming "no fat," "no cholesterol," "no salt," "no sugar," and the like. But I predict it won't be long before you start to see labels heralding the *presence*, rather than the absence, of something: phytoestrogens. Phytoestrogens are plant hormones found in soy products and some other foods that mimic estrogen's beneficial effects on the human body, including the bones. This is a health fad I hope will last. Including phytoestrogens in your diet regularly will protect your bones as well as your heart and breasts, among other things.

Asians in Asia have lower rates of just about all the serious diseases Americans suffer from, and the amount of soy in the Asian diet is one of the main reasons why. Of course, soy foods in an Asian diet are part of a generally low-fat way of eating that includes lots of vegetables, all of which help keep you healthy. Heart disease and many kinds of cancer, including breast and colon cancer, occur less commonly in Asia than in the United States. Osteoporosis is rare in Asia, even though the typical Asian diet contains little calcium (though Asian women in this country are at relatively high risk of developing it). Asian women living in Asia generally don't get hot flashes and other menopausal symptoms. The easy transition to lower estrogen levels—including maintaining bone density—happens because of the large amount of soy foods in their diets. Their bodies stop making as much estrogen, but the phytoestrogens they take in provide able backup.

Research in this country confirms a range of health benefits from phytoestrogens, and in particular isoflavones (phytoestrogens from soy). The most solidly established is *protection against heart disease*, thanks to lowered total cholesterol levels and increased HDL "good cholesterol" and lowered triglyceride levels. For example, one study linked eating lots of soy foods with a 20 percent drop in elevated cholesterol levels. Since heart disease is the #1 killer in the United States, the potential health benefits of soy are vast.

Another study showed that eating one bowl of miso soup a day lowered the risk of stomach cancer among Japanese people by 30 percent. Soy is often said to *prevent cancer*, particularly of the breast, colon, prostate, ovaries, endometrium, and uterus, probably thanks to the action of phytoestrogens in making and metabolizing estrogen. Though the evidence behind those claims is not as strong as that for heart disease, there's essentially no harm in increasing your intake of soy foods, so I'd say the information we do have should already be enough to motivate you to change your diet.

The third major category of health benefits of eating soy is the one that relates the most to this book: *alleviating menopausal symptoms and improving bone density*. The two are linked in my mind because phytoestrogens address them both in much the same way supplemental estrogen does. More work has gone into looking at menopause, generally, than bone density, probably because results are available in a shorter time frame and follow-up is cheaper. Anything that alleviates symptoms like hot flashes and vaginal dryness is working with the body's estrogen levels, and so will be affecting bone mass at the same time. (Men's bones probably also benefit from the hormonal effects of soy, and at the very least see improvement from using more nonanimal protein.) One study did connect a diet rich in soy protein with increases in bone density in the spine in women after menopause—in just six months with 90 mg of isoflavones (40 g of soy protein) a day. The women in the study started with high cholesterol levels, and the same diet increased the level of "good" cholesterol, and so would offer protection against heart disease after menopause as well as osteoporosis. An animal study showed soy could increase bone density at the hip, as well.

Soy builds bone mass and slows bone loss. It causes much less calcium loss than animal sources of protein do, and even seems to increase calcium absorption. So with a diet rich in soy you are ahead of the game even before taking isoflavones into account. But it is the phytoestrogens that really pack the power. They act basically the same way in the body as estrogen does, but with a fraction of the potency (about .1 percent), and they play a clever dual role. When estrogen levels are low (as after menopause), phytoestrogens step in to take over some of the important functions and to boost the effect of whatever estrogen is there. When estrogen levels are too high (as in PMS), however, phytoestrogens are still helpful. Because they compete for the same sites to bind on to in the body, phytoestrogens will prevent some other estrogens from taking effect. Phytoestrogens also spur production of a protein that binds with estrogen and makes it ineffective. Those are probably the mechanisms responsible for lowering breast cancer risk, since estrogen makes breast cells grow faster. Phytoestrogens, because they are weaker than the other estrogens they are blocking, would minimize growth.

So when your body is no longer making all the estrogen it once did, soy and phytoestrogens can smooth your course. One study showed improvements in American women's bone density in just six months on a diet rich in soy protein. Another showed women who eat soy regularly have fewer hot flashes and night sweats, and are less likely to complain of vaginal dryness or irritation. Research currently under way will give us better information about isoflavones' and other phytoestrogens' effect on bone density and menopausal symptoms. But the case is already compelling, especially given the lack of a downside to a diet rich in soy.

Soybeans have also been lauded as helping prevent and break down gallstones, relieving constipation, regulating blood sugar and insulin levels (and so helping heal diabetes), helping with symptoms of shingles, and even eliminating warts and dandruff. (Not all of that is thanks to phytoestrogens. In the last case, biotin is the active ingredient, as is lysine in the case of shingles.) The (scientific) jury is still out on most of these topics, and you can be sure you'll have to wait quite a while before someone funds an authoritative soy-and-warts study. Further research *is* being done to pin down the effect of phytoestrogens on various areas of the body. That's important to tease out, because they are still estrogens, and as we've seen, estrogens come with risks as well as benefits. There are enough good reasons to incorporate soy products and other phytoestrogens into your diet that I see no need to wait for further evidence before recommending action. Perhaps you'll get some of these other benefits as helpful side effects. But keep an eye on developments in the health news for future discoveries in this area. If you harbor any concerns about phytoestrogens—they are still estrogens, after all, if extremely weak ones in comparison to what the human body makes—just steer clear of supplements (see Chapter 19), and focus on getting them in your diet. As with all nutrients, that's the best way to get the highest quality anyway.

BUT I DON'T KNOW HOW TO USE SOY!

Soybeans are high in fiber and protein, and low in fat. They are a good source of calcium and magnesium (double your bone benefits!), folic acid, vitamin B_6, zinc, and the cholesterol-lowering omega-3 fatty acids made famous by fish—only this way, sans cholesterol. So soybeans are a great nutritional package before you even get to the chemicals with the hormonal effects: genistein, daidzein, and equol (in case you run into those terms on supplement packages now, or food packages in the future).

Almost all soy products—along with beans and legumes, some nuts and a handful of other fruits, vegetables, and grains—contain significant levels of phytoestrogens (see boxes on page 198). After soy, the richest source is probably flaxseeds, which contain a phytoestrogen called lignans. Flaxseed can be a very convenient way to

---

HOW TO GET YOUR SOY

How Much Is One Serving?

½ cup tofu

1 cup soymilk

¼ cup TVP (texturized vegetable protein) or soybean flakes, as a meat extender or substitute

⅓ cup soy flour

1 soy burger

2 soy hot dogs or sausages

½ cup soybeans (canned, frozen, or dried)

½ cup green soybeans

⅓ cup soy nuts

2 teaspoons flaxseed

½ cup tempeh

½ cup miso

1–2 tablespoons soy protein powder (concentrations vary widely by brand, so read the labels)

---

get the estrogenic effects you're after, because you get so much in such a small quantity (1 tablespoon of ground flaxseeds can give a day's supply of phytoestrogens). At first, getting high levels of soy and other phytoestrogens in your diet will take some doing,

---

OTHER SOURCES OF PHYTOESTROGENS

Many other foods have phytoestrogens, though not at levels comparable to soybeans and flaxseeds. But phytoestrogens give you one more healthy reason to enjoy apples, pomegranates, dates, peanuts, cashews, almonds, oats, corn, wheat, alfalfa, celery, brussels sprouts, beets, beans and legumes, and bean sprouts (especially black beans, chickpeas, pinto beans, yellow split peas, lima beans, anasazi beans, red kidney beans, red lentils, black-eyed peas, mung beans, adzuki beans, and fava beans).

In addition, many herbs are rich sources of phytoestrogens (see Chapter 21).

because most Americans are not exactly on intimate terms with soy foods. But as you'll see, there are a wide range of options for increasing your intake, even if you are not ready to switch over to daily miso-soup breakfasts, Japanese style.

First, a few pointers about eating soy foods. You should increase the amount of soy in your diet gradually to avoid intestinal upset and gas. Buy organic products when you can, since soybeans are often treated with heavy-duty chemicals if they are not grown on an organic farm. The good stuff is in the soy protein, so soy products without protein (soy sauce, soybean oil) won't count in your daily tally of isoflavones, whatever else they may have to recommend them. Processing may reduce the amount of isoflavones in products like soy hot dogs and soy burgers, so don't rely on only those things for your daily support (check the labels, as some list the amount of isoflavones). Keep an eye on how much fat you are taking in. Flaxseed, and many soy products, are higher than many other beans and seeds in fat and calories. Even though it is a good form of fat, at 10 g in 3 tablespoons of flaxseeds, and 7 g in 4 ounces of tofu, it can add up when you're aiming for as many servings as you'll need to protect your bones. Choose "lite" products when you can, and pay particular attention to how much fat you get from other sources. A low-fat diet is probably the most important single thing you can do for your overall health (aside from stopping smoking), so it doesn't pay to ignore it in your quest for phytoestrogens.

DON'T KNOCK IT UNTIL YOU TRY IT

If you haven't tasted *soymilk* since its first popularity in this country during the hippie era, you should know that the modern version is healthy and delicious (as opposed to its original healthy but unpalatable incarnation). Usually you'll see it sold in boxes, which is good for long-term storage, though you may also be able to find fresh soymilk, too. You can choose from a variety of flavors. Soymilk does not compare to cow's milk when it comes to calcium content, so look for fortified brands rather than compromise your calcium intake. If you choose reduced-fat soymilk, keep in mind that you'll get less in the way of isoflavones.

RECIPE: MARINATED TOFU

Slice firm tofu, press out any excess liquid, and marinate in soy sauce or tamari and garlic and ginger. Coat in sesame seeds and pan-fry in olive or peanut oil until golden brown on both sides. Use to fill a sandwich or top a salad, or with rice and steamed vegetables, or just as it is with your favorite dipping sauce on the side.

The gold medal for versatility goes to *tofu*. Don't limit yourself to using it in salads or stir-fries. Use it (mashed) as a base for smoothies, dressings, soups, and puddings. Marinate it, slice thickly, and broil it for a simple alternative to a burger. Or mash it and mix with bread crumbs and spices to form a burger. Use marinated and baked or broiled tofu at the center of a sandwich. Tofu takes on flavors easily. By itself it is very bland, which is why it is a good thickener for just about anything. But you probably won't want much to do with it if you only eat it plain. Use your imagination. Experiment with different kinds (extra-firm, silken, light, etc.) to find the textures you like best. Firm is better for stir-frying, for example, while silken is better for blending. Four ounces of tofu has about 100 mg of calcium your bones will thank you for, in addition to the phytoestrogens. Check the labels when possible, as not all tofus are created equal, and look for "calcium processed" brands, or brands that list significant calcium content, to take advantage of the two-in-one nutritional benefits.

❀ ❀

RECIPE: BASIC TOFU SPREAD

  4 ounces silken tofu
  ¼ cup olive oil
  1 garlic clove (optional)
  ½ teaspoon salt

Combine all ingredients in a food processor or blender until smooth and thoroughly mixed. Experiment with the proportions according to your taste and to change consistency and texture, depending on your planned use of the spread. Add flavors of your choice (see below); anything you have a taste for or your family can dream up will work in this versatile, creamy spread or dip. Combine in the blender or food processor for a smooth spread, or stir in after blending if you want it chunky style.

Use as a sandwich spread, dip, or salad dressing or anyplace else you need a creamy sauce, such as with poached fish or in baked potatoes or over brown rice or pasta with steamed vegetables.

Top 10 Tofu Spread Flavors
sun-dried tomatoes and basil
lox and scallions
horseradish
chopped fruit or vegetables
sesame seeds and honey
basil and pine nuts
jalapeño peppers
caviar, onions, and capers
mustard and honey
garam marsala and grated ginger

❀ ❀

One cup of *soybeans* gives you the rough equivalent of the estrogen dose in one pill of prescription estradiol, like Premarin. Use them in soups, stews, chilies, and casseroles as you would any other bean, or mash them for use as a basis for a burger or faux meatloaf. Try eating fresh (or fresh frozen) green soybeans in the Japanese style: boiled, drained, and cooled, and popped from the pods one by one. *Bean sprouts*—of this or any other bean—are an even better source of most nutrients than the beans themselves. That holds for phytoestrogens in particular, because the one known as genistein is increased during the germination process.

❈ ❈ ❈ ❈ ❈ ❈ ❈ ❈ ❈ ❈ ❈ ❈ ❈ ❈ ❈ ❈ ❈ ❈ ❈

RECIPE: TOFU MAYONNAISE

    8   ounces firm tofu
    1   garlic clove
    ¼   cup olive oil
    ½   teaspoon salt
    1   teaspoon Dijon mustard
    2   teaspoons cider vinegar

Place all ingredients in a food processor or blender and blend until creamy. Mayonnaise will keep refrigerated for 1 week.

Bonus: For your own "special sauce" for sandwiches, mix tofu mayo, tomato paste, minced onion, and sweet pickle relish.

❈ ❈ ❈ ❈ ❈ ❈ ❈ ❈ ❈ ❈ ❈ ❈ ❈ ❈ ❈ ❈ ❈ ❈ ❈

THE CORNELL FORMULA

For a nutritional triple play whenever you are baking, use the Cornell Formula, developed at the university during the Depression. When measuring flour, start with 1 tablespoon each of soy flour, powdered milk, and wheat germ at the bottom of a 1-cup measure, then fill the rest of the way with white or—even better—whole wheat flour. Use it for making whichever cookies, muffins, cakes, or breads you like the best and reap a dividend in calcium, phytoestrogens, and other nutrients.

Tempeh is an Indonesian staple made from fermented soybeans mixed with grains and cooked. You'll find packaged varieties in a range of flavors in the health food store. Its meaty taste and texture may placate devoted carnivores, and it takes well to just about any savory marinade you can dream up. Steaming it makes it softer and milder.

Another strategy is to start using *soy flour*. You can replace a fifth of any wheat or white flour called for in a recipe, as long as you up the amount of liquid you use a bit and bake whatever you're making at 25° less than otherwise called for.

So-called *soy nuts* are just roasted soybeans, and a nice alternative to less nutritious crunchy snacks. Eat a handful with a piece of fruit for a good balance of protein, fiber, and carbohydrates. You can also get "soy nut butter" to use in place of peanut butter for an extra nutritional punch.

❊ ❊

RECIPE: SALAD DRESSINGS
Make your salads even healthier by topping them with creamy tofu-based dressings like these.

Green Goddess Dressing
¼ cup olive oil
2 garlic cloves
4 ounces silken tofu
6 green peppercorns
1 large ripe peeled and pitted avocado
1 tablespoon lemon juice

Put oil, garlic, tofu, and peppercorns in a blender or food processor and blend until smooth. Add avocado and lemon juice and blend until thick and smooth.

Cucumber Dill Dressing
¼ cup olive oil
2 garlic cloves
¼ small white onion, chopped

    4 ounces silken tofu
    1 small cucumber, peeled, seeded, and chopped
    2 tablespoons fresh dill (or 2 teaspoons dried)

Put the oil, garlic, onion, and tofu in a blender or food processor
and blend until smooth. Add the cucumber and dill. Blend for 1
minute.

❋ ❋ ❋ ❋ ❋ ❋ ❋ ❋ ❋ ❋ ❋ ❋ ❋ ❋ ❋ ❋ ❋ ❋ ❋ ❋

FUN WITH COMPUTERS

Check out "The Cook's Thesaurus" for short definitions of
many foods, including soy products, and appropriate
substitutions if you don't have the exact item a recipe calls
for on hand. Go to *http://www.northcoast.com/~alden/
cookhome.html*, or search for the site by name with your
favorite browser.

Soy protein powder is an easy way to boost your phytoestrogen intake. Because it is so concentrated, you get a lot of isoflavones in just a small amount of it. The best thing to do is to
add it to a smoothie (make it with soymilk to double your fun).
Try drinking your breakfast, and you'll be well on your way to
your daily total before you even leave the house. As you know,
I'm an advocate of whole foods, generally, and the same goes for
soy products. The closer you are to the soybean itself, the more
complete nutritional package you'll be getting. But because it
is so easy to get soy in your diet—and to know just how much
you're getting—and is more like a food than a supplement, I'm a
fan of soy protein powder. Aim for 35 to 60 g of soy protein a day.
Labels on any soy protein powder should tell you how much it
contains.

Miso, a concentrated soybean paste, is another great way to
get isoflavones and is also high in iron, calcium, phosphorus, and
B vitamins. It takes only a minute to mix a dollop into hot water
for—*voilà!*—miso soup (garnish with a bit of diced tofu and, if
you want to get fancy, thinly sliced scallions). Add chopped greens

to the basic broth for a soup that is more substantive—and even more nutritious. You can also use miso broth as stock for any other soup. Or try it as a substitute for coffee or tea (see recipe below). Miso paste keeps for a long while in the refrigerator, so keep some on hand. Check out the different kinds (red, brown, and white) to discover what you enjoy the most.

❊ ❊

RECIPE: RED MISO TEA

    2 cups water
    2 tablespoons red miso
    1 squeeze of lemon or lime

Bring water to a boil and add the miso. Remove from the heat. Stir until miso is dissolved, pour into 2 mugs, and add citrus juice.

❊ ❊

Texturized vegetable protein (TVP) is another simple way to add soy to your diet. Just follow package instructions and use it to replace ground meat in any of your favorite recipes. In chili with beans, for example, you'll never know the difference, so this might be an especially good way to please your kids.

A range of other products, including the many kinds of *faux meats* (like burgers and sausages) extend your options even further. Processing can sometimes destroy isoflavones, so don't count on, say, soyburgers as the only source of soy in your diet. Check labels, as some will indicate the phytoestrogen content. At the very least, you'll get a low-fat, low-cholesterol source of protein that won't leach calcium from your bones.

Flaxseeds are, as I mentioned, an easy way to slip phytoestrogens into your diet. Use them instead of nuts when you are baking. Sprinkle them on salads for some added crunch. Look for flaxseed cereals, or use flaxseeds in making your own granola (then eat a bowl full with soymilk for a double whammy). Use a tablespoonful in a smoothie or shake, making sure to blend thoroughly for an even texture.

You should be able to find all of these products, along with a variety of prepackaged foods like soy cheese, yogurt, cream cheese, and sour cream, at your friendly neighborhood health food store or food co-op. Experiment to discover what you enjoy the most and find the easiest to prepare.

❁ ❁ ❁ ❁ ❁ ❁ ❁ ❁ ❁ ❁ ❁ ❁ ❁ ❁ ❁ ❁ ❁ ❁ ❁ ❁

RECIPE: ROASTED RED PEPPER DIP

1 12-ounce jar roasted red peppers, drained
2 8-ounce packages soy cream cheese
Plain soymilk or vegetable stock, as needed

Pat excess oil from peppers with a paper towel. Place peppers and soy cream cheese in blender or food processor and blend until smooth. Add soymilk or stock to thin to desired consistency, if necessary.

❁ ❁ ❁ ❁ ❁ ❁ ❁ ❁ ❁ ❁ ❁ ❁ ❁ ❁ ❁ ❁ ❁ ❁ ❁ ❁

HOW MUCH DO I NEED?

If you want to equal prescription estrogen's positive effects on your bones with phytoestrogens, you need several servings a day. As few as three might do it, but you may need up to eight. Menopausal symptoms should diminish with two servings a day, but you'll need more to protect your bones. But don't wait until menopause to enjoy the benefits of soy. Men as well as women benefit, of course, given the wide range of health concerns improved by a diet rich in phytoestrogens, and women before menopause surely will. If high cholesterol is your main concern, you'll need at least two servings each day, and perhaps as many as five, to bring it down. Breast cancer protection comes with about two servings a day.

If you don't want or need the phytoestrogens in soy, you can still benefit from the soy amino acids (protein) by using a soy powder with the plant estrogens removed. That will provide most of the benefits of whole soy foods, particularly the protection of your heart, without the hormonal effects.

The FDA recently began to consider a proposal to allow health claims about soy on food labels. The standard put forth is based on getting 25 mg a day of soy protein, and would require a food to have a quarter of that per serving before it could make any claims. If that goes through—and I hope it does—you'll see a blossoming of new products as well as new labels on old products, and it will get even easier to know what's best for your bones.

Chapter 12

Good Digestion

The most nutritious diet imaginable won't do you any good if you are not digesting and absorbing the bounty therein. Any gastrointestinal upset makes it more likely you're not getting all you should from your food. Given the plethora of products to address various digestive difficulties featured in big-bucks prime-time television advertising, I'd say there are plenty of people who should be recognizing themselves by this point in the chapter. In addition to gas, bloating, nausea, constipation, diarrhea, heartburn, and all the other pleasures the gastrointestinal tract produces when it doesn't like the way you're running the show, low stomach acid levels make it difficult to get the nutrients you need out of what you take in. That's a problem that grows more and more likely as you get older, but it is also rather subtle and goes undetected all too often.

The very first thing to do to ensure good absorption of nutrients is to make your digestion as problem-free as possible. But not with the aforementioned variety of products on the market. They just mask the underlying problem by making the symptoms more bearable. The idea is to not get to the point where you need them in the first place. A generally healthy diet high in fiber, like the one described in this book, should help you maintain good digestion. The simplest solutions are sometimes the best: chew your food well, and don't eat too much of it at any one time. That means no eating on the run, or while standing over the sink, or while rushing to catch your connecting flight. First get on the plane, then sit down and eat something in a (somewhat) civilized manner.

MINDFUL EATING

Try paying attention to what you are actually doing while you eat (getting a little ahead of ourselves here, into the "mind/body" portion of our program). *Mindful* eating—if you're ready for a rather Zen approach to your plate—means noticing your food, appreciating it for its nutritional and sensual value, and generally staying in the present as you eat. Not reading the paper, arguing politics, or balancing your checkbook while you dine. Did you ever have to think hard to recall what you ate for dinner last night? I bet you ate it in front of the television in 6.2 seconds flat, or before you made it home from the drive-through window. Make an effort to eat in calm and pleasant surroundings, sharing food you enjoy with people you enjoy. Soon you'll be able to call the pharmacy and cancel your standing order for the latest thing being hawked as a surefire way to settle your stomach.

FOOD ALLERGIES AND FOOD SENSITIVITIES

If settling your mind isn't enough to settle your stomach, check the amount of sugar, white flour, fried foods, caffeine, and alcohol you eat. You already know that many of these things are not good for your bones in the first place. Well, they are also difficult to digest, and in large quantities wreak havoc with your system. If you're body isn't cooperative on the diet you provide, it may have a good point: those foods are low in nutritive value, anyway, and surely you could choose high-test fuel for the most precious vehicle you own (irreplaceable as it is): your body. Smoking may also interfere with digestion, so if you smoke, you can add that to your enormous list of reasons to quit.

Food allergies or food sensitivities are often the culprits in digestive disorders. Foods that form a regular part of the average daily diet are frequently to blame, particularly dairy products, wheat and other grains, corn, and eggs. You might also want to watch out for reactions to citrus fruit, strawberries, kiwifruit, and tomatoes. Aged food (like wine, beer, soy sauce, and sauerkraut), or other foods with mold (like blue cheese), can also be problematic. Additives and preservatives are also common problems, which brings most packaged foods into the ring. If you notice improvement when you are *not* eating those things (or any other food you've come to suspect), or symptoms when you do, you have a clear path open to you: avoid that food.

THE CAVEMAN DIET

Up until the last 10,000 years or so, humans' diets were much different from how they are now, consisting of just what our ancestors could hunt or gather. So from an evolutionary perspective, our bodies have not had enough time to become accustomed to many of the things we eat in the modern world, and that disconnect can show up as a food sensitivity.

If you can't tell which particular food is bothering you, consider undertaking an elimination diet. That means, basically, eating a very narrow diet for a week or two, then gradually adding in one kind of food at a time over the next weeks. When you introduce a new food, eat it every day for four days before you try the next one, in order to observe any effect. If anything bothers you, you'll know to avoid it down the line. Talk with your health care professional before trying something like that, and find a good book or article explaining in detail how to do an elimination diet. It may seem like a lot of trouble, but once you've identified the foods you are sensitive to (and commit to avoiding them), you'll clear up your chronic symptoms *and* help your bones (by allowing full absorption of necessary nutrients). And there's an additional piece of good news. Once you've cut a food out of your diet for a while and your symptoms have abated, you may be able to tolerate the food in the future—in small quantities and infrequently—so the ban doesn't have to be a life sentence. (Just in case chocolate shows up on your list, I thought you'd like to know.)

HOW DO *YOU* SPELL RELIEF?

If you do need to take an antacid, why not rely on one made of calcium? Chewable tablets like Tums and Rolaids are made from calcium carbonate. Read the labels carefully to make sure there's no aluminum or sodium sneaking in. You should be getting nothing but calcium and the colorings and flavors that make it palatable. (As we discussed in Chapter 6, you absolutely must avoid antacid with aluminum—again, read the labels carefully.) But the only reason to take these antacids regularly is if you are using them as your calcium supplement. If you need them more than infrequently to ease your digestion, take a closer look at what and how you are eating to try to get to the root of the problem.

An excellent alternative for easing heartburn is a licorice root extract called DGL (or, sometimes, "deglycyrrhizinated licorice"). This is gentler on your body than standard licorice root, but as always, "natural" does not mean "completely safe." If you experience loose bowels while using DGL, lower the dose or switch to something else. Don't use it at all if you are taking corticosteroids unless your doctor approves, as it may interfere with those medicines.

There are also many homeopathic remedies for relief of heartburn, indigestion, bloating, and gas. Look for them in your health-food store or drugstore and follow package directions. Several

---

TOP 5 HERBS TO AID DIGESTION

Peppermint
Chamomile
Dandelion
Anise
Fennel

TOP 4 HOMEOPATHIC REMEDIES FOR DIGESTIVE TROUBLE

Nux vomica
Lycopodium
Carbo vegetabilis
Bryonia alba

herbs may also help, like the anise seeds you sometimes see offered on your way out of Indian restaurants where you might otherwise see mints—chewing them will freshen your breath along with aiding your digestion. A cup of peppermint tea after dinner instead of coffee might be just the ticket. Ginger and cloves stimulate acid production, making them good choices for easing nausea and aiding digestion, though you shouldn't take them if you have or ever have had an ulcer or are at increased risk of ulcers. Chew or suck a small piece of candied ginger, or, if the taste is too strong for you, look for ginger candies. Suck on a couple of whole cloves, or buy or make ginger tea.

BONE BOOSTERS

Make your own ginger and clove tea by steeping grated fresh ginger and whole cloves in hot water. Both ginger and cloves have very strong flavors, so use more or less according to your own taste.

THINGS TO THINK ABOUT

Forty percent of postmenopausal women don't make enough stomach acid to absorb all the calcium they take in.

LOW STOMACH ACID

A bigger risk to your bones than any chronic digestive symptoms is having insufficient stomach acid to thoroughly digest and absorb nutrients—because most often, you are unaware you have a problem and so do nothing to resolve it. Making insufficient stomach acid—actually hydrochloric acid, or HCl—is a very common problem. About 15 percent of Americans have low levels, and it occurs more frequently with age. By 60, about 40 percent of people don't make enough to properly absorb calcium, for example. Without sufficient stomach acid, you absorb just 4 percent of a calcium supplement (compared to 22 percent under normal conditions). Not only won't you be getting the cal-

THE ACID TEST

If you want to prove to yourself the importance of having enough acid to make use of the calcium you take, try this little test: when you're checking your calcium supplement for how well it dissolves in vinegar (see Chapter 9), fill a second glass with water, and drop another pill in there. If you have a good supplement, it will dissolve in the vinegar within half an hour. But even a good supplement won't change much in the water. Without acid, that calcium isn't going to be available in your body, either.

cium your bones need, but also you'll be wasting the money you spent on supplements (or swallowing truly obscene numbers of pills)! Besides calcium, you'll come up short on folic acid, copper, iron, and chromium, and probably magnesium, zinc, and manganese as well. All of those are important for optimum health, and, as we saw in Chapter 10, most are crucial for strong bones.

BONE BOOSTERS

Your calcium supplement will dissolve in vinegar (an acid) if it is going to dissolve in your stomach. Now consider the other side of the coin: no matter how well your supplement does in vinegar, it won't dissolve in your stomach if you don't have enough acid there to do the job.

One common sign of having low acid levels is bloating at the end of meals or within a half an hour, though that can also be a sign of a food allergy. The sensation of food just sitting in the stomach, especially rich, high-protein food like beef, can also indicate low stomach acid levels. Many things cause constipation, and low stomach acid is one of them. Diarrhea, too, is sometimes a result, especially if you experience it in the morning. Just to make this all the more complicated, you may well have no abdominal complaints at all with low stomach acid. Some additional signs to take note of are soft or easily breakable fingernails, hair loss, and visible small blood vessels on your face. No one thing is a sure indicator of low levels of stomach acid, but the symptoms described here should be enough to make you suspicious, especially if you experience more than one of them.

> **THINGS TO THINK ABOUT**
>
> Calcium in the mouth does not mean calcium in the bones.

Low stomach acid has been connected to many other illnesses, so if you have any of the following conditions, you should be paying attention to your HCl levels, as well as your other health concerns: allergies, arthritis, asthma, gallbladder disease, lupus, rosacea, thyroid disorders, and vitiligo.

Having your hair analyzed for mineral levels can give you some insight into how well you are digesting and absorbing some key nutrients—and low numbers may point to low stomach acid. Another option is to have stool analysis, looking for undigested food, which, again, might indicate a lack of HCl. You can have your serum gastric levels checked to see if you produce too much acid. There are several other direct and indirect ways to measure your stomach acid levels you can discuss with your doctor. Despite a range of complexity and reliability, there is no widely available "easy" lab test that can tell you exactly how you're doing in terms of stomach acid. So when it comes down to it, you'll probably have to . . . go with your gut!

If you fear you may not be making enough stomach acid, but believe the deficiency to be mild, taking nutritional supplements, particularly calcium, is the most important first step. Switching to an easily digestible calcium supplement, like calcium citrate, and taking it with meals, may be enough to correct the situation as far as your bones are concerned. Almost half of citrate is absorbed in people with low acid (and even more so in people with normal acid levels, of course).

BONE BOOSTERS

Simply taking in more acidic foods, like grapefruit, or vinegary foods, or orange juice (or having them along with a supplement) may also help in mild cases of low stomach acid. (Don't start taking any medicines with grapefruit juice without checking first with your doctor or pharmacist about potential interactions.) Using ginger or cloves increases acid production, so it may be worth trying a 500 mg capsule of ginger, or half a ginger candy, or sucking on whole cloves, or making clove and ginger tea (a delicious remedy, as long as you like the strong flavors). Hot, spicy foods also increase release of acid.

DIGESTIVE ENZYMES

You'll be shortchanging your bones, and throwing money away, to boot, if you are taking even very digestible supplements and don't have enough stomach acid to dissolve and make use of them. One way to correct the problem is by taking HCl supplements. The most common ones are betaine hydrochloride or glutamic acid hydrochloride, which are sometimes sold in combination with pepsin (an enzyme that digests protein) and pancreatic enzymes (which help with nutrient absorption).

Pepsin is a valuable addition. In the stomach, HCl makes nutrients more soluble (and therefore more likely to be absorbed through the walls of the intestine). But it is the pepsin that breaks down foods containing protein to release the nutrients in the first place. They work best together as a team.

The pancreatic enzymes help absorption of vitamins D and K, and zinc, valuable nutrients in general, and for bones in particular.

Case in Point: Alex

*A*lex, in her mid-30s, came to see me because the collection of symptoms she called "indigestion" (diarrhea, constipation, nausea) was getting to the point where it was interfering with her life. She was young enough that she was not yet focusing on her bone density, but I feared she wasn't digesting nutrients properly and so her bones may not have available all they need to maintain as much density as possible.

I treated her with a radical change in diet—eliminating sugars and simple carbohydrates, and increasing fiber from vegetables and whole grains to at least 25 grams a day—supplements of probiotics, an herbal supplement to decrease bowel permeability that included anti-inflammatories, and comprehensive digestive enzymes. She also started exercising as an outlet for her chronic stress, and increased her water intake dramatically, aiming for at least twelve glasses a day (or enough to make her urine clear, not yellow).

In her first trip to the health food store, Alex dropped a lot of money, and avoiding simple carbohydrates took some doing at first. But two weeks later she called to thank me. Her symptoms were completely gone.

But you're less likely to be deficient in them, and if you're not, there's no reason to take them. Alcoholism and pancreatitis can cause low levels of the enzymes, so if you fall into either of those categories, the addition makes sense. Bloating about an hour after eating, or after eating fatty foods, may signal insufficient pancreatic enzymes, as may oily or smelly stools and dry, flaky skin in some circumstances. Supplements made from pineapple (bromelain) and papaya (papain) are another way to boost your levels of these enzymes. Either way (in combination with HCl or on their own), you should consult with your health care provider.

The point bears repeating that "natural" or nonprescription does not mean there are no risks or side effects. Using HCl supplements puts you at risk of giving yourself an ulcer, so even though they are available over the counter, use them only with your doctor's supervision. The common recommendation is to start with 600 to 1,800 mg taken at the beginning of each meal. Heartburn is a common side effect. If you get it, decrease your dose or try switching from tablets to capsules. HCl supplements taken at the same time as aspirin, ibuprofen, or any NSAIDs can raise your risk of getting an ulcer, so be sure not to mix these medicines. If you are using drugs like Prilosec, Pepcid, and Zantac, you should not take HCl. (Discovering and correcting the underlying problem so you can get off the prescriptions is well worth the time and effort, however!) And you should use HCl supplements only if you are medically proven to have low stomach acid. The potential risk is too large to take a "try and see" approach.

A better option is to use digestive enzymes, which are probably safer and more effective than pure HCl supplements. Your stomach, salivary glands, pancreas, and bowel all make various enzymes that aid in digestion, and over-the-counter or prescription pills increase the levels in your body and so improve absorption of nutrients. You should be medically evaluated before you begin taking anything, so work with your health care provider to determine which ones are best for you. You could take a "shotgun" approach with one of the many brands of mixed enzymes, which may or may not work and may or may not have side effects. But it is better to be scientific about just where your problem is, and take the specific type of enzyme that is relevant.

This is not meant to be a long-term treatment, though the enzymes are valuable in righting a current imbalance. But true healing means finding the root of the problem and addressing the issue there. Very few people have an actual, permanent, physiological level of stomach acid (or digestive enzymes) that is abnormal. Almost always, abnormal readings are secondary to some other health problem that needs to be addressed, not smoothed over. Your best weapon for good digestion is simply good nutrition and an all-around healthy diet. Just about everyone should expect normal bowel function, without chronic constipation, diarrhea, bloating, or gas—provided you eat a variety of nutritious foods and avoid anything you are particularly sensitive to. Just trading in a prescription treatment for something else, no matter how "natural" or easily available, is not real progress.

PROBIOTICS

Another function of stomach acid is to protect your stomach against abnormal bacteria, viruses, and fungi. With an abnormal amount of acid, your stomach and small intestine won't allow any microorganisms to grow normally, even if you ingest them. Low stomach acid may allow them to take hold and multiply, with possible negative consequences to your health and well-being.

Your stomach and intestines are also populated by "good bacteria," which help keep you healthy by releasing chemicals that are necessary for digestion and for limiting the effects of harmful bacteria. Antibiotics kill these friendly bugs while they are killing the bad guys. (That's the reason so many women suffer from yeast infections when they take antibiotics—the good bacteria help keep the yeast under control, and when they are decimated, the yeast take advantage.) So after a course of one of these medicines, you should help the good guys stage a comeback by taking some lactobacillus or bifidobacterium *probiotics* (helpful bacteria) to get your digestive tract back to normal. They are also helpful for intestinal infections, diarrhea, and other digestive disorders, including diarrhea caused by antibiotics, yeast infections, and urinary tract infections. Probiotics help lower cholesterol and generally support the immune system. Some kinds make lactase, the enzyme you need to digest the milk protein lactose, and some kinds produce several B vitamins.

If you have food sensitivities, probiotic supplements will be particularly helpful to you. But anyone will benefit from taking them regularly, as they help digest food, absorb nutrients into the body, and decrease the amount of toxins allowed to pass into your body from your bowel. Use a combination of lactobacillus (the bacteria in yogurt or acidophilus, normally made in the small intestine) and bifida sporins (normally made in the large intestine) with colony counts around 20 million up to 20 billion (read the labels). That's about ten to twenty to a hundred or more times more potent than yogurt, to give you a little perspective. These helpful bacteria won't grow without a good supply of fiber, another reason to make sure your diet has enough of it, whether or not you take the supplements. Probiotics must be alive to do you any good, and the label will tell you if they are.

You already know I have a bias toward healthy bones as the basis for general good health. Digestion makes a good showing in that same race. Good digestion is crucial for getting your body all it needs in the way of nutrients for fueling every transaction it makes. You've heard the saying "Garbage in, garbage out." That's one of the guiding thoughts behind eating a well-balanced, low-fat, high-fiber, vegetable-based diet. But the scary part is, without the ability to properly process what you give it, your body may as well be subsisting on Twinkies. Don't let your good work in other aspects of your diet go down the tubes because of an easily correctable problem.

Chapter 13

Eating Well and Eating Right: Bone Density Recipes

This chapter provides recipes for many of the dishes in the Bone Density Diet. There are limitless ways to incorporate calcium-rich foods and good sources of phytoestrogens into your diet, so these are just to get you started. The menus in the next chapter include all these recipes.

Making meals has come to seem such a burden that most homes could do without a kitchen, as long as they had a freezer, a microwave, and nearby fast-food restaurants with drive-through windows. But preparing a delicious and healthy meal should be a sensual experience as pleasant as eating it. Of course, we're all busy, so the recipes here are not time-consuming and include no Martha Stewart–style froufrou touches. But several of these dishes would do just fine for company. Haul out the good china, light some candles, and perhaps share a bottle of wine. On second thought, don't wait for company to take out your nice things and gather those you love around the table. You might not be able to meet the *Leave It to Beaver* ideal of dinner on the table at 5:30, with all the nuclear family present every night. But make cooking and eating (and, yes, cleaning up) together a regular part of your routine. A meal should nourish both body and soul.

BREAKFAST RECIPES

❀ ❀

ANYTIME BREAKFAST BURRITOS

SERVES 4

    6 large eggs
    ¼ cup nonfat milk
    1 teaspoon canola oil
    1 3-ounce can fire-roasted chopped green chiles
    ½ cup grated cheddar or Monterey Jack cheese
    4 flour tortillas

In a mixing bowl, beat the eggs with milk. Heat oil in a large frying pan over medium heat. Add eggs. After the eggs have begun to set, add the chiles. Mix gently. When eggs are still slightly wet, remove from heat and sprinkle cheese over the eggs. Cover to allow cheese to melt. Spray the tortillas with vegetable oil spray and toast them on the burner you were using for the eggs a few seconds on each side. Watch them carefully! Divide eggs among the tortillas, wrap, and serve immediately. For a complete dinner, add a side of refried beans and fresh fruit or a tossed salad.

NUTRITIONAL INFORMATION PER SERVING:
Calories: 275
Carbohydrates (g): 18
Protein (g): 21
Fat (g): 14
Calcium (mg): 210

❀ ❀ ❀ ❀ ❀ ❀ ❀ ❀ ❀ ❀ ❀ ❀ ❀ ❀ ❀ ❀ ❀ ❀ ❀ ❀

❀ ❀

STRAWBERRY BANANA SMOOTHIE

SERVES 1

1	8-ounce container nonfat plain yogurt
1	small banana
½	cup frozen strawberries
1	cup nonfat milk or soymilk
	Stevia (herbal sweetener) to taste (optional)

Combine all ingredients in a blender and blend until smooth.

NUTRITIONAL INFORMATION PER SERVING:
Calories: 270
Carbohydrates (g): 62
Protein (g): 22
Fat (g): 1
Calcium: 617

❀ ❀

HEART'S DESIRE MUFFINS

MAKES 1 DOZEN

1½	cups all-purpose flour
½	cup toasted wheat germ
¼	cup poppy seeds
⅓	cup sugar
1	tablespoon baking powder
½	teaspoon salt
1	cup buttermilk
1	egg
¼	cup (½ stick) unsalted butter, melted
¾	cup whatever jam wins your heart

Preheat the oven to 375°F. In a large bowl, combine the dry ingredients and set aside. In a small bowl, whisk together the buttermilk, egg, and melted butter until smooth. Add to large bowl and stir until just blended. Fill standard-size muffin cups less than halfway. Place a dab of jam in the center of each cup, and then add more batter until the cups are two-thirds full. Bake 15 to 20 minutes. Cool in a pan for 3 minutes before removing.

NUTRITIONAL INFORMATION PER SERVING (1 MUFFIN):
Calories: 210
Carbohydrates (g): 45
Protein (g): 2
Fat (g): 16
Calcium: 67

❁ ❁

CORN GRIDDLE CAKES WITH MAPLE YOGURT TOPPING

SERVES 4

Cakes

¾ cup cornmeal
½ cup all-purpose flour
½ cup whole wheat flour
1 teaspoon baking powder
2 tablespoons sugar
½ teaspoon salt
1¼ cups nonfat milk
¼ cup nonfat plain yogurt
2 tablespoons vegetable oil
4 egg whites

Combine the dry ingredients in a large bowl and set aside. In a small bowl, mix the milk, yogurt, and oil. Stir into the dry ingredients until just blended. In a cool stainless steel bowl, beat the egg whites to stiff peaks and fold into the batter. Cook on a hot griddle that has been sprayed with vegetable oil spray. Serve hot, with maple yogurt topping (see below).

NUTRITIONAL INFORMATION PER SERVING:
Calories: 289
Carbohydrates (g): 73
Protein (g): 17

Fat (g): 11
Calcium: 104

Topping:

  1 cup nonfat plain yogurt
  ¼ cup maple syrup

Combine and spoon over hot griddle cakes.

NUTRITIONAL INFORMATION PER SERVING:
Calories: 80
Carbohydrates (g): 17
Protein (g): 3
Fat (g): 0
Calcium: 100

❊ ❊

SALADS AND SIDE DISHES

❊ ❊

WAKAME CUCUMBER SALAD

SERVES 4

  1 large English cucumber (seedless)
  1 lemon, juiced
  ¼ teaspoon sea salt
  1 large red bell pepper
  ½ medium red onion
  6 strips wakame
  ¼ cup brown rice vinegar
  2 teaspoons sesame seeds

Cut the cucumber in half lengthwise and thinly slice. Cover with cold water with the lemon juice and salt added. Thinly slice the red pepper and onion into half-rounds. Bring about 1 quart of water to a boil and add the wakame. Remove from heat and let stand 5 minutes. Drain, then cut wakame into small pieces. Cool. Drain cucumbers. Toss vegetables with vinegar and sprinkle with sesame seeds.

NUTRITIONAL INFORMATION PER SERVING:

Calories: 63

Carbohydrates (g): 12

Protein (g): 3

Fat (g): 1

Calcium: 114

❈ ❈ ❈ ❈ ❈ ❈ ❈ ❈ ❈ ❈ ❈ ❈ ❈ ❈ ❈ ❈ ❈ ❈ ❈ ❈

GREENS AND GARLIC

SERVES 4

1 pound mixed greens (kale, collard, mustard, and turnip greens)

½ pound spinach

1 tablespoon olive oil

4 large garlic cloves, minced

Salt and freshly ground pepper to taste

2 tablespoons chopped and toasted walnuts or pine nuts (optional)

Wash the greens and spinach thoroughly, and remove tough stems. Place in a large pot, cover, and cook over high heat for 2 minutes (the water still on the leaves from washing them will provide enough moisture). Stir and continue cooking for 2 to 3 more minutes, or until just wilted. Drain and chop coarsely, pressing on the greens gently to remove excess liquid. Heat the olive oil in a skillet, add the garlic, and sauté over medium heat for 2 to 3 minutes. Add the greens and sauté until heated through. Season with salt and pepper. Transfer to a serving bowl and sprinkle with nuts, if desired.

NUTRITIONAL INFORMATION PER SERVING:

Calories: 113

Carbohydrates (g): 13

Protein (g): 4

Fat (g): 4

Calcium (mg): 209

❈ ❈ ❈ ❈ ❈ ❈ ❈ ❈ ❈ ❈ ❈ ❈ ❈ ❈ ❈ ❈ ❈ ❈ ❈ ❈

❀ ❀ ❀ ❀ ❀ ❀ ❀ ❀ ❀ ❀ ❀ ❀ ❀ ❀ ❀ ❀ ❀ ❀ ❀ ❀

AROMATIC YELLOW RICE

SERVES 4

2	cups basmati rice
2⅔	cups water
1	teaspoon salt
¾	teaspoon turmeric
4	whole cloves
1	1-inch stick cinnamon
3	bay leaves
¼	cup pistachios, chopped
¼	cup dried fruit, chopped (prunes, apricots, apples) or raisins or currants
1	tablespoon butter

Rinse the rice in cold water and drain. Combine all ingredients in a heavy pot with a tight-fitting lid. Bring to a boil, turn heat to low, and cook for 25 minutes. Remove from the heat and let stand, covered, for 10 minutes. Remove cloves, cinnamon stick, and bay leaves before serving.

NUTRITIONAL INFORMATION PER SERVING:
Calories: 338
Carbohydrates (g): 66
Protein (g): 6
Fat (g): 5
Calcium: 20

❀ ❀ ❀ ❀ ❀ ❀ ❀ ❀ ❀ ❀ ❀ ❀ ❀ ❀ ❀ ❀ ❀ ❀ ❀ ❀

CONFETTI SALAD

SERVES 4

1	beet, peeled
1	carrot, peeled
1	apple
1	cup pecans, toasted and chopped
½	cup dried coconut
1	tablespoon minced fresh ginger

2 tablespoons white wine vinegar
1 tablespoon canola oil

Grate the beet, carrot, and apple in a food processor, and transfer to a mixing bowl. Add the remaining ingredients and mix gently. Chill before serving.

NUTRITIONAL INFORMATION PER SERVING:
Calories: 134
Carbohydrates (g): 15
Protein (g): 1
Fat (g): 9
Calcium: 14

❀ ❀

HUMMUS

SERVES 4

1 15-ounce can chickpeas, rinsed and drained
2 garlic cloves
1 12-ounce box light soft tofu
3 tablespoons lemon juice
2 tablespoons tahini
1 tablespoon olive oil
1 tablespoon cayenne pepper

Combine the ingredients in a food processor and purée until very smooth. Let stand at room temperature for 30 minutes before serving. Can be stored in the refrigerator for 3 days.

NUTRITIONAL INFORMATION PER SERVING:
Calories: 290
Carbohydrates (g): 31
Protein (g): 15
Fat (g): 13
Calcium: 169

❀ ❀

❁ ❁

TZATZIKI

SERVES 8

  1 large cucumber, peeled and diced
  2 cups plain nonfat yogurt
  3 large garlic cloves, minced
  ¼ teaspoon dried dill or ½ teaspoon minced fresh
  ½ teaspoon minced fresh mint

Combine all the ingredients in a medium mixing bowl, and refrigerate for an hour before serving.

Note: This traditional Greek condiment is a wonderful accompaniment to poached and grilled fish, or salmon cakes.

NUTRITIONAL INFORMATION PER SERVING:

Calories: 37
Carbohydrates (g): 6
Protein (g): 3
Fat (g): 0
Calcium: 95

❁ ❁

DINNER

❁ ❁

KOREAN BEAN THREADS

SERVES 6

     10 garlic cloves, chopped
      4 tablespoons olive oil
     10 carrots, cut into matchsticks
      2 heads bok choy, coarsely chopped
      2 bunches scallions, cut into 1-inch lengths
  16–20 ounces firm tofu, drained, cubed, and marinated
         in 2 tablespoons tamari

4 ounces bean or rice threads, cut in half
2 tablespoons tamari

In a large skillet, sauté half of the garlic in the olive oil over medium heat. Add the carrots and bok choy and stir-fry for 5 minutes. Add the scallions and continue stir-frying until they are just tender. Add the tofu along with the rest of the garlic, cover, and remove from heat. Bring about 1 quart of water to a boil and add the bean threads. Remove from the heat and let stand for 5 minutes, or until noodles are soft. Drain and return to pan with the tamari, stirring until color is even. Gently stir the bean threads into the vegetables and serve immediately.

Note: If you don't have bean threads, this dish is good with brown rice, too.

NUTRITIONAL INFORMATION PER SERVING:
Calories: 358
Carbohydrates (g): 30
Protein (g): 22
Fat (g): 22
Calcium: 504

❁ ❁ ❁ ❁ ❁ ❁ ❁ ❁ ❁ ❁ ❁ ❁ ❁ ❁ ❁ ❁ ❁ ❁ ❁ ❁

POACHED FLOUNDER WITH CAPER SAUCE

SERVES 4

Fish
1 medium onion, peeled and halved
1 carrot, washed and halved
1 celery stalk
1 bay leaf
6 black peppercorns
1½ pounds flounder fillets (4 pieces of fish)

Sauce
3 tablespoons olive oil
⅓ cup finely chopped fresh parsley
3 tablespoons capers, rinsed and chopped
3 tablespoons dry sherry

 2 tablespoons fresh lemon juice
 1 tablespoon fine dry unseasoned bread crumbs

Place the vegetables and spices in a large sauté pan with 1 quart of water. Bring to a boil, lower the heat, and simmer for 20 minutes. With a slotted spoon, remove and discard vegetables, peppercorns, and bay leaf. Add the fish and simmer gently over low heat for 3 minutes. Remove from heat and let stand for 5 minutes, or until fish is done (opaque). Lift fillets from the pan with a slotted spoon, draining well. Arrange on a warm serving platter.

In a small saucepan, heat the oil over low heat. Add the remaining sauce ingredients and stir until the mixture has a sauce-like consistency. If too thick, add 1 tablespoon warm water. Spoon over poached fish fillets.

NUTRITIONAL INFORMATION PER SERVING:
Calories: 280
Carbohydrates (g): 8
Protein (g): 33
Fat (g): 12
Calcium: 56

❁ ❁ ❁ ❁ ❁ ❁ ❁ ❁ ❁ ❁ ❁ ❁ ❁ ❁ ❁ ❁ ❁ ❁ ❁ ❁

TOASTING NUTS AND SEEDS

Nuts and seeds are an excellent addition to a bone-healthy diet, since many are rich in calcium, phytoestrogens, and other important nutrients. Toasting them before you use them brings out their wonderful aroma and nutty flavor. Just heat a skillet over medium-high heat, add the nuts or seeds, and toss gently until they release their lovely scent, 2 to 3 minutes. For even less labor-intensive (if less fragrant) preparation, spread them in a single layer on an ungreased baking sheet, and place in the oven, or toaster oven, at 350°, until just slightly browned, about 5 minutes for most nuts, and just a minute or two for seeds.

❊ ❊

RED AND GREEN FRITTATA

SERVES 6

1½	tablespoons olive oil
3	bunches kale, thoroughly washed, stems removed, and chopped
4	garlic cloves, minced
½	teaspoon salt
	Black pepper to taste
2	roasted red bell peppers, seeded and diced
2	scallions, thinly sliced
⅓	cup grated Parmesan cheese
¾	cup crumbled feta cheese
2	teaspoons finely chopped rosemary
2	teaspoons fresh lemon juice
8	eggs, beaten

Preheat the oven to 325°F. Heat the olive oil in a large skillet. Wilt the kale (still damp from washing) over high heat with the garlic, salt, and pepper. Drain and cool. Squeeze out excess moisture. Place the kale in a bowl with the red peppers, scallions, both cheeses, rosemary, and lemon juice. Stir the eggs into the mixture and pour into a lightly oiled 9-inch square baking dish. Bake for 25 minutes, or until the eggs are set and the frittata is golden. Serve warm or at room temperature, cut into wedges.

NUTRITIONAL INFORMATION PER SERVING:
Calories: 267
Carbohydrates (g): 10
Protein (g): 16
Fat (g): 18
Calcium: 306

❊ ❊ ❊ ❊ ❊ ❊ ❊ ❊ ❊ ❊ ❊ ❊ ❊ ❊ ❊ ❊ ❊ ❊ ❊ ❊

❀ ❀

EAST TEXAS CHICKEN STEW

SERVES 4

- 2 teaspoons cumin seeds
- 1 tablespoon vegetable oil
- 4 skinless and boneless chicken breasts, cut into bite-size pieces
- 1 10.5-ounce can chicken stock
- 1 large yellow onion, chopped
- 1 teaspoon sugar
- 2 tablespoons all-purpose flour
- 1 tablespoon chili powder
- 2 garlic cloves, minced
- 4 cups cubed butternut squash (about 2 pounds)
- 2 cups water
- 1 15.5-ounce can yellow hominy, drained
- 1 green bell pepper, seeded and finely chopped
- ¼ cup minced fresh cilantro

Toast the cumin seeds in a large saucepan over medium heat for 1 minute. Remove from pan and set aside. Heat the oil in the saucepan over medium heat. Add the chicken and cook just until browned. Put a splash of chicken stock in the pan if it gets too dry. Add half the toasted cumin seeds, along with the onion and sugar. Sauté 5 minutes or until onion is tender. Stir in the flour, chili powder, and garlic and stir to combine. Add the squash, water, hominy, and remaining broth. Bring to a boil, reduce the heat, cover, and simmer 10 minutes. Uncover and simmer another 10 minutes, or until the squash is very tender and the stew thickens. Stir in remaining toasted cumin seeds and the green bell pepper. Garnish with cilantro.

NUTRITIONAL INFORMATION PER SERVING:
Calories: 443
Carbohydrates (g): 32
Protein (g): 57

Fat (g): 10
Calcium: 81

❀ ❀

STUFFED RED PEPPERS WITH CREAMY PECAN SAUCE

SERVES 4

4 tablespoons olive oil
1 large onion, chopped
4 garlic cloves, minced
1 6-ounce package fresh mushrooms, sliced
1 28-ounce can diced tomatoes, drained
3 cups cooked brown rice
4 large red bell peppers
1 15-ounce can vegetable juice or tomato sauce
   Pecan Sauce (recipe follows)

Preheat the oven to 325°. Heat the oil over medium heat. Add the onion and cook until just soft, then add the garlic and mushrooms. Cook, stirring occasionally, for 4 minutes. Add the tomatoes and simmer for 5 minutes. Add the rice and stir gently to combine. Cut each pepper in half lengthwise and remove the seeds. You may leave the stem attached if you like. Add the vegetable juice to a glass baking dish. Fill each pepper half with some rice mixture and place in the baking dish. Cover with foil and bake for 40 minutes. Serve the peppers with some sauce from the baking dish and a large dollop of Pecan Sauce.

NUTRITIONAL INFORMATION PER SERVING:
Calories: 410
Carbohydrates (g): 24
Protein (g): 64
Fat (g): 16
Calcium: 136

❀ ❀ ❀ ❀ ❀ ❀ ❀ ❀ ❀ ❀ ❀ ❀ ❀ ❀ ❀ ❀ ❀ ❀ ❀ ❀

❀ ❀ ❀ ❀ ❀ ❀ ❀ ❀ ❀ ❀ ❀ ❀ ❀ ❀ ❀ ❀ ❀ ❀ ❀ ❀

PECAN SAUCE

½ cup light sour cream
½ cup toasted pecans
8 ounces nonfat cream cheese
¼ cup nonfat milk
1 teaspoon ground cinnamon

Purée all the ingredients in a food processor or blender until smooth.

Note: This sauce is also wonderful over steamed vegetables. Use it over plain steamed broccoli for a delicious—and calcium-packed—side dish.

NUTRITIONAL INFORMATION PER SERVING:
Calories: 122
Carbohydrates (g): 10
Protein (g): 12
Fat (g): 4
Calcium: 92

❀ ❀ ❀ ❀ ❀ ❀ ❀ ❀ ❀ ❀ ❀ ❀ ❀ ❀ ❀ ❀ ❀ ❀ ❀

GETTING RID OF "GARLIC HANDS"

Here's a trick I learned in New Orleans, where they know a thing or two about garlic: to get the smell out of your hands after chopping fresh garlic, wash your hands, then rub them along the faucet. Don't dismiss this as some kind of voodoo until you try it: something about the metal reacts with the garlic juices and neutralizes them. Experienced cooks know soap and water alone is never enough to do the job.

❋ ❋

PASTA WITH ESCAROLE AND CHICKPEAS

SERVES 4

1 pound pasta (penne or rigatoni)
3 large garlic cloves, minced
1 medium yellow onion, chopped
1 tablespoon olive oil
1 14.5-ounce can diced tomatoes with juice
1 15-ounce can chickpeas, drained and rinsed
2 teaspoons dried basil, or 4 fresh leaves, sliced
2 heads escarole, washed and coarsely chopped
2 tablespoons grated Parmesan cheese

Prepare pasta according to package directions. Sauté the garlic and onion in the oil in a large skillet over medium heat until tender. Add the tomatoes, beans, and basil and mix. Place the escarole on top of this mixture. Cover the pan and increase the heat to high. Cook for about 5 minutes, or until escarole is limp. Drain the pasta, transfer to a serving platter, and top with sauce. Sprinkle with cheese and serve immediately.

NUTRITIONAL INFORMATION PER SERVING:
Calories: 220
Carbohydrates (g): 36
Protein (g): 9
Fat (g): 6
Calcium: 120

❋ ❋

❀ ❀

BULGUR, TOMATOES, AND CHICKPEAS

SERVES 4

2	tablespoons canola oil
1	large onion, chopped
1	14-ounce can diced tomatoes, drained
2	15-ounce can chickpeas, drained and rinsed
½	teaspoon salt
2	tablespoons minced fresh parsley
1	cup coarse bulgur wheat
1	cup water
	Freshly ground black pepper

Heat the oil over medium heat in a 3-quart heavy saucepan with a tight-fitting lid. Sauté the onion until tender, then add the tomatoes, chickpeas, salt, and parsley and simmer for 5 minutes. Stir in the bulgur wheat and water. Return to a simmer, cover, turn heat to low, and cook for 35 minutes. Add pepper to taste and serve.

NUTRITIONAL INFORMATION PER SERVING:
Calories: 165
Carbohydrates (g): 24
Protein (g): 4
Fat (g): 7
Calcium: 50

❀ ❀ ❀ ❀ ❀ ❀ ❀ ❀ ❀ ❀ ❀ ❀ ❀ ❀ ❀ ❀ ❀ ❀ ❀ ❀

CAN O' BEANS

Since most dried beans and legumes take so long to soak and cook, you can save a lot of time by using canned beans. Most are acceptable substitutes for cooking your own, though you'll sacrifice some texture. Check the labels to make sure you get beans canned without any added sugar. You'll see that a lot of salt is almost always used, which is one of the reasons to rinse canned beans thoroughly before adding them to a dish—you'll get rid of much of the salt. Draining them thoroughly, then rinsing them, also helps make them easier on your digestive system (they'll cause less gas), particularly if you are not used to using a lot of beans in your current diet.

❁ ❁ ❁ ❁ ❁ ❁ ❁ ❁ ❁ ❁ ❁ ❁ ❁ ❁ ❁ ❁ ❁ ❁ ❁

SALMON CAKES

SERVES 6

    1   small onion, finely chopped
    1   celery stalk, finely chopped
    1   tablespoon butter
    1   1-pound can salmon, drained and flaked (bones
        included)
    2   cups bread crumbs
    2   teaspoons dried dill
    2   teaspoons lemon pepper
    2   eggs

Preheat the oven to 325°F. Sauté the onion and celery in the butter over medium heat until just tender. In a medium mixing bowl, combine all of the ingredients and mix thoroughly. If mixture is too dry to hold its shape, add a little nonfat milk. Form into 6 patties and place on a nonstick baking sheet. Bake for 20 minutes.

NUTRITIONAL INFORMATION PER SERVING:
Calories: 158
Carbohydrates (g): 3
Protein (g): 18
Fat (g): 8
Calcium: 176

❀ ❀ ❀ ❀ ❀ ❀ ❀ ❀ ❀ ❀ ❀ ❀ ❀ ❀ ❀ ❀ ❀ ❀ ❀ ❀

TANDOORI-STYLE CHICKEN

SERVES 6

2½ pounds skinless chicken pieces (on the bone)
    Juice of 1 lemon
1 teaspoon salt
2 cups plain nonfat yogurt
1 small onion, peeled and quartered
2 garlic cloves, peeled
    1-inch piece fresh ginger, peeled
2 teaspoons garam masala

Rinse the chicken and pat dry. Rub the lemon juice and salt into each piece and place in a large (nonmetal) bowl. In a food processor or blender, combine the yogurt, onion, garlic, ginger, and garam masala and purée until smooth. Stir into the chicken. Cover and refrigerate. Let marinate 2 to 6 hours. Preheat the oven to 400°F. Arrange the chicken on a baking sheet and bake for 25 minutes. (Discard remaining marinade.)

NUTRITIONAL INFORMATION PER SERVING:
Calories: 238
Carbohydrates (g): 8
Protein (g): 40
Fat (g): 4
Calcium: 140

❀ ❀ ❀ ❀ ❀ ❀ ❀ ❀ ❀ ❀ ❀ ❀ ❀ ❀ ❀ ❀ ❀ ❀ ❀ ❀

❀ ❀ ❀ ❀ ❀ ❀ ❀ ❀ ❀ ❀ ❀ ❀ ❀ ❀ ❀ ❀ ❀ ❀ ❀ ❀

BLACK-EYED PEAS AND SMOKED FISH SALAD

SERVES 4

    1 cup frozen or canned artichoke hearts (*not* packed
       in oil)
    2 15-ounce cans black-eyed peas, drained
    1 medium red onion, diced
    ¼ cup red wine vinegar
   1½ tablespoons olive oil
    1 tablespoon chicken or vegetable stock
    1 teaspoon whole-grain mustard
    6 ounces smoked fish, such as salmon or tuna, flaked
    2 bunches arugula, washed, dried, and stemmed
       Freshly ground black pepper

Quarter the artichoke hearts and combine them in a large bowl
with the black-eyed peas and onion. In a small bowl, whisk together the vinegar, oil, stock, and mustard. Pour over the black-
eyed peas and toss to mix. Gently stir in the fish. Place the arugula
on a serving platter and mound the salad on top. Grind black pepper over the top to taste.

NUTRITIONAL INFORMATION PER SERVING:
Calories: 223
Carbohydrates (g): 27
Protein (g): 17
Fat (g): 8
Calcium: 116

❀ ❀ ❀ ❀ ❀ ❀ ❀ ❀ ❀ ❀ ❀ ❀ ❀ ❀ ❀ ❀ ❀ ❀ ❀ ❀

DESERT

❋ ❋

HONEY NUT FROZEN YOGURT

SERVES 4

1 cup hazelnuts
16 ounces plain nonfat yogurt
½ cup honey
2 tablespoons Frangelico, or hazelnut liqueur

Toast the hazelnuts in a dry skillet until fragrant, then coarsely chop. Mix all ingredients in a large bowl. Transfer to an 8 × 8-inch pan and freeze until set, then cut into squares to serve. Or, process in an ice cream maker, according to product instructions.

Note: Use your imagination on this one. Substitute any flavor yogurt or liqueur, and/or replace nuts with a cup of blended frozen berries. (You may want to reduce the amount of honey accordingly if you use presweetened yogurt or add fruit.) Have fun with this dessert!

NUTRITIONAL INFORMATION PER SERVING:
Calories: 293
Carbohydrates (g): 52
Protein (g): 8
Fat (g): 7
Calcium: 196

❋ ❋

RICE AND COCONUT MILK PUDDING

SERVES 6

1 cup white basmati rice
2 cups water
  Salt
3 cups vanilla fortified soymilk
  2-inch piece of cinnamon stick
¼ cup sugar
14 ounces light coconut milk
8 unsalted pistachio nuts, chopped

Rinse the rice, then combine with the water in a saucepan with a tight-fitting lid. Add a pinch or two of salt, the soymilk, cinnamon, and sugar. Bring to a boil, lower the heat, and simmer slowly, stirring occasionally, for 45 minutes. Stir in the coconut milk and let the mixture cool. Serve warm or chilled, garnished with pistachios.

NUTRITIONAL INFORMATION PER SERVING:
Calories: 122
Carbohydrates (g): 20
Protein (g): 4
Fat (g): 4
Calcium: 10

❁ ❁

Once you've cooked these dishes a few times, tinker with the ingredients to create your own favorite variations. A bit of creativity in the kitchen is the best way to keep yourself interested in making and eating food that is good for your bones—and you. Use your imagination. Consider what you have on hand. No kale? Try another leafy green or broccoli. Bought a pound of mushrooms that will go bad in a couple days if you don't use them up? Sauté them and add them to the chicken stew or the bulgur with tomatoes and chickpeas. Want to add more phytoestrogens to your diet? Purée tofu to add to your creamy pecan sauce, or crumble it into your scrambled eggs (or use it instead of the eggs) for breakfast burritos, or dice it and add it to sautéed greens and garlic to boost it into a main dish. Or add flaxseed, whole or ground, to your muffins. Can't stand the sight of red peppers? Stuff zucchini "boats" instead. Now that you're familiar with the best sources of calcium, you'll be able to keep your intake up without being chained to the particular foods provided in these menus and recipes. Your bones and your waistline will show improvements—and your taste buds will thank you.

Chapter 14

The Bone Density Diet

Now that I've bombarded you with so many "musts" for good nutrition and good health, it is only fair I show you how to put it all together. This "diet" is low in saturated fat, high in fiber, rich in calcium, and moderate in calories. It also includes a number of foods with phytoestrogens. This is not a get-thin-quick plan, but it will allow you to attain and maintain a healthy weight if you combine it with an exercise plan along the lines of what is described in next week's section. Whatever your current and ideal weight, what eating this way will definitely do for you is help you build healthy bones. (Just as with weight loss, diet and exercise must go hand-in-hand to reach that goal.) There are twenty-one menus here, designed to get you through three weeks—long enough to cement the habit of eating this way—but this week's action plan will start you out gradually. This chapter is just to introduce the diet, and let you plan your meals and stock up on what you need to spend the last three weeks of this program actually on the diet.

The menus were designed with the help of Abby Greenspun, a registered dietitian for a leading national center for the study of bone health. They are meant to get you started eating this way for a lifetime. For simplicity's sake—eliminating the amount of thinking you have to do about just which foods to eat to get the right

amount of calcium and everything else—I recommend following this reasonably closely for the first three weeks. But there is
nothing magical about the order of the menus listed or about the
combinations of foods. If you don't like the sound of one of the
recipes, or don't want to learn to cook something new on a particular day, just skip it and choose another meal. If you don't have the
makings of one of the meals, try it later, after you've been to the grocery store, or when the coffee shop near your office offers a good
approximation. You can mix and match breakfasts, lunches, dinners, and snacks however you'd like. The calorie counts for each
meal and snack are roughly equivalent, so while you won't hit the
exact numbers given at the bottom of each day's menus if you switch
meals around, you'll still be in the ballpark. (If swapping meals and
recipes seems easier than restocking the fridge or preparing new
dishes, by all means do it your way right from the start.)

FUN WITH COMPUTERS

Check out "The Kitchen Counter" online, where you can
create your own menus and get an instant tally of the
calories, protein, fat, carbs, cholesterol, sodium, and
calcium in your food. Go to *http://homearts.com/helpers/
calculators/caldocf1.htm*, or try typing "Kitchen Counter"
into your favorite search engine.

By the end of three weeks, you'll have a feel for what goes into
a balanced, nutritious diet, and you'll be able to choose wisely on
your own. There's enough variety here that at the end of three
weeks you could just start the cycle over again without getting
bored. But better you should ultimately take what you like best
from these meals and add some of your personal favorites, to create an individual, ever-changing mix for you and your family.

These meal plans give you three meals a day, along with a
total count of the calories, fat grams, cholesterol, protein, complex carbohydrates, simple carbohydrates (sugars), fiber, and
calcium content. Meals marked with an asterisk have recipes included in the previous chapter. At the end of the chapter, you'll

find a list of calcium-rich snacks, *and you should include one or two of these each day to meet your calcium requirements.* Check the day's calcium totals against your own requirements, and pick up any slack as necessary with the snacks. You should never go hungry on this plan. Eating enough (without eating too much) is important to maintaining a healthy metabolism. Cutting your calories too low ultimately slows your metabolism, undercutting any attempt to burn off more calories and fat.

As you look over these menus, you'll see that specific portion sizes are usually given. If you like the sense of control that gives you, by all means use the information. It will allow you to keep careful track of the calories—along with the levels of other nutrients—you're taking in, which can be useful if you are trying to control your weight. But the foods included here are all healthy ones, so don't feel restricted in how much you can eat. If half a cup of quinoa doesn't satisfy, eat a cup. If the lunch menu doesn't fill you up, add carrot sticks and salsa, or bean salad, or a handful of nuts. In any event, there's no need to weigh or measure your portions constantly. Learn to estimate. As long as what you're eating is good for you, how much you eat, precisely, isn't critical. (Don't take that as a license to subsist on cheese alone. It's good for you, but not in unlimited amounts or to the exclusion of other things. Everything in moderation.) The one exception is with meat. You may want to measure your portions a few times—or just pay attention to how much is in a package and how many servings it yields—since we all tend to eat much larger servings, as a matter of habit, than are good for our bones.

The specific foods in these menus come in at around 1,200 calories a day, which is less than you should be eating. They are designed that way so that you can see it is possible to get all the nutrients you need that way. *Adding in one or two snacks will take you up to 1,500 calories or so, a more reasonable number.* So the only "optional" part of those snacks is opting for which ones you like. *But don't opt out of snacking all together—or not only won't you be getting all the calcium you should but you'll also be slowing your metabolism and interfering with your ability to maintain a reasonable weight* on a reasonable number of calories.

You can eat your snacks anytime you are in the mood for them—between lunch and dinner, or breakfast and lunch, or after dinner. You can also spread out foods from your other meals, if you like. Save your breakfast fruit for a midmorning snack, for example, then add calcium-rich snacks in the late afternoon and the evening.

The menus here provide you with the nutrition you need for healthy bones (though you should still consider supplements as insurance), and are easy to prepare and tasty to eat. They offer a variety of foods, all of which are healthy choices, so it is infinitely flexible within the guidelines we've set up in this book. I wanted to show you *examples* of bone-healthy menus to get you started on a new way of eating. But the idea is for you to decide what you like, and use that as an equally important guide to what you eat. If you are going to do this over the long haul (and as far as your bones are concerned, there's little point to doing it any other way), you're going to have to do it so you enjoy it.

If you dislike any of the foods included here, make a reasonable substitution. But keep an open mind. Mustard greens may not sound exciting to you, but don't dismiss them if you've never had them—or never had them deliciously prepared. Tempeh may look strange in the package, but don't knock it till you've tried it. The final rule of this diet is to enjoy what you eat.

We spend a lot of our lives preparing and consuming food, and in addition to fueling the machine, we should also find sensual pleasure in the experience, along with (healthy) psychological sustenance. Leaning on food as a cover for other, unaddressed feelings is one road to ruin. But delicious, beautiful food is a delight, and food can build and cement bridges between people (feasting together, sharing traditional foods, toasting with a nice glass of wine before a meal, joining hands in a blessing before eating, or even just two straws in one ice cream soda). There's a wonderful bounty of foods available to us, so indulge in the healthy ones you love. Not only will you feel better, but you'll actually be getting better nutrition. Research shows that when you like a meal, you absorb many more of the nutrients in it.

Though the recipes and menus are presented here, right now I want you to just familiarize yourself with them. Use this week to make some gradual changes, as outlined in the Action Plan. Then go on in the final three weeks of the program to follow the specific diet. Especially if your diet is in for a major overhaul rather than a tune-up, you don't want to make radical changes all at once. If changing your diet seems too hard, or scary, or strange, it will be that much harder to stick with. Since the goal here is not to drop 5 pounds in time for your high school reunion, or whatever other unrealistic dream so many of us embark on diets for, you have time to ease into this. Get it right, so it will last. You have the rest of your life to benefit.

General Guidelines: Make oatmeal with milk instead of water to increase the calcium content. When choosing a cold cereal, look for ones with at least 5 grams of fiber per serving (e.g., Total, Raisin Bran, and a lot of cereals found in health food stores). Most cereals are low in calories and fat (except for regular granola).

All breakfasts and lunches should include a fruit. It can be any fresh fruit or canned in its own juice. The best choice is whatever is in season. Aside from fruit canned in syrup, there is no bad fruit choice. The fruits that are on these menus are just suggestions. Eat what you like, what's in season, what you have on hand, what the cafeteria has out. Calcium-fortified orange or grapefruit juice are good choices, but don't get all your fruit in juice (unless you're using a modern juicer), as it lacks fiber and has concentrated levels of sugar.

All dinners should include a large mixed green salad with a variety of vegetables and 1 tablespoon of low-fat dressing.

Fresh, organic vegetables are best, but if it's easier to use canned or frozen veggies, they are a good second choice. Look for low-sodium canned veggies and plain frozen ones (not in sauces). Again, the choices included on these menus are just suggestions. Eat what you like, include dark green and orange vegetables frequently, and be sure to get a variety over time.

How to Make the Most of a Salad: Choose dark lettuces and include a variety of vegetables to keep it interesting as well as to maximize the nutrients you're getting. Sprinkle every salad with about 2 teaspoons of sesame seeds, poppy seeds, or flaxseeds (whole or ground) to add some calcium and/or phytoestrogens.

FIRST WEEK

Don't forget to add 2 snacks and a salad *every* day.

Menu 1

BREAKFAST

1 cup oatmeal made with ½ cup nonfat or reduced-fat enriched soymilk, ¼ cup chopped figs, and 1 teaspoon honey

6 ounces calcium-fortified orange juice

LUNCH

2-egg omelet with ¼ cup each mushrooms and spinach and 1 ounce diced mozzarella cheese (cooked with vegetable cooking spray)

1 cup cantaloupe cubes

DINNER

Poached Flounder with Caper Sauce*

½ cup wild rice with 2 tablespoons chopped toasted pecans

½ cup steamed brussels sprouts

Large mixed greens/vegetable salad

NOTE:

* means that there is a recipe for this dish in Chapter 13.

NUTRITIONAL INFORMATION FOR THIS MENU:
Calories: 1,150
Carbohydrates (g): 110

Protein (g): 70
Fat (g): 35
Calcium (mg): 840

Menu 2

BREAKFAST
---

1 cup raisin bran cereal with ½ cup nonfat milk or soymilk
1 cup strawberries

LUNCH

English muffin pizza with ½ cup veggies of your choice
and 2 slices low-fat mozzarella cheese (2 ounces)
Fresh fruit

DINNER

East Texas Chicken Stew*
Large mixed greens/vegetable salad

NUTRITIONAL INFORMATION FOR THIS MENU:
Calories: 1,110
Carbohydrates (g): 135
Protein (g): 88
Fat (g): 25
Calcium (mg): 810

Menu 3

BREAKFAST
---

1 Heart's Desire Muffin*
1 cup nonfat milk
1 banana

LUNCH

Large salad with 1 cup romaine lettuce and ¼ cup each
carrots, cucumber, red pepper, and mushrooms (or any
other veggie that you like) topped with 3 ounces sardines
(with bones) and 2 tablespoons low-fat salad dressing
Fruit

DINNER

Eggplant Parmesan

1   cup whole wheat spaghetti with ¼ cup marinara sauce
Large mixed greens/vegetable salad

NUTRITIONAL INFORMATION FOR THIS MENU:
Calories: 1,240
Carbohydrates (g): 190
Protein (g): 60
Fat (g): 35
Calcium (mg): 1,200

Menu 4

BREAKFAST

Strawberry Banana Smoothie*
Whole wheat English muffin with 1 teaspoon margarine
or butter

LUNCH

1½   cups mixed bean soup
Whole-grain roll
Fruit

DINNER

Tandoori-Style Chicken*
½   cup rice pilaf
1   cup steamed green beans
Large mixed greens/vegetable salad

NUTRITIONAL INFORMATION FOR THIS MENU:
Calories: 1,310
Carbohydrates (g): 200
Protein (g): 100
Fat (g): 15
Calcium (mg): 1,140

Menu 5

BREAKFAST

> 2 whole-grain waffles with ½ cup Maple Yogurt Topping*
> 6 ounces calcium-fortified orange juice

LUNCH

> Red and Green Frittata*
> Fruit

DINNER

> Stir-fried tofu and vegetables (4 ounces firm tofu, ½ cup
> each broccoli, bok choy, mushrooms, and carrots,
> cooked with 1 teaspoon canola oil)
> 1 cup Aromatic Yellow Rice*
> Large mixed greens/vegetable salad

NUTRITIONAL INFORMATION FOR THIS MENU:
Calories: 1,270
Carbohydrates (g): 190
Protein (g): 55
Fat (g): 45
Calcium (mg): 1,200

Menu 6

BREAKFAST

> 1 cup oatmeal made with ¾ cup nonfat milk
> ½ cup applesauce spiced with cinnamon

LUNCH

> 1 veggie/soy burger on a hamburger bun with lettuce and
> tomato
> Tangerine

DINNER

> 2 cups Pasta with Escarole and Chickpeas*
> Large mixed greens/vegetable salad

NUTRITIONAL INFORMATION FOR THIS MENU:
Calories: 1,160
Carbohydrates (g): 195
Protein (g): 55
Fat (g): 15
Calcium (mg): 520

Menu 7

BREAKFAST

> 1 cup raisin bran cereal with ½ cup nonfat or soymilk
> 1 banana

LUNCH

> 2 cups mixed greens with carrots, cucumber, and tomato
> topped with ½ cup each black-eyed peas and chickpeas
> Whole-grain roll
> Fruit

DINNER

> 4 ounces broiled flounder filet
> Wakame Cucumber Salad*
> Baked potato topped with ¼ cup plain yogurt and
> chives
> Large mixed greens/vegetable salad

NUTRITIONAL INFORMATION FOR THIS MENU:
Calories: 1,130
Carbohydrates (g): 200
Protein (g): 75
Fat (g): 15
Calcium (mg): 860

SECOND WEEK

Menu 8

BREAKFAST

---

  1 Heart's Desire Muffin*
  1 cup nonfat milk
     Fruit

LUNCH

---

  1 cup vegetable soup sprinkled with 1 tablespoon grated
     Parmesan cheese
  3 ounces lean roast beef on whole wheat bread with
     lettuce and tomato
     Fresh fruit salad

DINNER

     Stuffed Red Peppers with Creamy Pecan Sauce*
     Large mixed greens/vegetable salad

     NUTRITIONAL INFORMATION FOR THIS MENU:
     Calories: 1,100
     Carbohydrates (g): 150
     Protein (g): 90
     Fat (g): 35
     Calcium (mg): 720

Menu 9

BREAKFAST

---

  1 cup oatmeal with 2 tablespoons chopped dried apricots
     and ½ cup nonfat milk or soymilk
  ½ cup calcium-fortified orange juice

LUNCH

     Anytime Breakfast Burrito*
     Fresh fruit

DINNER

Stir-fried shrimp and vegetables (6 medium shrimp and ½ cup each broccoli, bok choy, carrots, zucchini)

1 cup brown rice

Large mixed greens/vegetable salad

NUTRITIONAL INFORMATION FOR THIS MENU:

Calories: 1,060

Carbohydrates (g): 185

Protein (g): 60

Fat (g): 25

Calcium (mg): 850

Menu 10

BREAKFAST

Corn Griddle Cakes with Maple Yogurt Topping*

Apple

LUNCH

Whole wheat pita with ½ cup Hummus,* cucumber, roasted red pepper

Banana

DINNER

2 cups spaghetti with 3 ounces chicken breast and ½ cup broccoli in ½ cup marinara sauce

Large mixed greens/vegetable salad

NUTRITIONAL INFORMATION FOR THIS MENU:

Calories: 1,710

Carbohydrates (g): 300

Protein (g): 90

Fat (g): 30

Calcium (mg): 570

Menu 11
BREAKFAST

Strawberry Banana Smoothie*

2 slices whole-grain toast with 1 teaspoon margarine or butter

LUNCH

Large chopped salad with 1 cup romaine lettuce and ¼ cup each of cucumber, carrots, tomato (or any vegetables you like), and 3 ounces canned salmon

1 small sourdough roll

Orange

DINNER

4 ounces grilled chicken breast

Baked sweet potato

1 cup sautéed spinach and mushrooms (cooked in 1 teaspoon olive oil)

Large mixed greens/vegetable salad

NUTRITIONAL INFORMATION FOR THIS MENU:
Calories: 1,110
Carbohydrates (g): 170
Protein (g): 80
Fat (g): 20
Calcium (mg): 1,020

Menu 12
BREAKFAST

2 slices whole wheat toast with 1 ounce Swiss cheese

½ grapefruit

LUNCH

Black-Eyed Peas and Smoked Fish Salad*

Fruit

DINNER

3–4 ounces broiled beef tenderloin
Baked potato with ¼ cup plain yogurt
1 cup sautéed kale (cooked with 1 teaspoon olive oil)
Large mixed greens/vegetable salad

NUTRITIONAL INFORMATION FOR THIS MENU:
Calories: 1,090
Carbohydrates (g): 140
Protein (g): 70
Fat (g): 35
Calcium (mg): 650

Menu 13

BREAKFAST

1 cup plain yogurt with 2 tablespoons wheat germ and
1 teaspoon honey
1 cup mixed fruit salad

LUNCH

Turkey (3 ounces) and cheese (1 ounce) sandwich on
pumpernickel bread with lettuce, tomato, and mustard
Fruit

DINNER

Salmon Cakes*
½ cup quinoa
1 cup sautéed zucchini (cooked with 1 teaspoon olive oil)
Large mixed greens/vegetable salad

NUTRITIONAL INFORMATION FOR THIS MENU:
Calories: 1,170
Carbohydrates (g): 130
Protein (g): 85
Fat (g): 35
Calcium (mg): 1,100

Menu 14

BREAKFAST

Sesame bagel (whole wheat sesame even better) with
2 slices (2 ounces) low-fat mozzarella cheese
1 banana

LUNCH

Bulgur, Tomatoes, and Chickpeas*
Fresh fruit

DINNER

4 ounces broiled snapper
1 cup couscous
Greens and Garlic*
Large mixed greens/vegetable salad

NUTRITIONAL INFORMATION FOR THIS MENU:
Calories: 1,080
Carbohydrates (g): 150
Protein (g): 60
Fat (g): 25
Calcium (mg): 730

THIRD WEEK

Menu 15

BREAKFAST

Strawberry Banana Smoothie*
English muffin with 1 tablespoon jam

LUNCH

3 ounces turkey and 1 ounce provolone cheese sandwich
with honey mustard, lettuce, and roasted red pepper on
whole wheat bread
Fresh fruit

DINNER

2 cups three-bean chili
1 cup amaranth
Large mixed greens/vegetable salad

NUTRITIONAL INFORMATION FOR THIS MENU:
Calories: 1,300
Carbohydrates (g): 170
Protein (g): 75
Fat (g): 25
Calcium (mg): 1,510

Menu 16
BREAKFAST

Buckwheat pancakes with ¼ cup Maple Yogurt Topping*
6 ounces calcium-fortified orange juice

LUNCH

2-egg omelet with broccoli, mushrooms, and mozzarella
(1 ounce)
Oven fries (1 cut potato, sprayed with cooking spray
and seasoned with paprika, salt, pepper, and baked)
Fresh fruit

DINNER

2 cups cheese ravioli primavera with ½ cup marinara sauce
Large mixed greens/vegetable salad

NUTRITIONAL INFORMATION FOR THIS MENU:
Calories: 1,420
Carbohydrates (g): 215
Protein (g): 56
Fat (g): 43
Calcium (mg): 1,150

Menu 17

BREAKFAST

---

  1 cup plain yogurt with 2 tablespoons wheat germ and 1
teaspoon honey

1½ cups strawberries

LUNCH

Tuna salad (with low-fat mayo, shredded carrots, and
parsley) rollup (in a whole wheat tortilla)

Fresh fruit

DINNER

Korean Bean Threads*

  1 cup brown rice

Large mixed greens/vegetable salad

NUTRITIONAL INFORMATION FOR THIS MENU:

Calories: 1,180

Carbohydrates (g): 160

Protein (g): 70

Fat (g): 35

Calcium (mg): 1,020

Menu 18

BREAKFAST

---

  1 cup oatmeal made with ¾ cup nonfat or soymilk with
1 tablespoon chopped hazelnuts and 1 teaspoon
brown sugar

  6 ounces calcium-fortified orange juice

LUNCH

Bulgur, Tomatoes, and Chickpeas*

Fresh fruit

DINNER

4 ounces turkey burger with lettuce and tomato on a whole wheat bun
Baked sweet potato
Greens and Garlic*
Large mixed greens/vegetable salad

NUTRITIONAL INFORMATION FOR THIS MENU:
Calories: 1,210
Carbohydrates (g): 175
Protein (g): 50
Fat (g): 35
Calcium (mg): 990

Menu 19

BREAKFAST

1 Heart's Desire Muffin*
1 cup nonfat milk
1 cup mixed berries

LUNCH

1 cup gazpacho
Parmesan pita chips (1 whole wheat pita, sprinkled with 2 tablespoons Parmesan cheese and garlic, sprayed with cooking spray, cut into wedges, and toasted in the oven)
Fruit

DINNER

3 ounces lamb chop
Wakame Cucumber Salad*
1 cup basmati rice
Large mixed greens/vegetable salad

NUTRITIONAL INFORMATION FOR THIS MENU:
Calories: 1,060
Carbohydrates (g): 150

Protein (g): 55
Fat (g): 35
Calcium (mg): 760

Menu 20

BREAKFAST

Poppyseed bagel with 1 slice of low-fat cheese
6 ounces calcium-fortified orange juice

LUNCH

Whole wheat pita with ½ cup hummus, cucumber, and red pepper
Fresh fruit salad

DINNER

4 ounces poached salmon with ¼ cup Tzatziki*
1 cup rice pilaf
1 cup sautéed snow peas
Large mixed greens/vegetable salad

NUTRITIONAL INFORMATION FOR THIS MENU:
Calories: 1,260
Carbohydrates (g): 195
Protein (g): 65
Fat (g): 30
Calcium (mg): 850

Menu 21

BREAKFAST

Buckwheat pancakes with 2 tablespoons chopped pecans
1 cup blueberries
1 cup nonfat milk

LUNCH

>Red and Green Frittata*
>
>Fresh fruit

DINNER

>East Texas Chicken Stew*
>
>Large mixed greens/vegetable salad

NUTRITIONAL INFORMATION FOR THIS MENU:
Calories: 1,270
Carbohydrates (g): 125
Protein (g): 85
Fat (g): 40
Calcium (mg): 790

CALCIUM-RICH SNACKS

You need one or two snacks each day to give you enough calories to keep your metabolism running in high gear. To do the best by your bones, choose calcium-rich snacks like these, all of which have roughly 200 calories or less:

- *1 cup plain yogurt with 2 teaspoons honey, ½ cup cut-up fruit, 2 teaspoons maple syrup, 2 teaspoons molasses, 2 tablespoons wheat germ, or 2 teaspoons chocolate syrup*
- *½ cup hummus with 1 small whole wheat pita*
- *½ cup ricotta cheese sprinkled with cinnamon on a rice cake or graham cracker*
- *½ cup pudding made with nonfat milk*
- *1 cup of three-bean salad (black-eyed peas, chickpeas, and green beans)*
- *½ cup dried figs, apricots, prunes, pecans, or hazelnuts*
- *Baked apple with ½ cup yogurt topping*
- *½ cup plain yogurt mixed with salad dressing packet and raw veggies*
- *½ cup Tzatziki* with raw veggies or pita bread*
- *Rice and Coconut Milk Pudding**
- *Honey Nut Frozen Yogurt**

❁ ❁ ❁ ❁ ❁ ❁ ❁ ❁ ❁ ❁ ❁ ❁ ❁ ❁ ❁ ❁ ❁ ❁ ❁ ❁

WEEK 3 ACTION PLAN

1. Consider this week a warm-up period. Following the diet laid out in this chapter for the final three weeks of the Bone Density program will be enough to cement mostly good habits. For now, use this week to work on your biggest problem area. If you're a confirmed meat-and-potatoes type, try eating a vegetarian lunch each day. If you're a pasta junkie, go some days without and switch to smaller portions of whole wheat for a couple of meals. If you're living on fast food and other junk foods, throw out nonnutritious foods in your cupboards and commit to preparing a few healthy meals for yourself (or at least carefully selecting some take-out you know is healthful).

2. At the same time, add in a few foods that are good for you. Get at least one good calcium food each day and a serving of either soy or fish. Eat beans at least three times.

3. Clean house. Get rid of all the soda (except seltzer), and then limit it to special occasions. Rid your cupboards of junk foods with no nutrient value. Clear out your coffee supplies if having it in the house will tempt you to overindulge. Don't keep wine and beer in the fridge.

4. Now go shopping. Stock up on what you need for healthful meals and snacks, including all the nonperishables called for in the menus and recipes of the Bone Density Diet and high-calcium snacks.

5. From the Bone Density recipes, pick three new dishes to try this week, and add everything you'll need to have on hand to your shopping list.

6. Include a variety of soy products in your shopping cart, and experiment with a few

---

WEEK 3 FOCUS

- Introduce more soy into your regular diet.
- Prepare to follow the Bone Density Diet.
- Address any digestive complaints you have.

you haven't used before. Start with tofu if you are a rank beginner, as that offers the most possibilities. Or, if tofu is old hat, try tempeh or branch out to a different brand of soy burger or dog, or get some roasted soy nuts or some frozen soybean pods to boil up and snack on. Try something new this week, like tofu dip or soymilk smoothie or TVP chili, that you've never prepared before.

7. Buy a sampler of unfamiliar items that are good for your bones, like a sea vegetable or other leafy green you've never tried, or mineral water with a lot of calcium, or a can of salmon, or quinoa or another whole grain.

8. Make it easy to eat well and healthy. Make your kitchen, including your pantry, seasonings, and pots and pans, well stocked, organized, and easy to get at—and thus easy to use.

9. If you have any chronic digestive issues and use over-the-counter products with any regularity, investigate gentler, natural alternatives and turn your focus to getting to the root of the problem rather than managing symptoms.

10. If you have digestive complaints, look for patterns in your symptoms to see if you can pinpoint any foods that "disagree" with you. Avoid them all week and notice if you feel any improvement.

11. Do you have any of the signs of low stomach acid? If you decided it is right for you, try digestive enzyme supplements.

12. If probiotics sound right for you, experiment to find the supplements best for you.

13. Which of the Bone Density recipes do *not* sound appealing to you? What creative ingredient substitutions could make them more to your liking?

14. Go through your family's favorite dishes, picking out the ones that are bone healthy, and working out modifications to make others good choices for your bones.

15. Check your favorite cookbooks for some new recipes that are good for your bones, and test them out.

16. Talk to your family and friends about the changes you're making in the way you eat. This way of eating is healthy

for everyone, and should have enough variety to please every palate. Sharing what you've learned with those who express interest will encourage others to look after their own health as well. Ask for support in your new healthy habits—and be specific about what you would find helpful. (Don't make the people who love you guess!)

17. Schedule at least one full-family meal each week, starting this week, with everyone contributing to menu planning, preparation, and cleanup.

18. Share a meal with someone (or someones) you love—and don't say one word about weight or illness or nutrition. Let this meal—no matter what it is composed of—nourish your soul by giving you a brief respite from your day and a way of bonding with another human being.

19. Looking forward to starting on the full-scale diet next week, make any necessary revisions to the first seven menus to fit your individual needs. If you don't like a particular food, plan a reasonable substitution. If you cook only on weekends, and live on leftovers and takeout the rest of the week, arrange the order of the meals accordingly. Don't give yourself any excuses to fall off the train just as it is leaving the station!

20. Make a shopping list of everything you'll need for the first week's menus—and go get it.

❈ ❈ ❈ ❈ ❈ ❈ ❈ ❈ ❈ ❈ ❈ ❈ ❈ ❈ ❈ ❈ ❈ ❈ ❈

CREATE AN EXERCISE PLAN

The Bone Density Diet is only half the battle. As you've seen, good nutrition must be paired with regular exercise to make and keep your bones healthy. The first chapter in this section focuses on the various kinds of exercise you need for general good health, and which kinds are particularly important for your bones—and some of the surprising reasons why. This week you'll learn a strength-training workout and a yoga workout to help get you started. There are almost infinite variations you could learn within these two areas and many, many more kinds of exercise you would benefit from. These workouts are just two examples. They are not the *only* things that work. But they *do* work—if you work at them. This week's Action Plan will help you sort through your options to customize a plan that fits your life.

Chapter 15

Move It or Lose It

Exercise makes you healthier. It makes you look better. It makes you feel better. It makes you feel happier. It builds your bones. As they say at the sneaker shop, just do it.

But just in case you're among those *not* doing it, let me try to inspire you to get up and get moving. (You can read this book just as well on your exercise bike as you can lying on the couch. But if you feel you have to choose one or the other, by all means put this down right now.) Exercising lowers the risk of heart disease, stroke, Type II diabetes, and arthritis, and is an effective treatment or, even better, prevention for those conditions. It counters high blood pressure, depression, constipation, high cholesterol, back pain, poor circulation, anxiety, insomnia, and menopausal symptoms. It is crucial for losing weight and for maintaining a healthy weight, and doing so without losing muscle. It is a boon to the immune system, generally. It reduces stress. Exercise cuts the death rate at any age, and lessens the risk of disability.

People who exercise have higher bone density than those who don't. Women with more muscle strength also have stronger bones. Exercisers are less likely to fall, given their superior balance, coordination, reaction times, flexibility, and strength, and so are much less likely to break anything regardless of their bone

> ### YEARS IN YOUR LIFE *AND* LIFE IN YOUR YEARS
>
> *Regular exercise adds up to two years to your life* and improves the quality of your life no matter how long it is, not to mention decreasing the rate of osteoporosis and fractures, including hip fractures.

density. Exercise develops bones and muscles directly, and also triggers the release of hormones that do the same thing. Getting exercise throughout childhood and young adulthood allows you to reach your maximum potential bone density, then delays and slows the rate of bone loss once your body is no longer building up bone faster than it tears it down. Studies have shown that just three hours of moderate activity (including, say, gardening and going dancing, not just time on the treadmill or trips to the gym) per week is enough to prevent bone loss after menopause, and even build bone mass in some women—though the more you do, the more your bones benefit. Another study showed that just 20 minutes of aerobic activity every other day built bone. Exercise also improves bone quality, along with density.

Studies suggest that calcium helps build your bones *only* if you are also exercising properly (and exercise may only help if you are also getting sufficient calcium). Exercising three times a week built bone density over 6 percent in under two years in one study (compared to bone *loss* in sedentary women). That's about what many people get from the best drug treatments, and, unlike prescriptions, just about all the side effects of exercising are positive. Getting regular exercise, in combination with getting enough calcium and vitamin D, can cut your fracture risk 30 percent or more.

> ### BONE BOOSTERS
>
> Moderate exercise—walking, gardening, social dancing—helps prevent osteoporosis and reduce the risk of fractures, even in women over 65.

You don't have to run marathons to reap the benefits. The more hours spent actively, and the more vigorous the movement, the more protection you get. One study demonstrated that though you need two or more hours a week of reasonable exercise to give you the best results, even an hour a week made a significant difference. Just being on your feet, rather than sitting or lying down, helps: four hours a day off your duff, even if you are just standing there, is enough to lower your risk of osteoporosis. Of course, if you want to make your bones as strong as possible, don't just stand there—*do* something. As described later in this chapter, particular kinds of exercise are important for your bones.

THINGS TO THINK ABOUT
The more large muscles you work, the faster you will change your metabolism and the faster you will lose weight and/or fat.

It is never too late to start exercising. One study showed exercise brought increased endurance, expanded abilities, and decreased depression to nursing home patients averaging 87 years old! It is also never too early: studies show that how active a child is predicts how dense his or her bones will be as an adult. Exercise is for every person, at any age and any initial ability level. Even if you are inexperienced with exercise, or haven't exercised in a long time, or have never tried a particular kind of exercise, or have chronic health concerns, you can start now to work exercise into your life. Start slowly with a plan that's right for you, and get expert guidance to start you out if necessary. No matter who you are, you'll benefit from a program like the ones described in this section. When you're trying something new, no matter what your level of fitness, learn proper technique to protect yourself from injury and maximize benefits, and add it gradually to your usual routine.

Be sure to discuss it with your health care advisor first if you are starting exercise for the first time or haven't been active for the last two years, or if you are overweight, over 45, or haven't had a checkup in a couple of years. Anyone with high blood pressure, heart disease, or high risk of heart disease, diabetes, or other chronic illness, or on regular medication, should also check with

My Story: Deborah

I'm one of the most sedentary people who ever lived. I've never had a weight problem, so I never bothered with working out. In fact, I used to laugh at my friends, teasing them about all the hopping and flailing about they did, or the stairways or bike trips to nowhere.

Then a bone density scan showed I had significant bone loss, though it wasn't yet officially osteoporosis. But I haven't even gone through menopause yet, so I got a bit worried about my future, and I took a lot of steps to prevent any further deterioration, including doubling the amount of calcium supplements I took and taking Fosamax. But the big change for me has been exercising. Now I lift weights, though I'm not religious about it. And I started to walk three miles a day at least four times a week. Last month I hurt my foot, and have had to stop for a while. Don't tell anyone, but I miss it!

a doctor before beginning to exercise. If your bone density is already low, or if you are at increased risk of fractures, you should seek professional advice about safe exercise strategies in order to avoid injury at the same time you are building bone.

WHAT KIND OF EXERCISE DO I NEED?

The type of exercise is less important than *that* you exercise, and you should focus on the kind of exercise you like best, since that's what you are most likely to actually do. Still, we know that exercising for optimal health entails developing strength, flexibility, balance, heart and lung capacity, and endurance. Everyone should get aerobic exercise for a healthy heart and weight control, as well as exercise that increases flexibility, builds better balance, and reduces stress to live longer and better. To build and protect your bones, you must do weight-bearing exercise (see page 272). Many forms of exercise combine these elements, so don't give up before you start for fear of having to learn too many new things and devote too much time. Stay in shape overall by choosing one or more of the types of exercise described here each day, or every other day. Vary how you work out, and combine at least a few different forms of exercise in your plan. Cross-training is important because it ensures you include all the various components of overall fitness—and all-around good health—and prevents overuse or abuse of a particular set of muscles and joints. Many forms of aerobic exercise, for example, leave the upper body more or less out of it—and half your muscles are above your waist. Focusing on just one form of exercise—running, for example—will give you lopsided results.

You should get at least half an hour of aerobic exercise at least three times a week to protect your heart and maintain a healthy weight. (If you do it five or more days a week, 20 minutes at a time would do it.) To burn fat (and lose weight), you'll need to work out longer each time or work out more times.

> **BONE BOOSTERS**
>
> Get at least 30 minutes of aerobic exercise, three times a week, or 20 minutes five days a week.

Make sure not to turn your aerobic ("with oxygen") workout into an anaerobic ("without oxygen") workout by becoming out of breath. If you can't hold a brief conversation without huffing and puffing, you are out of breath—and working anaerobically. If you are out of breath, your body is not getting the oxygen it needs in order to burn fat and relies on sugars instead. You should exert yourself enough to know you're working, but you should also feel you could keep at it for quite some time. Even if you walk briskly for half an hour, for example, you should feel like you could go another 15 minutes or more when you reach your endpoint. If you are exhausted when you are done, or get so tired you have to stop before you planned to, you were most likely working anaerobically. Duration is more important than intensity. The key is to keep moving at a fairly constant rate. Stopping and starting means you won't get enough aerobics—or, if you're working so hard that you *have* to stop before starting again, you're working anaerobically.

So ignore the chart on the wall of the room where you take a step aerobics class, as it will tell you how to calculate your target heart rate: 85 percent of your capacity. To be working truly aerobically (no matter what they call the class you're in), you should aim for more like 70 percent of your capacity. (A very rough rule of thumb would be that your maximum pulse is 220 less your age. So if you are 50, for example, your maximum pulse rate would be 170 beats a minute, and your target should be about 119. Count your pulse for ten seconds—watching a clock—then multiply by 6 to find out if you are near your target.)

BONE BOOSTERS

For a rough estimate of your target heart rate to ensure you're working aerobically (not anaerobically), subtract your age from 180.

You won't burn as many calories per hour of exercise this way, but you'll burn more every hour thanks to speeding up your metabolism. The more muscles you involve in exercise, the more calories you burn, and the more muscle you have the more calories you burn even when you are asleep. You'll lose inches and drop clothing sizes, though you may not see the pounds fall away as quickly. You may even put on some weight, since muscle weighs more than fat—but takes up less space.

Getting regular aerobic exercise is the only way to speed up your body's metabolism. The faster your metabolism, the more food you need to maintain your weight and the more calories you burn while at rest. Over the long term, it isn't the calories you burn *while* exercising that help you stay slim, it is the calories you burn while *not* exercising. After all, even the most avid athletes among us spend more time not exercising than exercising.

DON'T BE A SLAVE TO THE SCALE

If you're trying to "lose weight," keep track of your waist, hip, and chest measurements to monitor your progress. With a good exercise plan, you might be surprised to find you're losing inches even if your weight is steady.

BONE BOOSTERS

Weight-bearing exercises include:
Walking
Running and jogging
Hiking
Stair climbing
Dancing
Skiing (cross-country or downhill)
Aerobic dance
Step aerobics
Basketball
Soccer
Tennis and other racquet sports
Volleyball
Ice-skating
In-line skating
Strength training with machines or weights
Treadmills and the other aerobic machines

WEIGHT-BEARING EXERCISE

While everyone should get aerobic exercise, the key to healthy bones is *weight-bearing exercise*. That doesn't mean you have to lift weights, though that is an excellent way to build your bone strength as well as your muscles. Rather, weight-bearing exercise is anything requiring your muscles to work against gravity in moving the various parts of your body. You should get *30 minutes* of weight-bearing exercise *three to five times per week* to protect your bones. As you can see, in most cases, that requirement will overlap with your body's need for aerobic exercise. Tennis, however,

---

BONE BOOSTERS

Get 30 minutes of weight-bearing exercise three to five times a week. Most choices will also be aerobic, so you'll be killing two birds with one stone.

Myth: Running can "pound the calcium into your bones."
Fact: The high-impact activities often touted as good for bone density can do more harm than good, damaging joints and generally creating more stress than your body can absorb.

and other activities with mostly stop-and-go movement give you a better weight-bearing workout than an aerobic one, so don't count them double.

Impact (like jumping) and strain (like moving something heavy) both spur bone growth, but you want to be careful of anything high-impact—anything pounding—which is very hard on the body in general and the joints in particular. If you favor jogging or *non*-low-impact aerobics, be sure you do them with good form. If you've never had formal instruction, the investment in time and money will be worth it when you consider the real payoff: reduced wear and tear on your body. You should also alternate with gentler forms of exercise. Die-hard runners might enjoy the new elliptical running machines for a similar movement without the stress on the joints.

The party line is that *swimming* is not a weight-bearing exercise (since the water is bearing most of your weight), and so, whatever its other benefits with respect to your cardiovascular system and muscle tone, it isn't of any particular use to your bones. But studies have proved that swimming can increase bone density in your spine. And since water provides twelve times the resistance of air, and swimming uses all your big muscles against gravity, I think it is safe to assume your entire skeleton will benefit. Exercising in water, including swimming, makes your muscles stronger (which makes your bones stronger), and does not stress your joints, since it is as close as you can get to a *no*-impact workout. If

Myth: Swimming is a good cardiovascular workout, but does nothing for your bones.
Fact: Anything that works your muscles against your bones triggers bone growth and development.

Case in Point: Lynn

*I*deally, your doctor is your equal partner and advocate for your health. But sometimes, even a doctor you generally respect prefers different approaches than you do. That can be intimidating, but remember no one knows more about your body than you do. An insurance company or HMO policy can also complicate matters. You have to take the best advice and information from your health care providers, and work within the insurance system as best you can, but then make your own decisions according to what feels right to you. That's just what Lynn did when she found herself facing a gynecologist who was a great believer in prescription hormones for almost every woman, and an insurance company that wouldn't pay for the bone density testing that could help her make crucial decisions about what, if any, drug therapy her bones needed.

Lynn was already a decade into menopause, and had long ago decided against hormone replacement therapy, when she began to get worried about her bone density. She'd never been bothered by any other menopausal symptoms, but now it seemed like she was reading more and more about the dangers of low bone density every day, and it was a topic of much discussion among her friends. Each time she went to the gynecologist, he urged her to reconsider taking estrogen, reeling off its benefits to bones and the heart. Then, at her last annual exam, the doctor told her she'd be a good candidate for the newest drug for low bone density, Evista, which had estrogenlike protective effects on the bone, without the increased risk in breast cancer that makes HRT unacceptable to many women.

Lynn's insurance plan wouldn't cover a bone density scan. Her doctor was satisfied with a standard x-ray from an old knee injury from when she was perimenopausal that showed she had "good bones" (in a general sense). He just assumed she'd been steadily losing density since, given her age and her refusal of HRT. He sent her home with an Evista sample and a prescription slip.

Instead, she had a bone density screening at a health fair at her neighborhood community center, where it cost only $35 for a DEXA scan *of her wrist. She never even broke the seal on that Evista sample because the scan showed only a tiny loss in density compared to average. And who knew if a −.01 standard deviation even meant any loss at all in her particular case? She knew she was past the years when bone loss is usually most rapid, so she decided that she'd keep on with what she'd been doing for her health for years, with no pharmacological intervention. After all, it appeared to be working!*

Lynn has been a competitive synchronized swimmer for over twelve years, and counted her bone density as a bit of proof that swimming can help develop your bones, just as traditional weight-bearing exercises can. She knew the party line was that in the water you don't have the same gravity pulling against your bones, and that without it, your bones wouldn't be building in the same way. While she did believe that water workouts were much easier on the joints, she agreed with the articles in her swimming magazines about how anything that worked muscle against bone would build both muscle and bone. She knew for sure that it took a lot of strength and hard, hard work to make graceful water ballets look effortless.

She began lifting weights twice a week years ago to build her strength for the lifts required in her sport. She is on the treadmill three or four times a week—any day she doesn't swim—for half an hour. She swims at least three times a week, for an hour to an hour and a half each time, which would include 3/4 mile of laps just for warm-up. *This combination keeps her limber, strong, and aerobically fit so she can keep up with the much younger swimmers on her team without batting an eye.*

To control high cholesterol levels, Lynn started eating a largely vegetarian diet, with chicken or fish once or twice a week, and meat a handful of times over the course of a year, and she believes that plays a large role in keeping her bones healthy as well. She's careful to get three major sources of calcium in her diet every day, usually milk on her morning cereal, a yogurt or cottage cheese with lunch, and something dark green and leafy with dinner. She takes 500 mg of calcium in a supplement to get up to the 1,500 mg total recommended for menopausal women not taking HRT, along with vitamin E (for her heart) and a multivitamin with trace minerals to cover all the bases.

After such an encouraging bone scan, the only change Lynn made was to add even more soy to her diet to reap the benefits—to both her bones and her cholesterol level—of phytoestrogens. She's long been a fan of tofu—in fact, goes out of her way to get to a particular store where they sell excellent fresh tofu—but now is using a soy protein powder regularly, sprinkled on her cereal and in her yogurt-fruit smoothies. The only other major thing she's done as a result is to encourage her friends to get their bone density tested and to talk to her swimming buddies about how much the sport has done to keep her healthy.

swimming is your workout of choice, I think you can rest easy knowing you're doing the right thing for your bones, as well as the rest of your body. Everyone should do cross-training, however, and including other types of exercise will ensure you have all your bases covered. Enjoying exercise is the key to sticking with it over the long haul, so unless you are faced with a medical reason, never stop doing what you like best.

The same party that put out the party line on swimming holds a similar one about *biking*: that it isn't weight-bearing exercise (because your rear end, not your legs, is holding most of your weight). Newer thought puts biking (and swimming) just behind walking and running in effectiveness in building bone density— and any of the other three are easier on the joints than running. I agree riding a bicycle *is* effective, whether on a stationary or regular bike, as long as you feel resistance on the pedals. Then you know you're working your muscles, which in turn strengthens your bones. So again, if this is your preferred way to go, don't stop. Cross-training will still be important, and that variety will balance anything bicycling misses. Biking doesn't give your upper body much in the way of a strength workout, so you should include something that does in your routine. The various big muscles in the upper body all affect the back and spine, so you don't want to overlook them if you are concerned about avoiding or countering low bone density.

Dancing is a wonderful form of exercise. Since swing dancing is all the rage, you'll be able to find a class or club easily, and if you're doing it right, it'll probably be aerobic as well as weight bearing, not to mention fun. But you don't have to *learn* any particular steps (unless you want to). Just get up and boogie at the next wedding or bar mitzvah you're at, or go out with your friends—or turn up the volume on your favorite CD and cut a rug all by yourself in the privacy of your own living room. More structured dance is also an excellent way to get fit, especially if it is aerobic. Take a class in any style you like—jazz, tap, ballet, modern. Good dance instruction will emphasize elongating the spine, and dancing improves your balance, strength, and coordination. You may get an aerobic workout, too. Take care to use proper form, particularly in some of the not-exactly-natural postures of ballet. Assuming you are not aiming to dance professionally, there's no need to suffer for your art! Once you've mastered the basics, dancing can cross the line into "moving meditations" (see page 282), as you lose yourself in the music.

WALKING

The best way to start exercising, especially if you've been sedentary, is simply to walk. You don't need any particular equipment and you don't have to learn any particular technique. Walking is a weight-bearing exercise, so your bones will benefit. And walking regularly helped women in one study lower their risk of heart disease by up to 75 percent. Consider this comparison: lowering your cholesterol level 1 percent decreases your risk of heart disease 2 to 3 percent. If we all embrace walking (or exercise in general) with the enthusiasm we now have for low cholesterol, we'll be a much healthier species.

Walking is good for everyone, no matter what your fitness level. It isn't just a way to break yourself in to exercise—it is a way to stay fit and healthy for the long haul. Walking for exercise should be moderately aerobic. If you are just starting out, begin with walking 10 minutes a day, and take a break every few days. Each week, increase the length of time you walk by 5 minutes, and keep building up until you reach the point where you can walk three-quarters of an hour at a time—or up to an hour. "Brisk" walking should put you at or near 4 mph eventually. But the time spent is far more important than the distance involved. If you are a precise or high-control person, feel free to check the length of your path with your car odometer, or estimate it with a pedometer calibrated to the length of your stride. Or perhaps, observing how far you can go (in addition to how long) will be an additional motivation for you. Otherwise, don't get hung up on distance. Just make sure you work long enough and hard enough. But not too hard; as mentioned above, you should be able to hold a conversation while you walk, but not speak a lengthy monologue. Your heart rate and breathing should be faster than normal. If you are an experienced exerciser, you may want to swing your arms as you walk to get some upper-body involvement and to make it more aerobic.

Walking can also be an ideal form of "moving meditation," as discussed below, and in Chapter 21's section on mind-body medicine. At the very least, you can increase the amount of stress reduction you reap from exercising. And you might even find, or enrich, a spiritual path along with your physical one.

STRENGTH TRAINING

Walking may be the best all-around exercise, but as far as bone building goes, strength training is the cream of the crop. The pull of muscle against bone stresses a bone, and that kind of stress is what makes a bone become stronger. Impact also strengthens a bone, but the impact that comes from running or jumping, say, can be otherwise harmful to the body. Muscle working against gravity provides another kind of impact for the bones, stimulating bone formation and slowing loss. Strength training with free weights (including light hand and ankle weights) or weight machines is the most direct way to provide that stress and impact of muscle on bone, which is what makes it ideal for building and preserving bone density.

We know that weight lifters have much denser bones in their back and legs than do runners, for example. Studies do show that walking prevents bone loss in the spine, but strength training has been proved to *build* bone mass in the spine *and* hip. One study that (deservedly) got a lot of media attention followed a group of postmenopausal women who were generally healthy—but sedentary. None were taking HRT, or any other bone-related medicines, or taking calcium supplements. Half performed a simple weight-lifting routine twice a week, while the other half stuck with their couch potato ways. After one year, the weight lifters built their bone mass 1 percent on average, at both the hip and spine. That compares favorably to what you'd see with HRT alone. To give you perspective, consider this: the women who did not lift weights lost up to 2.5 percent of their bone mass over the same time period— and also lost muscle mass and gained body fat and weight. The weight lifters became much more active in general (as the researchers calculated it, a 27 percent increase), while the sedentary group became *less* active. The weight lifters lowered their body fat, gained muscle, and had better balance and more strength. And here's a wonderful bonus: the researchers had the daughters of the women who lifted weights come in and do the tests their mothers were acing. In every case, the weight-lifting women outperformed their own daughters!

I only wonder how much better they might have done if they also took calcium. Or HRT: another study looked at women taking HRT after surgical menopause, and found that after a year of strength training the average increase in bone density was 4 percent in the wrist and 8 percent in the spine!

Building muscle also increases your metabolic rate—that is, how fast your body burns calories *at rest*. Think of your metabolism like a fire: a large fire produces more heat and uses more fuel than a small fire. Exercise stokes the flames of your metabolism. That is increasingly important as you age, because your metabolism usually slows as you get older, partly because of muscle loss. Muscle mass begins to decrease in midlife unless you are active. Strength drops, on average, about 15 percent during your sixties, and another 15 percent in your seventies, and 30 percent each successive decade. This is not a result of aging, but of inactivity.

Muscle uses more calories to maintain itself than fat does. The stronger you are (the more muscle you have), the more calories you will burn at all times and the easier it will be to control your weight—and the more you will need to eat to stay at the same weight. Weight-loss diets typically fail because you don't *permanently* change the way you eat *and* work. Restricting the number of calories you take in results in *muscle* loss, not fat loss. You also end up in double jeopardy because if you just reduce the calories you take in (as opposed to increasing your body's caloric requirement, with exercise), your metabolism slows to accommodate only the lower number of calories. So when you increase them again (going "off" the diet), all you will have done is set yourself up for immediate weight *gain*.

Muscle also helps the body use sugar efficiently, so strength training is an important addition to a diabetes treatment or prevention program. Losing muscle reduces your sugar tolerance. Strength training has been shown to prevent weight gain, fractures, and injury, and to lower the risk of heart attack and colon cancer in ways aerobic exercise alone does not. Loss of muscle impairs your body's ability to regulate its temperature, too. Just one strength workout a week is enough to prevent the muscle loss that accompanies aging, even in devoted athletes who focus only on cardiovascular exercise. Increasing your strength lowers the risk of injury to joints and muscles. It also improves your balance and so reduces your risk of falling, which in turn reduces the risk of fracture.

As with every other strategy in this book, it is never too late to benefit from strength training. One study of people in their 80s and 90s living in nursing homes who exercised with weight machines three times a week for just eight weeks showed improvements in strength, balance, and walking speed. Even people who are already frail can, with proper exercise using light weights, build up enough leg strength to walk without a cane. I've no doubt of the bone benefits that went along with these results, even though they weren't tracked by the researchers.

Studies show that two 15-minute strength workouts a week is enough to build bone density. As you'll see in the next chapter, you can target all the major muscle groups with a very compact routine, which should take you no more than about 20 minutes once you've got it down. If you prefer machines to hand weights, a thorough workout may take a bit longer just because you need time to adjust each piece of equipment properly before you use it. You should rest at least one day between sessions to allow your muscles to recover, because it is during the recovery period that muscle actually grows. If you want to exercise every day, just alternate which group of muscles you work on which days—that is, do upper body one day and lower body the next. Once you start a regular routine with weights or weight machines, your bones will be denser before a year is up. But if you stop, you'll start losing bone again immediately. As with dieting, you have to think of embarking on a fitness program that includes strength training as a lifetime plan, not a solution you achieve in a set time period, then don't have to work on anymore.

> **DID YOU KNOW?**
>
> Hip fractures require nursing home care for almost a third of patients—usually long-term care (averaging about seven years).

STRETCHING

Stretching relaxes the mind as well as the body, so you get the benefit of stress reduction as well as better balance and coordination, increased range of motion, reduced tension, fewer injuries, greater body awareness, and improved circulation. No matter what else you do in the way of physical activity (or even just everyday motions), stretching will make it easier for you. That's all generally good for you, plus it will decrease your chance of falling, and so your risk of fracture, no matter what your bone density. Stretching after exercise will also lessen later soreness and stiffness—thereby making exercise more pleasant and easier to stick with.

Many of us are stuck with old stretching habits picked up long ago, and odds are they are, at best, not maximally effective. At worst, they could be making you *less* flexible and *more* prone to injury. Whatever you do, no bouncing! Just about every weekend jogger I see stretching is bouncing up and down trying to get that nose a little closer to the knee with each bounce, but in reality that's the worst possible approach. The muscles knot up tighter with each rebound, and the rapid pace doesn't allow the muscle to stretch at all before it is contracted again.

If this sounds like you—or if you have only dim memories of high school gym class lessons in stretching to go on—I recommend taking a stretching class or checking a recent book or video out of the library to update your technique. I favor "active-isolated" stretching, or AI in fitness parlance, which holds that to stretch a muscle, it must be relaxed. Relaxing a muscle requires contracting the muscle or muscles that work in opposition to it. That is, to stretch the hamstrings (back of the thigh), you should be in a position that relaxes them by requiring contraction of the quads (front of the thigh.) In AI, you hold each stretch for just two seconds, but repeat it, slowly, several times. This is the best kind of stretching to use pre-exercise.

You should devote 15 to 20 minutes at a time to stretching to cover all the major muscle groups. For the benefit of your bones, be sure to stretch your back and hips well. The abdominals and thigh muscles all participate in rotating your hip, so they should be targeted as well. Make stretching a regular part of your routine, and you should be able to see a difference within three weeks.

The second most common stretching mistake—after The Bounce—is using it as a warm-up. The best *pre*-exercise warm-up is to simply do the exercise you will be doing at a much slower rate to ease the muscles into it. If you are doing just a stretching workout, you will need to warm yourself up a bit first—walk briskly around the block or march in place for a few minutes, swinging your arms— to get your muscles warm before you stretch them. Or try stretching after a warm shower. The best time to stretch is as a cool-down after another form of exercise, when your muscles are already warm and easier to stretch. Then you may want to use a longer, larger stretch than AI techniques provide, with slow progression.

MOVING MEDITATIONS

For all the wonderful benefits of the types of exercise described above, none can compare to the full range of benefits you get from the kind of exercises I think of as moving meditations. You are more than bones. You are more than just your body. And while aerobic dance or power walking or lifting weights may strengthen and tone the physical part of you, moving meditations do all that *and* develop mental, emotional, and spiritual fitness. That's a desirable end in and of itself, but in addition, research shows that nurturing a spiritual sensibility (whether or not that means religion for you) prevents illness and assists in healing.

Yoga, tai chi, and qi gong by definition combine movement and meditation. But you can also meditate while doing any kind of exercise, once the physical activity itself has become automatic. Walking is probably the best way to start if you want to do both at once, since the movement comes naturally. You could do the same when lifting weights or on the treadmill or stationary bike. Many people complain that exercise is boring (especially on machines in the gym), and if that includes you, try fully engaging mentally while you do it. Turn off the TV, take off your headphones, put down the magazine, and focus your mind intently on what you are doing, letting go of all other intruding thoughts. Voilà! You are meditating.

FINDING "THE ZONE"

High-level athletes—and dedicated hobbyists, too—describe being in "the zone," or reaching a place of mental clarity and ease of movement. Successful moving meditation produces the same result, but with the focus on yourself rather than an outside activity. After an exquisite match, a tennis player may call it "a spiritual experience." And it no doubt was one. You don't have to reach peak physical performance to elicit that state, however; you can conjure the state of mind yourself, with movement as the background.

As low-impact, weight-bearing exercise, yoga, tai chi, qi gong, and similar schools of movement increase flexibility, promote good balance, and reduce stress. Though they are usually not aerobic (though yoga and qi gong can be), I believe these forms of exercise can also change your metabolism for the better—partly because of the physical exercise and partly because they tap into the powerful connection between the mind and the body.

Mindful walking, as described in the section in Chapter 21 on mind-body medicine, provides similar benefits. Turning what might otherwise be a pleasant stroll, or perhaps a grueling work-out, into an inner pilgrimage helps counter the many distracting stresses of modern life, returning you to your own center. Some reluctant exercisers will find a mind-body approach is just what they need to engage them with exercise. Whatever brings you to it, integrating the physical and nonphysical aspects of your individu-ality is the truest sense of holistic health.

Qi gong looks much like tai chi, though the movements are somewhat more complicated and are generally performed more quickly. This ancient tradition has long been known to support good health, but the news is just sinking in across the United States. My brother was recently raving to me about the exercises his physical therapist taught him, about how many different ways they worked the body all at once and how energized he felt doing them. Of course, I wanted to know more about this wonderful new technique, and as he started to demonstrate it, I realized he was showing me a variation of the qi gong routine I do! As Westerners are discovering this Eastern movement and meditation system, classes are becoming easier to find, so if you are interested, look for one in your community.

Myth: Yoga and tai chi are good for stress reduction, but won't really contribute to fitness.

Fact: You'll most likely have to get aerobics elsewhere, but with development of strength, balance, and flexibility, these other "gentle" movement forms are excellent workouts in their own rights.

A typical yoga class or workout begins and ends with relax-ation, meditation, visualization, and stretching. Breathing exercises are an integral part of traditional yoga, though many classes give them a more limited role. The main "workout," then, as we think of it from our modern gym-focused exercise mind-set, would be the series of poses, many of which have by now been adapted into other types of exercise. The poses emphasize strength, flexibility, and balance—all the key components of exercising for bone health. The next chapter provides a number of poses selected especially to target the hips and back, along with general balance and strength, for you to try at home. I suggest taking an introductory class, or checking out a good book or video from the library, to familiarize yourself with some of the basics of yoga. The exercises this book provides will work best if you incorporate them into a full-length yoga workout. Since they are targeted, you could also use them as part of your other routines, including them when you stretch, for example, and reap much the same physical benefit, if the whole yoga package doesn't appeal to you.

PAIN MANAGEMENT

Any kind of stress reduction is good for ebbing chronic pain, and any "moving meditation" will help you accomplish that. In fact, since exercise in general is stress reducing, anything that gets you moving (as long as it doesn't aggravate your condition) will help. Deep breathing helps, too, and all these forms of exercise incorporate breathing exercises. You can do it on your own by focusing solely on your breathing, inhaling through the nose and exhaling through the mouth, watching your abdomen rise and fall with each breath.

Yoga is an excellent technique for managing chronic pain, so it may be a good choice for you if you have back pain from low bone density. If you do have low bone density, however, be sure to talk it over with your health care provider before starting yoga, since some of the classic spine movements may not be a good idea for you. If you do have low bone density, you should at least begin with a class, as a good instructor will help you tailor a workout to your own health concerns, even in a group setting, giving you alternatives to postures that might exacerbate your condition, and providing additional movements to focus on your problem areas.

The brain controls everything in your body, and you can learn to tap into that connection consciously. The brain tells you when to breathe, and how to sleep, and what to do with the food you eat, and how much pain you feel, and countless other things—almost always on autopilot. Anything you can imagine, your brain has a role in, so use your imagination to see how you can use your brain. When you harness the power of the brain, your possibilities are endless.

POSTURE

An often overlooked component of good health and fitness is proper posture. Posture is the balance struck between the unrelenting force of gravity pulling down on you and the valiant effort of your body structure to hold you up. The path of least resistance between these forces is what we call posture. Good posture causes no pain or problems and helps you use your muscles, tendons, and bones optimally. "Bad" posture actually uses more energy, though it is often thought of as laziness. That's a mistake, because poor posture may indicate an underlying structural problem that is not your fault at all. And if you try to correct a structural problem without knowing exactly what it is, you will probably exacerbate the situation.

Say you have one leg that is significantly shorter than the other. To compensate, in an attempt to keep your eyes level (a real priority for your brain), you'll probably hold your shoulders unevenly, creating a scoliosis in your spine. Your mother's advice to "straighten up" will be useless—you literally can't. A doctor without appropriate training might advise you to do some back-strengthening exercises to even out your shoulders, but getting stronger while you are still uneven will just exaggerate the tilt. If you made an appointment with me, your checkup would reveal the different lengths of your legs as the cause of your problem, and I'd prescribe a gradually adjusting series of heel lifts and several sessions of osteopathic manipulation to fix the cause of your problem. Now you have a physical support to help keep you level, and your muscles and bones will no longer have to contort themselves. Of course, this is a very simplistic explanation and an exaggerated example, but I think you get the idea: address the cause of the problem, not the result.

Your posture is your posture, and you can't will it to be different. If your shoulders are rounded, no amount of throwing them back or thrusting your chest out is going to "fix" them. You can make your posture work as well as possible for you, but you can't make it into something it is not. So make sure your posture is maximally efficient, and get any permanent "bad" posture evaluated to discover if there is a correctable underlying problem. You'll need an appropriate therapy program to make any changes necessary for optimal body positioning.

Simply maintaining good posture no matter what you are doing in the course of your day is an excellent defense against kyphosis, the spinal curve commonly called "dowager's hump" or "hunchback" that is a hallmark of osteoporosis. Keeping the head, shoulders, spine, and hips in alignment protects the spine, so you need to be conscious of how you walk, stand, sit, lie, climb stairs, sleep, drive, type, and everything in between. Stick with the natural curves of your back. If you stand against a wall, your heels, buttocks, upper back and shoulders, and back of your head should touch the wall. With a side view, you should be able to draw a straight line from your ear to your shoulder to the middle of the curve of your lower back to your hip, knee, and ankle. From the front, it should be clear that your eyes, shoulders, chest, and hips are all level and parallel to the floor.

That is the alignment you should strive for at all times.

If this is not your normal or comfortable posture, you may have a structural problem that should be evaluated by a professional. I recommend an osteopathic structural evaluation, as most nonspecialists tend to recommend strengthening exercises that may be good for posture in general but will actually exacerbate a structural problem. But for most people, conscious effort and increased strength will be able to help posture, barring a medical issue.

A major pitfall to good posture is working at a desk. Proper alignment is crucial when typing or working at a computer in order to avoid carpal tunnel syndrome or other repetitive motion injuries to nerves and joints—and just to eliminate the achiness you feel at the end of a long day at your desk. When you're at your desk, not using your computer, prop your work on a stand at an angle in front of you, so you don't have to hang your head forward over flat papers to read them. Use a footrest, especially if you need one in order to keep your thighs parallel to the floor when your chair is otherwise adjusted to the proper height. Your chair should support the curve of your lower back, and if it doesn't, use a pillow or rolled-up towel to do the job. When you are driving (which puts you in much the same position as sitting at your desk), use the headrest.

Lifting anything without injury also requires proper posture: bend at the knees and hinge at the hips, not the waist, so your legs, not your back, are taking the heavy load.

Sleep on your back or side, as sleeping on your stomach places a strain on your lower back.

The first key is to be aware of your body position no matter what you are doing. It may require conscious attention at first, but eventually you'll develop good habits and will align yourself properly automatically. The second key is to build your flexibility, balance, and strength (particularly of the front of the thighs, buttocks, and stomach), all of which are important to support good posture. The exercises in this chapter will do just that.

SUGGESTED WORKOUT SCHEDULES

	Minimum	Basic Bone Health I	Basic Bone Health II	Daily Plan Health III
Monday	Weight-bearing aerobics	Aerobics	Aerobics and weight training	Aerobics and weight training
Tuesday		Weight training		Moving meditation
Wednesday	Weight-bearing aerobics	Aerobics	Aerobics	Aerobics
Thursday		Weight training		Moving meditation
Friday	Weight-bearing aerobics	Aerobics	Aerobics and weight training	Aerobics and weight training
Saturday				Moving meditation
Sunday	Comprehensive stretch	Comprehensive stretch	Comprehensive stretch	Comprehensive stretch

PUTTING IT ALL TOGETHER

Three weekly sessions of weight-bearing aerobic exercise are enough to give you general good health, including reasonably dense bones. But the benefits to be gained from strength training and stretching should not be overlooked. The simplest approach to working out that encompasses all those is probably to do aerobic exercise three times a week, with weight training after at least two sessions. Stretch after each workout, with at least one intensive, full-body stretch each week. You could put together any number of combinations and arrangements that would also work, so experiment until you find a setup you like and will stick to.

The more you get into it, the longer your workouts will last, and you should build up to at least an hour workout each time. If you are so inclined, by all means, do something every day (just remember to alternate the muscle groups you focus on if you are strength-training every day). In moving beyond aerobics three times a week, I recommend filling in with "moving meditations" like yoga, tai chi, and qi gong because they combine many aspects of fitness.

Start with shorter and/or less frequent workouts, and build up gradually to your goal. Get whatever support you need to stick with it. Join a group, take a class, recruit a partner, hire a baby-sitter (or take turns with another parent looking to carve out some time for exercise). Dress comfortably and appropriately. Stick to a regular place and time at first, until you've formed a habit. If you usually exercise outdoors, have a ready-made alternate in mind if rain or cold threatens to keep you from your routine. Schedule your workouts as you would any other important appointment. Write specific windows for exercise in your calendar, and at first be very specific: "Monday: 7–8 A.M., aerobics class at the 'Y'; Wednesday: 6:30–7:15 P.M., meet Joyce at the gym to lift weights; Saturday: 10–11 A.M. biking," and so on. Get those dates on your calendar before you start setting up anything else. At least until you're in the groove, work haircuts and brunch dates *around* your exercise plans. Otherwise, it is too easy to let one workout after another slide, and that does your bones no favors. Once you are used to regular exercise, and realize how much better you feel when you do it (and how sluggish you feel when you don't), you'll no longer have to force those priorities. You may not believe me now, but once you find the forms of exercise that appeal to you, you won't *want* to go without. Just because you never could stick with jogging when that was all the rage doesn't mean you aren't cut out for exercise. You probably aren't cut out for *jogging* (and as far as I'm concerned, that's just as well), but there are many other op-tions you can experiment with until you find the one that really moves you (pun intended).

Starting slow, setting moderate and realistic goals, attending to injury prevention, and doing what you can to ensure success will keep your body physically safe as you introduce it to new ways of moving. It will also cement this most beneficial of all habits.

Bite off more than you can chew and nothing tastes good, and you'll never go back for seconds. Let your body be your guide. You should never have any pain while exercising, though sometimes discomfort is a sign you are pushing yourself, which is not necessarily a bad thing. You may get sore or stiff after a workout, but that shouldn't last for more than a day or two—if it does, scale back, at least for a while, because you're doing too much too soon. Making this a lifetime habit (just as you are not "dieting" so much as changing the way you eat, permanently) is very important. When you stop exercising, bone density will stop growing and begin to decline immediately (depending on your age). It will grow again when you start again, but you'll always be further behind than if you had never let it slide in the first place. What it comes right down to is: move it or lose it!

Chapter 16

Work Out with Weights

You know you should be getting 30 minutes of weight-bearing aerobic exercise three times a week. If you don't have a routine already, start with walking, as described in the previous chapter. Whatever you decide to do in the way of aerobics, strength training is a valuable addition because we know it builds bone more directly and efficiently than any other kind of exercise you can do.

Anyone can do this routine and the one in the following chapter, no matter what your previous experience with exercise. It may take a little while to learn them and make the movements familiar. But with proper form (and your doctor's OK, if necessary), both the strength training and yoga workouts are safe and effective at any fitness level. As your fitness increases, you'll be able to do each move better, or longer, or with more resistance, or in a more advanced format. The routines automatically grow with you, so both beginning and advanced exercisers will benefit from them.

For all the exercises here, there are a few ground rules that will help you get the most out of each movement and prevent injury. Before I start, let me warn you that these preliminaries—and the descriptions of the exercises themselves—will appear very mechanical as you read them over and will seem to involve a thousand tiny details. That's a hazard of describing physical movements in words. Keep in mind that the goal is to use your body as Mother Nature intended, with the full range of motion, with the appropriate muscles engaged, and with smooth, natural movements. Pinning them down on paper forces them into a string of picky steps. Read them, so you'll be able to check yourself if you work on your own. But the way to really know you're doing it right is that it will feel as if your body was meant to do it. Movements may feel unfamiliar at first, of course. Particularly when you are isolating a particular muscle, it may feel strange; in everyday life, we generally use a combination of muscles for anything we do. But once you are used to performing a particular move, it shouldn't feel awkward.

We need "exercise" precisely *because* we don't routinely use our bodies in a physical way. Thus the absurdity of a stair-climbing machine to nowhere. If we continually exploited and explored the physical possibilities and limitations of our bodies as a part of our daily lives, making a special trip to the gym would be laughable and unnecessary. If you're like me, and spend most of your day relatively stationary, you do have to make a point of moving it if you don't want to risk losing it. Even people who use their bodies a lot during the course of the day—delivering packages via bicycle, say, or loading heavy cargo onto trucks, or lifting, holding, and generally keeping up with infants and young children—don't achieve overall fitness doing that alone because they use a limited variety of motions and muscles. Parents don't get much in the way of aerobics; bike messengers don't develop their upper-body muscles.

Your body is a beautifully complex structure (consider just the elaborate interplay involved in creating and maintaining your bones), so just lifting your arm involves a whole host of actions, conscious and unconscious. Don't get bogged down in the conscious efforts of the exercises described here. Take your time to learn them properly, and to familiarize your body with how it is meant to move. Then go with the flow.

ABOUT STRENGTH TRAINING

In strength training, "flow" is built on a foundation of maintaining good posture and using the appropriate muscles to do the work. "Cheating," by letting another, more distant muscle take over, exposes you to the risk of strain or injury, and undermines building strength in the targeted area. You may go through the motions, striking the positions and diligently counting the repetitions, but all you'll achieve is finishing the workout. You won't be getting stronger, at least not in a healthy and efficient way.

So note the keys to correct body positioning. Your abdominal muscles are central to most of the movements you make with any part of the body—and are key for balance and for preventing back strain—so keep them engaged. Keep the natural curve in your back, and don't compensate for other muscles' work by arching or hyperextending. Anytime you lift your arms over your head, or do any other motion that strains the lower back, use a "pelvic tilt" to protect your back: draw your abdominal muscles gently in and up, pulling your tailbone down and as if to curve it forward slightly, rocking your hips forward just a bit. (This is a "I know it when I feel it" kind of motion, which no amount of description can really capture. You just have to try it for yourself and see.) Don't "lock" your joints (pushing an extension as far as it can go when straightening a limb). Keep them slightly soft instead. Keep your wrists in line with your forearms.

Good technique is equally important. Don't hold your breath! Exhale as you do the first part of a move that engages your muscles strongly, and inhale on the release. Use your full range of motion, but don't lock your joints. Move slowly, using a count of three for the first part of the exercise (tightening the muscles) and another three seconds to release. In the following exercises, muscle is actually built more in that release than in the initial movement, when it feels like you are working harder. Don't slack off in the second half, or you'll be getting less than half the full benefit.

Finally, use a sensible approach to resistance and repetition to get the most out of your strength training. You should do two sets of fifteen repetitions of each exercise below, separated by a minute's rest. Use enough resistance (whether from hand weights, free weights, a weight machine, exercise bands, or just your body and gravity) so that the last three or four of the second set are a little difficult, but not so much that you can't get to the end of that second set. Doing the full routine two or three times per week will give you a good bone-density workout as a complement to your weight-bearing aerobic exercise. When the last few reps in the second set are easy, step up the amount of resistance you are using. Increase the weight no more than 10 percent at a time, so you will still be able to perform two sets with the new, heavier weight. Rest a day between strength workouts. (If you want to do some every day, focus on lower body and abs one day, and upper body the next, so each muscle group gets a day of rest.)

The exercises given here will hit all of the major muscle groups, with a particular focus on your hips and back. Many of them require no more resistance than gravity and the weight of your own body, and some call for hand weights. (You'll find equivalent moves on weight machines at the gym. You can also use exercise bands, which are more portable but less precise.) Start with 1- to 3-pound weights (men, or anyone who already has significant upper-body strength, may begin with somewhat higher weights), moving up to heavier ones as you become able to. If an exercise doesn't need weights, start with more advanced options when you can. There are no prizes for lifting the heaviest weights or stretching the farthest. As long as your body is working—hard, but

---

GO WITH THE FLOW

To get the most out of your workout, no matter what exercises you are doing:

- Use easy, natural body positioning and posture.
- Learn proper technique.
- Move slowly.
- Keep breathing slow and steady. Let the breath help you.
- Listen to your body. Stop immediately if anything feels painful.
- Understand the purpose of your actions.
- Find your flow.

safely—you're benefiting. If you are still using 3-pound weights for the shoulder press months later because the next increment is just too heavy to complete your sets, who cares? If your shoulders don't clear the floor by more than ¼ inch in the crunch, so what? Keep at it and progress will come. But it looks different for everyone. Your body will show you what to do, and when to move on—and how much good you are doing yourself.

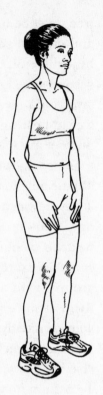

THE STRENGTH-TRAINING WORKOUT
Squat

PURPOSE: Strengthening your legs, especially hip and thigh muscles. This exercise also improves your balance.

START POSITION: Standing tall, with your legs body width apart and knees slightly bent.

THE MOTION: As if you are going to sit down in a chair. Keep your stomach, buttocks, and thigh muscles tight, and lower your body until your thighs are nearly parallel to the floor. Return, slowly, to standing.

STYLE POINTS: Don't let your knees get ahead of your toes—if they are, you're squatting too far and putting undue strain on your knees. As long as you feel your hip, thigh, and buttock muscles working strongly, it doesn't matter how far down you go, so if getting your thighs parallel to the floor is too uncomfortable, or forces your knees in front of your toes, or puts pressure on your joints, simply don't "sit" as far. If you feel unsteady, hold lightly on to the back of a sturdy chair, or a counter-top, as you squat.

TO INCREASE THE CHALLENGE: Do this exercise with a weight in each hand.

Leg Lifts

PURPOSE: Strengthening your legs, particularly the muscles on the outside of your thighs, and improving your balance.

START POSITION: Standing tall, with your stomach tight.

THE MOTION: Standing on one leg and pressing your foot into the ground, lift your other leg out to the side as far as you can without losing your balance or arching your back. Slowly return to standing on both feet (still using your muscles). Do all your reps on one side, then switch to the other.

STYLE POINTS: When you are just starting out, you may want to rest one hand on the back of a sturdy chair, or on a counter, for balance, until you feel stable on your own.

TO INCREASE THE CHALLENGE: Add ankle weights, or use an exercise band, looping one around the ankle of the moving leg, and standing on the loose ends with the other foot.

Calf Raises

PURPOSE: To strengthen your calves and improve your balance.

START POSITION: Stand next to a wall, with your feet hip width apart and one hand resting on the wall beside you for balance.

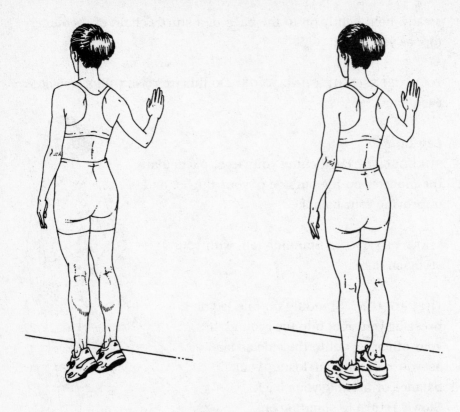

THE MOTION: Press up through your feet and toes to raise your entire body. Get as high on your toes as you can, then lower to standing.

STYLE POINTS: Hold for a moment at the top of the rise, to check your balance.

TO INCREASE THE CHALLENGE: Switch to single leg raises: wrap one foot around the ankle of the standing leg, then raise and lower as above. Do all your reps on one side, then switch to the other leg. To add yet another layer of work for your muscles—and a nice stretch—do this exercise on the bottom step of a staircase. Face the stairs, with the balls of your feet on the edge of the bottom step. Raise as above, and when you lower, keep going until your heels are just below the top of the step. Raise again from that position. You can also do this variation on one leg, when you are ready.

Crunches

PURPOSE: To strengthen your abdominal muscles, particularly the upper abs. The abs not only affect the front of your torso, but also protect your back from strain and play a central role in good balance.

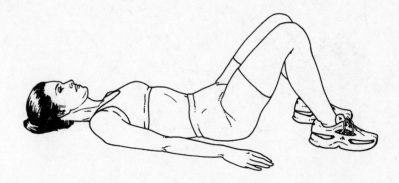

START POSITION: Lie on your back with your knees bent, body width apart, feet flat on the floor, hip distance apart. Position your hands in front of your hips, or, for more of a challenge, cross your arms in front of your chest or place your hands by your ears with your elbows out to the sides.

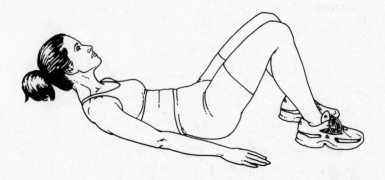

THE MOTION: Tighten your stomach muscles, as if you are pulling them up toward your head from below your belly button. Your lower back should flatten into the floor. As you exhale, lift your shoulders off the floor. That's a small movement—just 2 to 3 inches. Lower yourself slowly to the floor as you breathe in.

STYLE POINTS: Stop if you feel strain in your lower back, and make sure you are *not* holding your breath and *are* maintaining a pelvic tilt. Don't pull on your head or neck, as that may cause an injury.

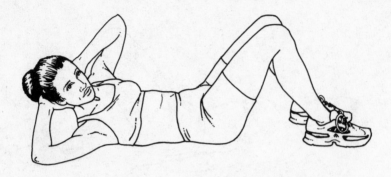

TO INCREASE THE CHALLENGE: Position yourself as above, and twist one shoulder toward the opposite hip as you raise your shoulders. Lower to the floor, and alternate which side you twist to.

Reverse Curl

PURPOSE: To strengthen your abdominal muscles, focusing on the lower abs.

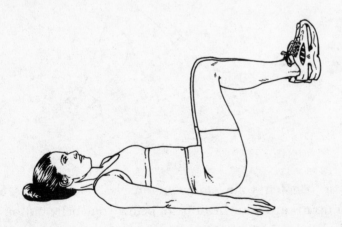

START POSITION: Lie on your back with your legs together and knees bent at about a 90° angle. Lift your legs so your calves are parallel to the floor.

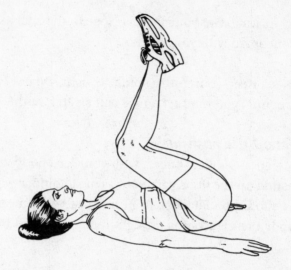

THE MOTION: By contracting your abdominal muscles, your lower back will press into the floor, and your knees will move closer to your chest as your hips roll (curl) up. Slowly lower back to the floor.

STYLE POINTS: Be careful of your lower back position.

TO INCREASE THE CHALLENGE: Combine with a crunch (see above).

Push-up

PURPOSE: To strengthen arm and chest muscles, both of which are key to back strength.

Beginner: Wall push-up

START POSITION: Stand at arm's length from a wall. Place both palms on the wall at shoulder height.

THE MOTION: Keeping your feet flat on the ground, lean toward the wall. As your arms bend, you should feel the muscles along both arms, and across your chest, working. Get your face as close to the wall as possible, then push out again with your arms.

STYLE POINTS: Keep your entire spine straight. Do not bend at the waist. As a bonus, you may get a nice calf stretch in this position.

Intermediate: Knee push-up

START POSITION: On your knees, with your legs body width apart and your hands on the floor with your arms shoulder width apart. Your hands should be far enough in front of your knees that you can keep your back and hips straight and your head in line with your spine.

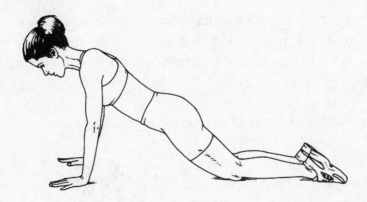

THE MOTION: Tightening your chest muscles, slowly lower your chest as close to the floor as you can by bending your elbows. Then push up to start position.

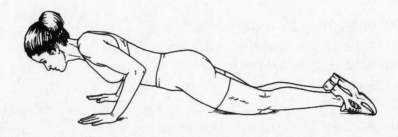

STYLE POINTS: Keep your back flat, and your neck and head in line with your back.

Advanced: Full push-up

START POSITION: Lying on the front of your body, tuck your toes under, place your hands under your shoulders, and push up on your arms. Your hands and toes support most of your body weight, though your abdominals should be engaged as well, to keep your body aligned and balanced.

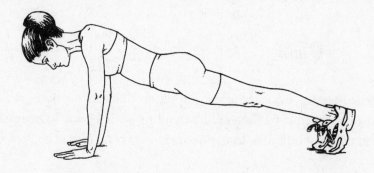

THE MOTION: Lower your chest slowly toward the floor, using your arm and chest muscles to control the movement. Get as close to the ground as you can, then push up again, straightening your arms to return to the start position.

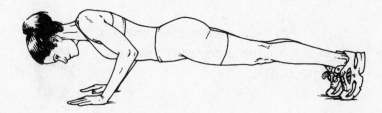

STYLE POINTS: Be careful to maintain your entire body (paying particular attention to the spine) in one long line.

Rows

PURPOSE: To strengthen your upper body, particularly your chest and back.

START POSITION: Lie on your stomach along the edge of a bed. Let one arm hang over the edge, holding a weight.

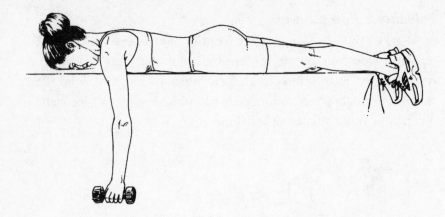

THE MOTION: Squeeze your shoulder blades together and lift your arm up toward the ceiling, bending your elbow to keep your forearm perpendicular to the floor. Slowly return to start.

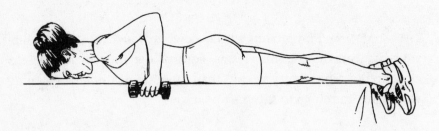

STYLE POINTS: After completing your reps on one side, switch to the other arm (and the other side of the bed).

Shoulder Press

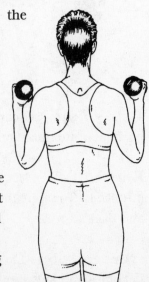

PURPOSE: Strengthening your shoulders and back.

START POSITION: You can do this one standing, or sitting on a chair or weight bench. Hold one weight in each hand close to your body at shoulder level, with your elbows bent and your palms facing your ears.

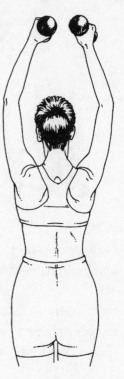

THE MOTION: Squeeze your shoulder blades together and push the weights up toward the ceiling until your arms are almost straight (but keep your elbows soft). Then lower the weights slowly back to shoulder level.

STYLE POINTS: Keep a natural curve in your back. You should feel this in your upper—*but not lower*—back.

Biceps Curl

PURPOSE: Strengthening your arms, particularly the front of the upper arm.

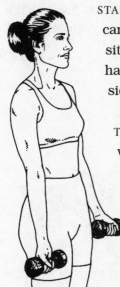

START POSITION: This one can also be done standing or sitting. Hold a weight in each hand with your arms by your side, palms facing forward.

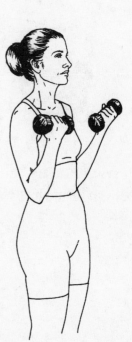

THE MOTION: Lift the weights to your shoulders by bending your elbow as you exhale. Then return them slowly to your sides while you breathe in.

STYLE POINTS: Not to sound like a broken record, but: watch your back.

Triceps Extension

PURPOSE: To strengthen your arms, particularly the back of your upper arm.

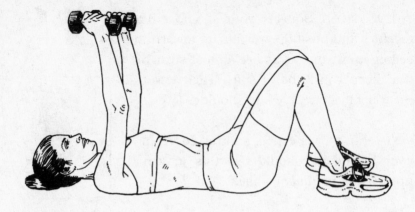

START POSITION: Lie on your back with a weight in each hand and your arms straight up in the air.

THE MOTION: Slowly lower the weights toward your head, bending your elbows until they reach a 90° angle. Then straighten back to start position, slowly.

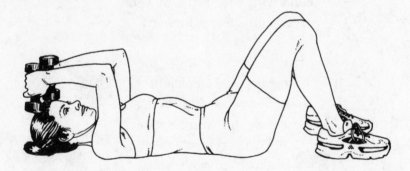

STYLE POINTS: In the starting position, do not lock your elbows; keep them slightly soft.

My Story: Doris

I started a new total-body weight-lifting routine after a bone scan before I was even in menopause showed I had serious bone loss. All my life, I have been small and slender (I've "bulked up" to 105 pounds). I grew up in a poor family, which meant poor nutrition for me in those critical years. After a near-fatal illness in my late teens, I got interested in fitness, and included in my workout some resistance work, largely focused on the upper body. I thought, wrongly as it turns out, that aerobics and stretches would be sufficient for the lower body.

I do not belong to a gym. I own a simple weight bench, three sets of dumbbells, a bar, and 180 pounds of free weights. (I got my husband into resistance work, too, which has shrunk his waistline, and, he says, given him more endurance in general.)

I entered perimenopause early. At 39, my periods began to be erratic. However, since I was sure I was not already menopausal, I gave no thought to issues of menopause until I was 47. By that time, my periods were coming 3–4 months apart, and I went to my internist to get information about HRT. He, as part of gathering information before making a recommendation, sent me for several hormone tests and a bone scan. The hormone tests indicated that I was not menopausal by the technical definition, but the bone scan showed a hip density almost three standard deviations below normal for my age.

It is worth noting at this point that my spine was fine—in fact, slightly above normal in density. According to my doctor, this is an unusual situation, and he put it down to my weight lifting. After discussion, we decided to go with Fosamax, calcium supplementation with vitamin D, and an expanded resistance routine. To be sure the exercises were providing optimum support for my whole skeleton, especially the hips, I went to a physical therapy clinic and developed a routine with their exercise specialist. (For me, learning the correct technique for efficiency and safety was well worth the money.) The exercises we added were very mild to avoid overstressing the hips, with the understanding that I could build up both weight and repetitions slowly, as the work became too easy. Being a bit of a fanatic, I work out four to six times a week, with a minimum of one day off a week, on the orders of my physical therapist, to allow the muscles to shed some chemical buildup and to heal any small tears.

After 14 months, I was doing all my lower-body work with 10-pound ankle weights on, and, in some cases, additional weights in hand. I went for a second scan, and the results were wonderful. I had regained 16 percent of the density I had lost! My doctor says that is about three times what I could have expected from Fosamax and supplementation alone. After another scan to confirm these results, and comparing me to other patients he was treating the same way, my doctor was convinced that the difference was, indeed, the weight work.

I spend most of my waking hours in front of a computer—not a very active lifestyle, I admit. I do walk almost everywhere I go when it isn't winter. Since I started this new weights workout I can, however, lift heavy objects more easily, have seen a noticeable improvement in my general mood and confidence, and have noticed that my endurance has definitely improved, as has my general health (I am just getting over my first cold in over a year, and it lasted only three days). For what it is worth, my bust measurement has increased as I've built up my pecs, and that sag that comes with age has lifted noticeably. As the shape of my body overall changed, a lot of my clothes stopped fitting, and I needed to get a new wardrobe—just a warning for anyone who becomes a fanatic like me!

Because I have some unfortunate reactions to Fosamax (especially reflux), I want to get off it as soon as possible. However, given the results, and some indications in the recent literature that simply quitting Fosamax results in a rapid loss of any gains seen from the drug, I am staying on it for another year, then will gradually cut down. I am also now fully menopausal, so have begun HRT, which I hope will be sufficient to maintain any gains after I stop taking Fosamax. In the meantime, I am also continuing my workouts. Whatever else I might be doing, the initial spine measurement and the increase in hip density—not to mention the new shape of my body—have convinced me that they are worth it.

Chapter 17

Yoga Workout

Yoga focuses on strength, balance, and flexibility, which are important not only for building bone but also for preventing falls and injury. (If you had low bone density, but never fell or broke a bone, you'd be able to maintain reasonably good health.) The added benefit of relaxation and stress reduction makes it a worthwhile addition to your repertoire. No matter what other kind of exercise you favor, strength training and yoga practice (or tai chi or qi gong, which provide similar benefits) will improve your performance—or prepare you for new kinds of movement.

Even at a very basic level, yoga is an excellent way to stretch. A simple routine is enough to increase your flexibility, balance, and strength, and following the directions here will get you that. But the ancient traditions of yoga include relaxation and breathing techniques, and the best way to learn about the full scope of yoga philosophy is to take a class. A good teacher individualizes each movement for each student, as necessary, which is particularly important if you already have low bone density. (In which case, you should consult with your doctor before starting any exercise program, including yoga.) Learning from an expert is the best way to work most effectively and safely. You might want to try a video or book, though of course they won't be personalized. You should never feel pain in any yoga posture, and if you do, you need to stop or adjust.

Below you will find a series of exercises recommended by yoga instructors Alice Cassman and Shelly Greenberg specifically for preventing low bone density and the risk of fracture. They are a good way to introduce yourself to yoga. They'd be ideal for practicing at home between classes or on their own.

The first three are aimed at your spine, and you should consider doing them daily, as they take just a few minutes and don't require any special clothing or equipment. You don't even need to warm up before doing these gentle movements. You could do them on your coffee break—and still have time to go down the hall to the water cooler afterward.

QUICK BACK ENERGIZER

To increase circulation in and promote the health of the spine, you should move all of it in six directions each day: bending forward and back; leaning left and right; and twisting left and right. The following set of exercises incorporates all those movements and can be done while sitting on the floor, or on a chair, preferably one without arms. Do this set on its own or incorporate it into a longer yoga workout. As with any exercise or stretch, you should move only to the normal limits of motion—never force it.

Forward and Backward Bends

PURPOSE: To keep the spine limber and strong.

START POSITION: Sitting on the floor in a comfortable cross-legged position or sitting on a chair.

THE MOTION:

INHALE: Raise hands in front of face, palms in.

EXHALE: Lower chin to chest.

INHALE: Raise face and arms, arching in upper back (elbows will point in front of you).

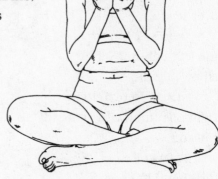

EXHALE: Return to start position. Repeat 3–5 times.

STYLE POINTS: Keep your torso erect and long, as if you were lengthening the spine from the crown of the head.

Side Leans

PURPOSE: To keep the spine limber and strong.

START POSITION: Sitting on the floor in a comfortable cross-legged position, or sitting on a chair, with arms at sides, palms on the floor or chair seat.

THE MOTION:

INHALE: Extend right arm to the side, reaching out through fingers, and raise it overhead.

EXHALE: Lean to the left, bending left elbow slightly.

INHALE: Return to upright position, with arm still raised.

EXHALE: Return hand to floor.

Repeat 3–5 times on this side, then do the same for the other side.

STYLE POINTS: Keep your torso erect and long, as if you were lengthening the spine from the crown of the head.

Twists

PURPOSE: To keep the spine limber and strong.

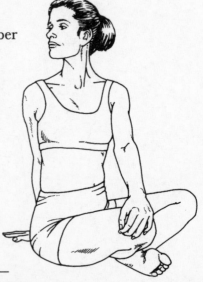

START POSITION: Sitting on the floor in a comfortable cross-legged position, or sitting on a chair with knees hip-width apart.

THE MOTION:

EXHALE: Bring right hand to left knee.

INHALE: Sweep left arm behind— place hand on floor palm down or fingers in a tepee with fingers pointed away from body.

EXHALE: Twist hips, ribs, and shoulders toward your left arm. Keep your head in line with your shoulders. You can press with your right hand to increase the twist once you are comfortable in this position. Stay and breathe.

INHALE: Turn head over right shoulder; stay and breathe.

INHALE: Look left—eyes in opposition to head; stay and breathe.

INHALE: Release and come back to center.

Repeat on the other side.

STYLE POINTS: Keep your torso erect and long, as if you were lengthening the spine from the crown of the head. Keep your chin over the center of your chest. Turning the head in the direction of the twist gives the illusion of more progress, but it doesn't really do anything for the spine.

RELAXING BACK WARM-UP

The next two exercises are good for warming up at the beginning of a yoga session or for relaxing the back anytime it is tense (including in the middle of a yoga routine). You'll probably want to work on a padded surface, like a carpeted floor or a mat.

Back Warm-up

PURPOSE: Releasing tension in the back.

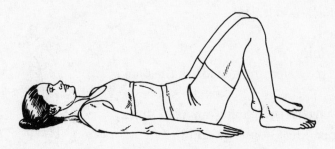

START POSITION: Lying on your back, with knees bent and apart, feet flat on the floor hip distance apart, arms extended by your sides so your hands are near your hips.

THE MOTION:

INHALE: As your chest fills with air, note that your back arches slightly. Just notice the natural movement—don't do anything else.

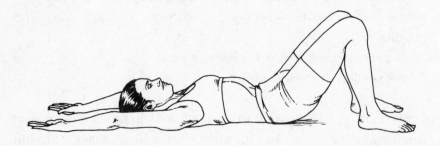

EXHALE: Notice how your back flattens against the floor as you breathe out, and again, just take note, don't do anything else.

Repeat several times, focusing on the breath, then add arm and hip movement:

INHALE: Lift both arms up and over your head

EXHALE: Lower both arms and contract abdominals and buttocks to lengthen spine and rotate hips upward (a "pelvic tilt"). This is a very small movement.

INHALE: Raise arms again, maintaining the pelvic tilt.

EXHALE: Lower arms and release.

Repeat several times. When you are done, move your feet slightly wider than hip distance apart, let knees lean against each other, and relax until any tension in your lower back is released.

Spine Roll

PURPOSE: Releasing tension in the back.

START POSITION: Lying on your back, bend one knee at a time and bring each in to your chest.

Cross your ankles, and place one hand on each knee, ankle, or foot.

THE MOTION: Begin a gentle rocking motion along the length of your spine:

INHALE: Lift hips (knees move toward chest).

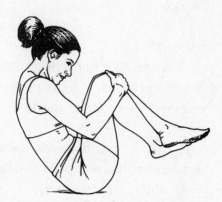

EXHALE: Lower feet toward floor.

Gradually increase the rocking motion, until eventually you rock forward into a sitting position, with your feet on the floor and the torso upright.

STYLE POINTS: Try to make the rocking motion as smooth as possible. Don't yank on your ankles and feet in an attempt to gather momentum.

YOGA WORKOUT FOR BONE HEALTH

The following exercises, combined with the basic poses, above, provide a complete yoga workout, with focus on your back, spine, and hips. They incorporate all six directions of spinal movement. With this workout, you'll be improving your strength, flexibility, and balance. Yoga is thousands of years old and encompasses a seemingly endless variety of poses. You can start with what is here, but, again, taking a class will make sure you use the correct technique for safety and effectiveness and will expose you to a wider range of yoga possibilities. If you do take a class, you might want to continue doing this series at home for additional focus on the areas that are so important when you have a particular concern about bone density. When working on the floor, use a mat or exercise in a carpeted room.

Chest Expander

PURPOSE: To open the chest and strengthen the back.

START POSITION: Can be done sitting or standing. If you sit in a chair, turn sideways so the back of the chair won't interfere with your movement. Or use a stool. Bring your palms together behind your buttocks and interlace your fingers.

THE MOTION:

INHALE: As your chest fills with air, you should feel the front of the chest expand; squeeze your shoulder blades together to increase the stretch.

EXHALE: Extend hands back, keeping elbows and wrists soft (that should bring shoulder blades closer together).

INHALE: Raise your hands, keeping shoulder blades squeezed.

EXHALE: Lower hands and arms.

Repeat three times. Keeping your hands behind your back, release your fingers and interlace them again with the other thumb on top. Repeat the movement sequence three times with the hands in this second, less familiar position.

Hip Opener

PURPOSE: To increase hip flexibility.

START POSITION: Lying on your back, bend your knees and bring them—one at a time—into your chest.

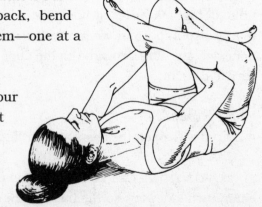

THE MOTION: Place your right ankle on your left knee, pointing your right knee out to the side. Clasp both hands behind your left thigh, next to the knee, and using gentle tension, pull the knee farther into your chest. Use your right elbow to push the right knee farther out to the side. Release.

Repeat several times, then switch to the other side.

STYLE POINTS: You should feel this stretch along the back of your left leg, and all along the outside of your right hip and leg.

Cat

PURPOSE: To promote back suppleness and strength.

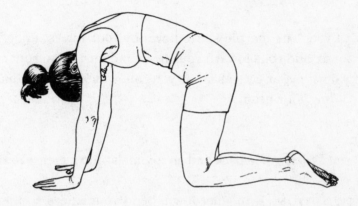

START POSITION: On hands and knees, knees slightly separated, hands slightly wider than shoulder distance apart with fingers spread and pointing straight ahead. The inside of the elbows should be facing each other.

THE MOTION:

EXHALE: Pull belly muscles in, round lower back, relax neck, and let head drop.

INHALE: Keeping the lower back rounded as much as you can, reach forward with your chin gradually, until you have an arch in the upper back.

Repeat five or six times.

STYLE POINTS: On the "inhale" portion of this movement, pretend to follow, with your eyes and head, a marble slowly rolling away in

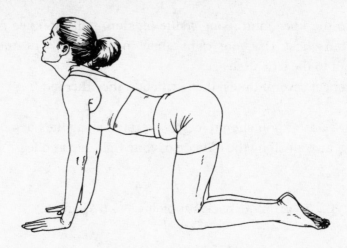

front of you. The marble starts down by your knees, underneath your torso, and rolls toward your head and past it, in front of you. Follow it with your eyes as far as you can, which will eventually require lifting your head.

Bow

PURPOSE: Strengthen back and abdominals, and increase flexibility.

START POSITION: Lying facedown, bend your knees so the soles of your feet are parallel to the ceiling. Reach back with your arms and hold on to your ankles.

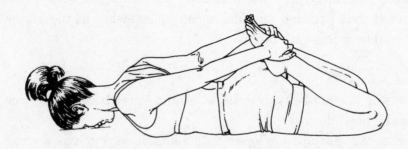

THE MOTION:

INHALE: Lift your knees and thighs off the floor; arch your upper back and raise your chest off the floor.

EXHALE: Release.

Repeat several times.

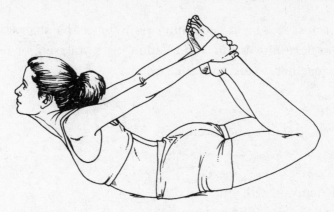

STYLE POINTS: Your chest and knees should be about equally lifted at the peak of this pose.

Cow Face

PURPOSE: Promote flexibility and strength in upper back.

START POSITION: Sitting on the floor in a comfortable cross-legged position on the floor, or sitting on a chair.

THE MOTION: Raise your right arm over-head, bend your elbow, and drop your hand behind your neck, with the palm facing your back. Use your left hand to gently pull your elbow behind your head, letting your right hand drop farther down your back. Lower your left hand and place it behind your back, bending at the elbow, reaching up toward your right hand, with the palm of your left hand facing out.

Try to connect the fingers of both hands in the center of your back.

Stay for several breaths.

Release on an inhale, and repeat on the other side.

STYLE POINTS: Aim for touching your fingertips at first, and as you gain flexibility, try to "hold hands" with yourself, or hook the fingers together, to increase the stretch.

Warrior

PURPOSE: Balance and strength.

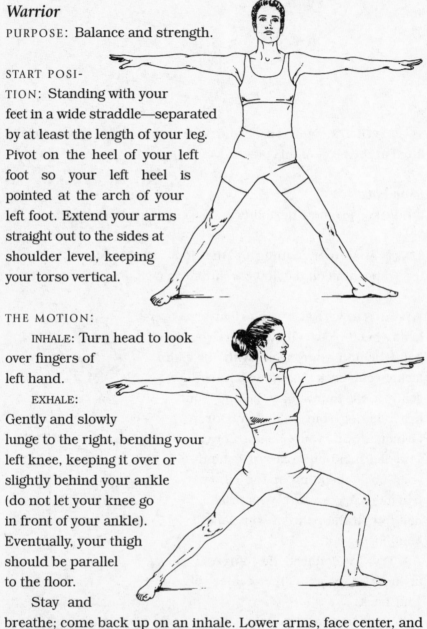

START POSI-
TION: Standing with your feet in a wide straddle—separated by at least the length of your leg. Pivot on the heel of your left foot so your left heel is pointed at the arch of your left foot. Extend your arms straight out to the sides at shoulder level, keeping your torso vertical.

THE MOTION:

INHALE: Turn head to look over fingers of left hand.

EXHALE: Gently and slowly lunge to the right, bending your left knee, keeping it over or slightly behind your ankle (do not let your knee go in front of your ankle). Eventually, your thigh should be parallel to the floor.

Stay and breathe; come back up on an inhale. Lower arms, face center, and step feet together on an exhale.

Repeat on the other side.

STYLE POINTS: If you can't get your thigh parallel to the floor without pushing your knee ahead of the ankle, step your feet farther apart. Keep your torso upright, and do not twist it. Keep the knee of the back leg pointing straight ahead, or turned slightly toward the ceiling; just don't let it collapse down toward the floor.

Tree

PURPOSE: Balance and strength. Hip flexibility.

START POSITION: Standing with your hands chest high, palms together, fingers pointing up.

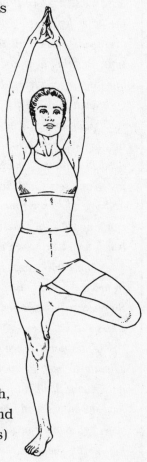

THE MOTION:

BEGINNER: Shift your weight to your right foot. Place the heel of your left foot on top of your right foot.

INTERMEDIATE: Standing on your right leg, bend left leg at the knee, place the sole of the left foot against the inside thigh of the standing leg, turning your knee to the outside.

ADVANCED: In the intermediate pose, raise your arms over your head, keeping your palms together.

Stay for several breaths. Repeat, standing on the left foot.

STYLE POINTS: Build your balance, strength, and endurance gradually until you can stand in the tree pose (any of the three variations) for 60 seconds on each leg.

Case in Point: Leah

*E*xperts who insist weight lifting and high-impact exercise are the only ways to build your bones should meet Leah, a swimmer and yoga student. Leah has been doing yoga for years and years, and though she cannot put her feet behind her neck, her flexibility and balance easily match those of the much younger women in her classes, including her granddaughter. Sitting cross-legged on the floor, with her torso twisted past 90 degrees? No problem. Standing on one foot, with the other foot resting against the knee of the standing leg, arms raised overhead? She's built up to holding this "Tree" pose for a minute at a time. Bending over to grasp her ankles, pulling her chest in closer to her knees for a good lower-back stretch? Piece of cake.

Leah is 87 years old. She stands straight and tall in her Birkenstocks, her long gray hair loosely piled on top of her head. She leads walking tours around the historic district every other weekend. She's a devoted gardener. She happily reports the tomato plants she started from last year's seeds are already up, but it is flowers that are her true pride and joy. The only time she misses her yoga class is for the two or three camping trips she takes each year. The last one she spent in a tent on the beach on a Caribbean island.

Along with yoga, Leah is a master swimmer and regularly competes in meets. "I don't always win," she admits, "but I do it for the fun of it." She keeps in shape for racing by swimming laps for 45 minutes three times a week.

She's never taken hormone replacement therapy, but she does take calcium to keep her bones strong. She watches what she eats, but "I'm not systematic about it," she says. She eats mostly wholesome, nutritious food she enjoys, and is a believer in moderation in all things. A bone scan years ago showed healthy bones, and since she hasn't lost a millimeter of her height, she hasn't worried about it since. She hands part of the credit to "good genes," but her active lifestyle, healthy diet, and vigorous exercise have clearly done their work.

RELAXATION

Many yoga classes end with a full-body relaxation, sometimes with guided visualization. You can learn the details of how to do that in a class or another book, but here I do want to give you the basic position. It is a wonderful way to relax because it allows your spine to be in a neutral position, and frees it from the usual direction of gravitational pull. In this position you can also release tension in muscles in every area of the body. This makes it a good choice before and after any workout or for a 5-minute "time-out" in the middle of a day.

Lie flat on the floor without a pillow. Extend your legs so they do not touch each other at any point, and place your arms slightly away from your body, resting your hands beside your hips, palms up. If this makes your lower back uncomfortable, bend one knee at a time and place your feet flat on the floor, slightly wider than hip distance apart, and lean your knees against each other. Stay for at least 5 minutes. Relax and feel your breath go in and out of all parts of your body. Focus on the breath and let the body reap the benefits—don't focus on the body parts or try moving them, but follow the breath. This is an ideal time to practice the "relaxation response" (see Chapter 21), or any other meditative or visualization technique that calms and centers you.

❈ ❈

WEEK 4 ACTION PLAN

1. Begin the Bone Density Diet, using the first week's menus (with any modifications you planned last week).
2. What exercise do you get in a typical week?
3. Try something new (new move, new class, new video, new type of exercise, new piece of equipment) each day this week. Add something into your usual routine, or switch for at least a day to something else, just to see how you like it. Or try walking the half-mile to the drugstore instead of driving, or climbing the stairs to your office instead of using the elevator, or going for a walk with a friend on your lunch hour instead of meeting at a fast-food restaurant.
4. If you don't have a regular exercise routine, or if what you

usually do doesn't include an aerobic component, take three 30-minute walks this week, or five 20-minute walks.

5. Do the strength-training workout twice this week, and for the remaining weeks of the program. In just those three weeks, you should feel a difference in how much weight you can handle or how many repetitions of each movement you can do.

6. Do the yoga workout at least once this week, and for the remaining weeks of the program. That should be enough for the movements to start to feel familiar, and if you do it twice a week, you should begin to notice some difference in balance and flexibility. If you like the movement, consider working it into your regular routine. Take a class to learn more, or check a video out of the library.

7. Clarify your general exercise goals. What do you want exercise to do for you? Help you lose weight? Maintain your current weight? Build muscle? Lose fat? Build bone? Improve balance? Increase flexibility? We all want some combination of these things, but zeroing in on your primary focus will allow you to choose your exercise program accordingly.

8. Figure out if you should have any restrictions (jogging is not good for an old knee injury, or whatever), given your medical history, and design around them. If your health care professional gives you the green light, just do what you enjoy most, and mix it up.

9. Make a general schedule of what sort of workout you will do and when. One of the samples at the end of Chapter 16 may suit you, but likely you'll want to make some adjustments to fit into your life.

WEEK 4 FOCUS

- Experiment with different types of exercise and different forms of movement to discover what is right for you.
- Create a fitness plan.
- Schedule exercise into your life.
- Begin the Bone Density Diet.

10. Now get specific. What kind of exercise will you do? For how long? On which days? At what time? Where? With whom? Will your aerobics be jogging or swimming? Will your weight training be full-body each time, or would you rather do upper body one day and lower the next? What kind of moving meditation will you choose on which day— qi gong or yoga or mindful walking? Will you ride the bike for 20 minutes? Forty? Will you be in a class or on your own? At the gym? Alone or with a partner? Who?

11. Create specific exercise goals (on the order of "walk three days a week, lift weights twice a week, take a weekly tai chi class"). Do what you like to do, so you will do it for a lifetime.

12. Block out the specific times for exercise on your daily calendar as you would any other appointment. Make specific dates with yourself for exercise in your regular calendar. Block out the times called for in your general schedule for at least the next month in your calendar. Then keep your appointments!

13. Spend some of your free time this weekend on a physical activity. Learning to incorporate movement into your usual life—not just as special "workouts" set apart from the rest of your day—is the best way to stay healthy over the long haul.

14. Explore other forms of moving meditation, even just plain meditation. Mindful walking you can do on your own, so try it at least once this week in addition to your regular workout or instead of what you usually do. Or try making one of your regular workouts mindful. Instead of reading or watching TV or listening to music on your headphones while you pedal the bike or use the stairclimber, try mentally focusing on what you're doing, keeping your mind in the present and calling it back from any attempts it makes to stray to the argument you had with your boss or the phone call you forgot to return or what you'll make for dinner. If tai chi or qi gong appeal to you, look into classes or books or videos to introduce yourself to a new form of movement.

15. Buy any equipment you need (weights, or a loose, comfortable workout outfit, or gym membership, or sign up for a class, or a notebook to log your results in, or a session with a personal trainer to show you the ropes, or a book or video to teach you a workout routine). Try out the equipment at a gym or in the store or at a friend's before you buy—the larger the purchase, the more important this is. To make a good investment, make sure anything you buy will (1) be something you will use and (2) will help you achieve your goals. If you want to build muscle, a bicycle won't help, but a Soloflex-type system can. If you want to lose fat, any aerobic exercise will get you there, so you don't need anything fancy unless that's what will motivate you. If you want to lose fat and increase muscle all over the body, a treadmill will leave out your upper-body muscles, but a rowing or cross-country skiing machine would fill the bill. Get the simplest things you need—spending more money or getting the most famous brand name or being loaded with electronic gizmos isn't going to get you any fitter if those things do nothing more than collect dust.

16. Start slow and work up to your goals gradually. This is a lifetime plan, not a one-week, how-far/fast-can-I-go test.

17. Looking forward to next week's diet, make any revisions to the second week's menus that you need to make the perfect fit. Make a shopping list of everything you'll need—and go get it.

❈ ❈ ❈ ❈ ❈ ❈ ❈ ❈ ❈ ❈ ❈ ❈ ❈ ❈ ❈ ❈ ❈ ❈ ❈

BALANCE YOUR HORMONES

Hormones have an important role in many aspects of overall health, and maintaining their delicate balance is key in keeping your bones strong. With the hormonal shifts of perimenopause and menopause, all women should carefully consider the full range of options for easing the transition. This section covers traditional prescriptions—and their benefits and drawbacks—as well as a range of alternatives.

Hot flashes or other more obvious symptoms, like night sweats and mood swings, may be uppermost in your mind when you begin perimenopause, but using hormones, whether they are "natural" or synthetic, is just as important for less obvious problems, including bone density. Keep in mind that the goal should be to balance *all* of the hormones, not just to get estrogen levels, or even the ratio of estrogen to progesterone, within normal ranges.

At the end of this section, the Action Plan helps you sort through all the information to customize a hormone balance plan that's right for your life.

Chapter 18

Hormone Replacement Therapy

For many women at high risk for osteoporosis, or who already have significant bone loss, or who had an early menopause (because of surgery or any other reason), HRT is the best regimen for health. When your bones are at risk, your entire life—and lifestyle—is at risk. Unless there is a medical reason, like having breast cancer, that trumps all other concerns, HRT is an extremely valuable adjunct to proper diet and exercise in the battle to keep your bones healthy. (Later in this chapter, you'll see that not even having breast cancer is a reason to avoid all traditional forms of HRT, or the alternatives described in the next chapter.)

Even with excellent nutrition and diligent exercise, the drop in estrogen at menopause presents a major challenge to your bones. The first line of defense against increased bone loss that every woman should consider is hormone replacement therapy (HRT). Its protective effect on bones is remarkable, especially when you are also following a healthy diet and exercise plan similar to the one laid out in this program. There are also very real—and really well publicized—risks associated with taking HRT, and it is not, medically speaking, for everyone. Many people have specific medical reasons *not* to take HRT. Many women have their own objections to a prescription drug meant to be taken for a lifetime for what is not, after all, a disease, but rather a natural part of the life cycle. So whether or not to take HRT is a very personal question that requires careful individual evaluation of your own situation.

BENEFITS OF HRT

The potential benefits of HRT are enormous. We have nothing else currently available that is anywhere near as effective at slowing or stopping the bone loss women experience as their periods stop. In addition, estrogen supplements offer protection against heart disease—still the number one killer for all Americans—lowering cholesterol levels, boosting "good cholesterol," and preventing arteriosclerosis ("hardening of the arteries"). It reduces your risk of stroke and cataracts, and relieves osteoarthritis symptoms. There is some good evidence it helps prevent, delay, or at least mitigate Alzheimer's disease, and it decreases your risk of colon cancer by 50 percent. It also relieves many of the unpleasant and disruptive symptoms of menopause, including hot flashes, vaginal dryness, difficulty sleeping, short-term memory decline, skin aging, tooth loss, and mood swings. And maintaining estrogen levels also keeps your skin younger looking. It is as close as we have to an elixir of youth, or so it seems from the marketing materials.

The drug companies are right to tout the fact that taking hormone replacement therapy can decrease bone loss by 30 to 100 percent. Taking it cuts your risk of fractures at least in half, not to mention cutting your risk of heart disease and death from heart disease in half, too. That's a powerful one-two punch, and accounts for why HRT is always near the top of the list when you look up the most commonly prescribed drugs, or which drugs bring the most money into manufacturers' coffers each year.

REALITY CHECK

But let's have a reality check about what HRT, which is starting to look like a magic bullet, can really do. Low bone density is about a lot more than low estrogen—hip fracture rates rise well before menopause for Caucasian women, when their estrogen levels are still high. About half your lifetime bone loss occurs before menopause begins, and taking estrogen around menopause won't do anything about that. Many, many of the more than a million fractures from low bone density that occur each year are in women who are taking estrogen. Up to 30 percent of women do not lose significant amounts of bone after menopause, and for them, the risks of HRT may outweigh the benefits. For women who do experience a dramatic drop in bone density, estrogen does slow bone loss, but the jury is still out about whether it can, on its own, do anything about increasing bone formation or even about limiting the slowdown in that arena. Your Z-score will eventually get back to normal—the level expected for someone of your age—but your T-score, the true measure of healthy bones, may never be reached using HRT alone. HRT can reverse the trend of bone loss, but it can't replace what is already gone. And despite what HRT can do for your heart and how it can prevent strokes, we also know that smart diet, exercise, and lifestyle choices can do equally well—or better.

Then comes the biggest downside: an increase in cancer risk. Estrogen ups the risk of endometrial cancer by *ten times* when it is prescribed on its own. That's why, for women who have a uterus, it should be taken together with a progestin. The combination of hormones puts the cancer risk back at normal, or is perhaps even protective.

The bigger (though less well documented) fear is of an increase in breast cancer risk. It isn't hard to find alarmists who want to lay every case of breast cancer in this country at the feet of HRT and birth control pills (which are also estrogen based). Some valid controversy does surround the degree of risk involved. Some studies have shown a negligible difference on HRT, but some have shown an increase of up to 30 percent (in women taking hormones for at least five years before age 65—just what most experts generally recommend you do). And some evidence indicates that women who get breast cancer while taking hormones actually have a lower mortality rate than those who get it while not on HRT. If there is an increase in the rate of breast cancer, it is a small one.

TALK TO YOUR DOCTOR

Until recently, everyone agreed that women with breast cancer or already at high risk should steer clear of taking estrogen, though experts make no one clear recommendation regarding everyone else. Now we know there are some forms of estrogen—and other hormones— safe even for breast cancer survivors.

But with the lifetime risk of breast cancer already so high—one in nine women in this country, or over 11 percent, will have it—even a 1 percent change puts the rate up over 14 percent. That's thirty-three more breast cancers detected per thousand women (on top of the 111 you'd already expect).

The key thing to remember—the fact most people overlook— is how much more common heart disease is in women than breast cancer. Breast cancer provokes a more visceral response, but the reality is that the average woman is much more likely to have serious heart disease than to have breast cancer, and far more likely to die from the former than the latter. One of every three women under 40 right now, and one in two women after menopause, will develop heart disease sometime in the future. That's at least *three times* the commonly quoted one-in-nine risk for breast cancer.

More American women die from heart disease each year than anything else (conservative estimates put the numbers at 233,000 of them, vs. 43,000 for breast cancer and 65,000 for hip fracture). Of course, that means different things on a statistical and an individual level. If you are the one with breast cancer, the smaller likelihood of that happening means nothing to you. But since most of us can't reasonably guess ahead of time if we are headed for breast cancer (setting aside those already known to be at high risk), the odds for large groups are the best we have to go on.

Even studies showing an increase in breast cancer in women taking estrogen do *not* show an increase in the death rate. In fact, women who take estrogen turn out to live longer on the whole, probably because of the many health benefits of being on HRT. Part

ISN'T MENOPAUSE SUPPOSED TO MEAN NO MORE PERIODS?

Taking estrogen also means you may resume having periods (if you have a uterus). Though that's not a major health factor, it is a real lifestyle consideration for women who had been eagerly awaiting no longer having to deal with a monthly cycle. Bleeding usually lessens over time, stopping eventually. Using a progestin in combination with estrogen for 12 to 14 days a month (cyclic therapy) for the first two years or so will at least make the bleeding predictable. Then, if you switch to taking a combination of estrogen and progestin every day (continuous therapy), you'll probably stop having periods altogether within a year (80 percent of patients do within six months, and 90 percent within a year). That seems like a reasonable compromise, for the greater good of your bones.

of the confusion may arise from the fact that on HRT, breast cancer seems to appear earlier, but then have a lower recurrence rate.

HOW ESTROGEN WORKS ON BONES

Estrogen controls the effect of parathyroid hormone on osteoclasts, so when estrogen dramatically decreases, the osteoclasts go about the business of breaking bone more rapidly than ever, releasing calcium from the bones back into the blood. A high level of calcium signals the body that no more vitamin D is needed, so no more is converted from the form it is stored in to the form the body actually uses it in. Without vitamin D, calcium from your diet can't be properly absorbed, so there may not be enough for proper bone formation. So this vicious cycle ensures that on top of resorption speeding up, formation also slows down. Your bones get a double whammy. (Osteoblasts, the bone-building cells, also have estrogen receptors, so the hormone probably plays a role there, too, but one that is not yet fully understood.)

Estrogen may play a role, but probably promotes breast cancer that is already there rather than causing a new cancer itself. The most alarming studies were on estrogen alone, so it remains unclear if the addition of progestins mitigates or intensifies any increase in risk. At least one study suggests that your risk will return to normal (if it in fact increased) within five years of discontinuing estrogen use, and other studies show that the higher the lifetime dose of estrogen, the higher the breast cancer risk is.

BONE FORMATION AND BREAKDOWN BY AGE

Depending on your stage of life, your bones will be building up more or less rapidly and breaking down more or less rapidly. As bone building is at its peak, the most important thing is to get bones what they need for healthy growth and density. As bone breakdown speeds up, therapies that slow bone loss and build bone are more important. Match your specific prevention and/or treatment strategies to where you are in the cycle (see chart). The idea is to never let bone breakdown outpace bone formation—or to keep formation as far ahead of breakdown as you can.

	Bone Formation	Bone Breakdown
Childhood	↑ ↑ ↑ ↑	↓
Adolescence	↑ ↑ ↑	↓
Age 30	↑ ↑	↓
Age 40	↑	↓ ↓
Age 50/menopause	↑	↓ ↓
Age 60	↑	↓ ↓ ↓
Age 70	↑	↓ ↓ ↓ ↓

You also have to throw into the mix the various potential side effects of HRT, which run the gamut from weight gain, nausea, vomiting, cramps, breast swelling and tenderness, hair loss, jaundice, irregular and uncontrollable vaginal bleeding, inability to wear contacts, yeast infections, dizziness, loss of sex drive, low blood sugar (making you crave sweets), bloating and headaches to increased risk of gallstones, higher risk of blood clots (which can lead to a stroke or heart attack), endometriosis, high blood pressure, fibrocystic breast disease, depression, liver problems, and fibroids. That's a disheartening list, and on top of that is what progestins can do to you. Even if you experience only a couple of these items, they can make your life miserable. Altering the kind of estrogen you take, the dose you take, the schedule of dosing, or the combination with a progestin may alleviate the side effects, but it may also require a lengthy trial-and-error period. Of course, many women take estrogen with no symptoms whatsoever. Keep in mind that most studies have been done with conjugated estrogen, so other forms, like estradiol, may not have the same side effects.

PRIORITIZE

My advice is to prioritize your own concerns and do your own risk-benefit analysis. Look at what runs in your family, paying particular attention to your mother, grandmother, and sisters. Evaluate all your risk factors. Factor in your attitude toward drugs in general and toward menopause. If you are already experiencing symptoms from menopause, rate how bad (or bearable) they are. Keep in mind all that you have learned in this book about the importance of good bone density to overall health, longevity, and quality of life. Consider your bone density screening results, if you have them (and get them if you don't!). Look at your family history of heart disease and your own risk of coronary artery disease. Be realistic about the possible increase in risk of breast cancer, but don't take an alarmist attitude. Finally, women in surgical menopause (having had their ovaries removed) lose bone twice as fast as other women at menopause, so estrogen would be even more beneficial to them. Women who have had a hysterectomy but kept their ovaries still experience accelerated bone loss (though not as rapid as without ovaries) and should also give extra consideration to taking HRT. When you've totted it all up, talk with your health care practitioner about what is right for you.

"Patient-Specific Decisions About Hormone Replacement Therapy in Postmenopausal Women," an article in the prestigious *Journal of the American Medical Association (JAMA)* published April 9, 1997, enumerates and weights each health risk to be considered in the decision of whether to use HRT. If that decision is plaguing you, it might be worth looking it up and matching your own situation to the article's formulas. Check through the *Index Medicus*, or ask your doctor to help you out. The article is as detailed and specific an approach to the subject as I've seen—and backed up by research, to boot! If you do look it up, bear in mind that the authors conclude that very few women should *not* take HRT and are ready to sign up the other 99 percent of the population immediately. (More aggressive even than the figure commonly bandied about that 10 percent of women either shouldn't take estrogen because of medical contraindications or won't tolerate estrogen when they do take it.) As they see it, even a lot of women with increased breast cancer risk would benefit from HRT, if you look at the statistical picture. Let's just say you shouldn't count on this article to talk you out of hormones, if that's what you're leaning toward.

The researchers conclude that HRT would increase longevity for just about every woman, adding three years (or even more) to her life, depending on her risk factors for heart disease and cancer. Particularly for anyone with at least one risk factor for heart disease (including high blood pressure, high cholesterol levels, or high ratios of "bad" to "good" cholesterol, diabetes, obesity, and smoking—which is more than half of women), HRT is beneficial, even for women with a relatively high risk of breast cancer. The only exception they make is for someone with no risk factors for heart disease or fractures, who has two relatives with breast cancer. Whatever vanishingly small portion of the population falls into that category (they estimate 1 percent) should steer clear of taking estrogen, they say.

My Story: Ann

I really wanted a "natural" menopause. I didn't want to put something into my body every day for the rest of my life that by Mother Nature's design wasn't meant to be there. Of course, my regular doctor recommended hormone replacement therapy to me as soon as my periods became irregular, though I don't remember her making any connection to bone density, or my family history of osteoporosis, and she certainly never sent me for a bone scan. But as I said, I was determined to let my body do its own thing, so I declined a prescription.

But after a couple years, when my periods stopped altogether, the fun really began. I had hot flashes, of course, and night sweats that drenched the sheets. I was gaining weight no matter what I ate or didn't eat. I became depressed as I never have been in my entire life. Worst of all, I couldn't sleep (no wonder I was depressed!), and developed the bad habit of lying awake and counting up all the days of my life ruined from lack of sleep.

I went to my chiropractor, and a homeopath he recommended, for help with my symptoms. You know, they always tell you what they do is good for everything. And truthfully, chiropractors have been an enormous help to me with other health issues. But nothing helped the symptoms I was having now.

After a year, I couldn't stand it anymore, and called up my doctor for a prescription. I was ready to try anything! Within the first month on a standard dose of estrogen and progestin, my insomnia was gone and I was sleeping through the night and generally feeling like my regular self again.

I never experienced any unpleasant side effects from taking the hormones. But after a while, I wanted to try taking lower doses, to make sure I was giving my body what it needed and nothing more. My doctor gave me the go-ahead to try taking my pills every other day, with a phytoestrogen supplement on the off days. I was pleased with the plan, but my sleeping problems came back right away. I'd already been through enough, and then found relief with HRT, that I didn't have patience now for enduring any more in an attempt to just lower the numbers on the prescription form. So I made my peace with the standard dose.

I figured if what I really wanted was what was right for my body, well, I had found it. Just not in the place I expected to. I also learned more about the benefits of HRT beyond relief of menopause symptoms, and in particular the protection estrogen seems to offer against Alzheimer's disease. My mother suffered for more than ten years with Alzheimer's, and if there was any way I could spare myself and my family that, I would do it. The protection for bones, too, was important to me, since my mom and grandmothers had osteoporosis.

After several years of taking hormones, I saw a sign at my local drugstore advertising a day where they would be doing inexpensive bone density screening. Because of my family history, I decided to get tested. Once I saw the results that said I still had the bone density of a 30-year-old, I never thought about giving up the hormones again.

And one thing, at least, is still the "natural" way: because I take estrogen and a progestin every day, I do not get a period.

The other risk factors for breast cancer they take into account include the age at which you gave birth for the first time, if ever (younger is better, for this purpose); your history of breast biopsies with benign results; and the age of your first period (older is better). The risks they considered for hip fracture include having a mother who fractured a hip, having elevated thyroid hormone levels (natural or synthetic), taking benzodiazepines, being sedentary, having a fast resting pulse, having lost a large amount of weight after age 25, and being very tall. They also considered rating yourself as having fair or poor health, and having low bone density, as major risk factors.

On her 50th birthday, the average woman can look forward to between twenty-two and thirty-four more years on this planet. HRT adds at least six months to that tally, and often more like three years. (This study only looked at women who began taking hormones right around the time of menopause, so it can't draw any conclusions about women who take HRT before menopause or more than five years after.) That's a 15 percent increase for those at greatest risk for heart disease and lowest risk of breast

Case in Point: Elise

*O*ne of my patients started on estrogen and progestin as she neared her fiftieth birthday and her periods became few and far between. After Elise went through menopause, a bone density scan showed her Z-score (comparing her to other women her age) was actually positive, and her T-score (comparing her to peak bone density) was just −.3. In the midst of what would otherwise have been the most rapid bone loss of her life, Elise was sitting pretty thanks to HRT.

In this case, I know HRT was largely responsible for Elise's relatively dense bones because although she took calcium supplements fairly regularly, her diet and exercise habits were otherwise far from ideal. Her job, in addition to being extremely stressful in general, required constant travel. Because of her schedule, she had long ago given up on the idea of a regular workout. Elise felt she couldn't really eat right, since so many of her meals came from vending machines or room service or while dashing through the airport.

For all these reasons, Elise had room for improvement. She began taking a range of other supplements along with her calcium, and starting paying attention to what she ate. She couldn't always get all the calcium and other nutrients she would like (which is where the supplements come in), but found it was just as easy to grab a yogurt as anything else to eat, and began carrying healthier snacks along with her in her travels. She also committed to a walking program she could do wherever she was, and began making inquiries about gym facilities at the hotels she was destined for.

If she sticks to those things, I've no doubt that her next bone scan will show her density to be right up there with the densest of 30-year-olds.

cancer. The only women who wouldn't reap increased longevity would be those at low risk for heart disease and high risk for breast cancer. The bigger the risk of heart disease, the bigger the benefit of HRT. But it has to be a long-term commitment. Half the increase in longevity accrues to you after ten years of taking hormones, and three quarters of it after twenty years. Trying it for a few months or a year, or until your hot flashes stop, won't give you the most important benefits.

HOW TO TAKE HRT

Most advocates recommend taking HRT beginning when your periods become irregular and continuing throughout your life. At the least, you'd want to be covered during the ten-year period following menopause, when bone loss is the fastest. (Women who have their hormone-producing ovaries removed experience a similar rapid rate of bone loss for four to six years after surgery.) If you start taking HRT after you've reached menopause, you'll still benefit, but your overall results will never be as good as if you had started a little before your last period. Impressive results have been proven after just six months of using HRT. But short-term use of HRT, while it may relieve your most troublesome menopausal symptoms as your body transitions, will not give you any of the major benefits of long-term use. In fact, when you stop taking hormones, bone loss starts up again right away. Within seven years (or sooner, depending on how long you've been on HRT), your bones will be the same as those of a woman similar to you who never took hormones.

> **TALK TO YOUR DOCTOR**
>
> Discontinuing HRT can bring about bone loss as dramatic as menopause with no supplemental hormones.

On the other hand, even women over 70 who have never before taken hormone replacement can benefit from starting on estrogen, as can women who already have osteoporosis (particularly when used in conjunction with one of the therapies described in the next chapter). In fact, some studies show the best results in women the farthest past menopause (setting aside the group that hands down does the best: those who take it immediately upon reaching menopause). After age 65, most breast cancers that occur are less influenced by estrogen levels generally, and so will be less affected by the taking of estrogen supplements. So once you are

Case in Point: Sophie

*S*ophie, in her mid-50s, came to see me because her menopausal symptoms were out of control. She had fibroids, and had heard that estrogen often caused fibroids to increase in size, so she hadn't wanted to take hormone replacement therapy. But she was having a rough time of it without supplemental hormones, so we discussed her options. I explained that fibroids would not grow with the over-the-counter phytoestrogen ipriflavone; or the natural progesterone cream sometimes recommended to combat menopausal symptoms; or testosterone, which sometimes relieves menopausal symptoms; or Evista, the newest drug being sold to treat osteoporosis, which had many estrogen-like properties. My belief is that fibroids are unlikely to grow with estriol and estrone, either, though I haven't seen any official studies on the matter as yet. Many of my patients with fibroids, or heavy uterine bleeding at menopause, or on Premarin, have had success by changing the type or form of estrogen they use, so I suggested that option to Sophie as well. I encouraged her to look for a way to balance her hormones that would relieve her symptoms and protect her heart and bones, as I was sure we could find one that wouldn't make her fibroids any worse, though it might take a bit of experimenting to hit on the best one. Finally, I explained that though estradiol (the usual prescription at menopause) is likely to make fibroids grow, not all fibroids are estrogen sensitive, so you could always try it and see, dropping estradiol if you did develop unwanted side effects.

Sophie—a nurse—was most comfortable with the most mainstream option, and decided to try an estrogen patch, with an oral progestin, despite the risk of aggravating her fibroids. She also started taking calcium and vitamin D, and took up a regular program of weight-bearing exercise to protect her bones. She had no side effects from the hormones, including no bleeding (a common sign of large fibroids). I monitored her fibroids via sonogram, which confirmed they did not change in size. And the menopausal symptoms that brought her into my office in the first place also disappeared.

far enough past menopause, your personal calculus of the risks and benefits of HRT may change. If you've avoided HRT to that point, but find you are still at high risk, you may want to reconsider.

SORTING THROUGH JUST WHAT HORMONES "HRT" MEANS FOR YOU

Several types and forms of estrogen are available (with and without several varieties of progestins or progesterone), in a variety of doses. There are no hard-and-fast rules about which way of taking estrogen is right for who, and you may have to experiment a bit to figure out what works best for you. Your needs may change as time goes on; what works, say, during your transition to menopause may not be the best thing for you a few years later, when a much smaller dose will probably do.

Estrogen comes in pills, patches, creams, and now even a ring that is placed inside the vagina. It can be synthetic or natural. Different forms may help some problems and symptoms more effectively than others. Pills and patches have FDA approval for osteoporosis prevention (give appropriate dosages— see below), but creams and the ring are localized and come in extremely low doses, so they are more targeted to specific issues and won't benefit bones as much. For that same reason, they are less likely to increase your risk of breast cancer. That won't do your bones any good, but may still allow you to relieve some menopausal symptoms.

Another of the twists and turns on the road to making decisions about using estrogen is that the more you take and the longer you take it, the more your risk of breast cancer goes up. The trick is to get enough estrogen to receive the benefits, but not so much that side effects become too risky or too unpleasant. For protection of bone in the hip and spine, the standard daily dose is .625 mg of "conjugated estrogen" (the kind made from horse urine, brand name Premarin), which is the most common prescription. For "micronized estradiol" (pill form, brand name Estrace) the usual dose is .5–2 mg, which is proven to protect the spine, with less clear results at the hip. For estradiol in a patch

TYPE OF ESTROGEN	FORM	BRAND NAMES	COMMON DOSE
Conjugated estrogen	Pills	Premarin	.625 mg daily (available in doses up to 2.5 mg daily)
	Vaginal cream	Premarin	.5–2 g daily (.3125–1.25 mg estrogen)
	Combination pill	Prempro, Premphase	.625 mg daily estrogen and 2.5–5 mg of a progestin
Micronized estradiol Estradiol	Pills Patch	Estrace Climara, Estraderm, Vivelle, Alora, FemPatch Estrace	.5–2 mg 0.05–0.1 mg once or twice weekly
	Combination patch	CombiPatch	.05 mg estrogen and .14–.25 mg of a progestin
	Vaginal cream		1 g 1–3 times weekly (.1 mg estrogen)
	Vaginal ring	Estring	1 ring every 3 months (2 mg estrogen)
Estropipate	Pills Vaginal cream	Ogen, Ortho-Est Ogen	.625–1.25 mg 2–4 g daily (3–6 mg estrogen)
Ethinyl estradiol	Pills	Estinyl (sold under many brands of birth control pills)	.03–mg
Esterified estrogen	Pills	Estratab, Menest	0.3–2.5 mg daily

TALK TO YOUR DOCTOR

On a standard dose of estrogen, there can be a tenfold difference between individuals in the resulting estrogen levels in the blood. That is, you might take Premarin at the usual dose and be just fine, and your neighbor may take the same thing and have ten times less—or ten times more—working in her body, and either still having menopausal symptoms unrelieved or side effects from the estrogen itself. That's why it is important to have your own hormone levels measured before you start taking any supplemental hormones, and why it is important to have them checked again once you've been on medication for a while, to make sure you're getting the effects you want.

(brand name Climara, Estraderm, Vivelle), .05–1 mg daily is the usual dose and is protective of both the back and hip. And 0.625 mg a day of estrone sulfate protects the spine but not necessarily the hip. Estropipate (Ogen and Ortho-Est) requires .625–3 mg to work in the vertebrae, but 1.25 mg to help in the hip. Ethinyl estradiol (Estinyl) is usually prescribed at .03–.1 mg a day for the spine, and "esterified estrogens" (Estratab) at .3–2.5 mg, though in both cases the results at the hip are unknown.

Heavy women may be able to use smaller doses because estrogen is made and stored in body fat, so their own supplies may be higher. Thin women and smokers, on the other hand, may need higher doses to realize all the benefits to their bones. Smokers should try the patches, as transdermal estrogen may be more effective for them than pills.

BONE BOOSTERS

I had one 40-year-old patient with the bones of a 20-year-old. Her secret? The many years she'd used "the pill" for contraception.

TALK TO YOUR DOCTOR

For HRT for women with a uterus, a low dose of progestin should be added to estrogen, usually 2.5–5 mg, and sometimes up to 10 mg, a day for at least part of each month. It definitely does not interfere with estrogen's bone protection abilities. It may even boost them, and progestins alone have been shown to build bone density. There's no good evidence yet about progestins' effect on estrogen's effect on blood lipid levels, but the level of overall protection does not seem to change when they are taken in combination. Most important, progestin prevents the increase in risk of endometrial cancer.

Take the smallest doses that work for you in order to limit side effects large and small. Taking calcium supplements will help you reap the full benefits of HRT even at lower doses. We know low doses can help your bones in part because of the effects on bone density seen in patients who have taken oral contraceptives for years. Birth control pills are estrogen based and use much smaller amounts than HRT. Even so, women get increased bone density as a side benefit.

No matter what hormones you are taking (or not taking), you should be following the other guidelines in this book to maximize the benefits and minimize any risks. Be sure to get enough calcium, magnesium, and vitamin D, as well as all the other nutrients described in Chapter 8, so your bones have enough of what they need to create healthy bone even as the rate of loss is slowing. Women taking (and absorbing) calcium and other supplements may be able to use half the dose of estrogen and still get the full benefit. That's good news for anyone who experiences side effects from the hormones (and might not at lower doses), and may also lessen the increase (if any) in breast cancer risk.

Case in Point: Ivy

*I*vy's mother and sister had breast cancer, so she was reluctant to take HRT. She is 60 now, and when she was perimenopausal a decade ago, her doctor warned her against it because of her family history. Now, with serious bone loss in her spine as well as loss in her hip, but a low NTX score indicating slow progression, she faced a real dilemma.

As more evidence has come in about estrogen and breast cancer, the possible link seems ever shakier, and general medical opinion has shifted to include HRT even for women with a family history of breast cancer. So now that she faced an immediate problem with her bones, Ivy was willing to try it, and I recommended a standard dose of Premarin, with a plan to have a mammogram every six months for three years, then annually after that. But the side effects—everything from weight gain and breast sensitivity to mood swings and depression—soon made her stop. She then asked me to try her on Evista, which set her mind at ease about the breast cancer risk, but she felt anxious and shaky, and started experiencing allergic-type responses (rashes and blotching) to things that had never bothered her before, so she stopped that, too.

Ivy is very detail oriented, and a perfectionist to boot, so she wasn't about to give up on finding a bone density treatment that would work for her. She knew her bones were fragile enough that she needed some intervention along with good diet and exercise. So I prescribed Fosamax, but she got terrible reflux from it. She started taking an additional medication to reduce acid, thereby cutting down on the reflux symptoms, but was then worried she wouldn't have enough stomach acid to absorb the calcium supplements and all the nutrients in her food.

So although reflux no longer bothered her, and she had reason to believe the Fosamax was working for her bones, Ivy still wasn't satisfied with that approach—or with doing nothing beyond lifestyle changes. A second bone scan just six months after the first showed no change, which wasn't a surprise given the short amount of time and the switching of medications. It was a reality check, however, and motivated Ivy to try Premarin again. This time, I started her with a lower dose, .3 mg daily, *less than half of what she had before, and it didn't give her the side effects she had with the standard dose.*

At the same time, I recommended she start taking selenium supplements to help reduce her cancer risk, along with the calcium and multivitamin she takes. She continued getting frequent mammograms. She has a sonogram of her breasts as part of her regular checkups, and does a monthly breast self-exam at home.

Ivy loves good food, but is mindful about what she eats, and is now careful to include some good nondairy sources of calcium in her diet every day. Her home is full of beautiful things, and she treats herself well, in general, but lives with a very high level of stress and currently has a lot of emotional turmoil in her life. She walks miles every day, and has for years, but is experimenting with adding a meditative element to the workout in an attempt to reduce her stress. I added trace minerals to the supplements she takes when she went off estrogen the first time, and now she's also selected some additional nutritional supplements recommended for coping with stress. She also eats flaxseeds for the healthful omega-3 oils and bone-boosting phytoestrogens they contain.

She recently started taking the phytoestrogen ipriflavone. With its proven bone benefits, it should back up the synthetic estrogen, in case the lower dose doesn't offer as complete protection. But ipriflavone has none of estrogen's side effects, and Ivy didn't get mood swings or sore breasts or an upset stomach with this combination.

With a solution finally in place, Ivy turned down my suggestion that she try estriol, a natural estrogen that generally has fewer side effects than Premarin, including no elevated risk of breast cancer. (In fact, some breast cancer patients even use it.) Unless her next bone scan reveals her strategy isn't working as well as expected, Ivy is comfortable with the precautions she's taken against breast cancer and satisfied with what she's done for her bones, and doesn't want to change anything.

This successful combination of the traditional (Premarin) and the nontraditional (ipriflavone) is what complementary medicine is all about. Neither avenue alone would have gotten Ivy the care she needed. The moral of the story is, with all the choices now out there for preventing and treating low bone density, if you look long enough, you'll find an approach that works and is right for you.

My Story: Evelyn

*W*hen a bone scan showed I had bone loss that was serious, but not yet osteoporosis, my family physician referred me to a menopause clinic with a whole team of care providers. I saw an endocrinologist, a pharmacologist, a breast health nurse, and a nutritionist. Everyone was very knowledgeable and supportive, and wanted to help me take steps that would fit in with my life. If you don't like the idea of one pill, they have ten other options to tell you about. The information I got was very individualized, and by the time I went back to my regular doctor, I felt confident in the plan I had in place. For me, that meant weight lifting, aerobic walking, calcium supplements, and Fosamax. HRT hadn't agreed with me, so I was surprised and relieved at how many other ways I could protect my bones.

Women have big choices to make about how to care for their bones, and I can't say enough about what it meant to me to have a network of people pulling together on my behalf, knowing I had the best information in each area available to help me decide what was right for me.

MONITORING YOUR PROGRESS

Estrogen effectively protects bones for 85 percent of users, especially when used for ten years or more, in particular right around menopause. Since it isn't enough for some women, you should monitor your progress with the tests described in Chapter 7, so you will know if you need to add another treatment (see following chapter) or discontinue this one. Studies are under way to determine the effectiveness of combining HRT with the more aggressive treatments described in the next chapter. Given what we know now, I recommended adding one of them if HRT alone is helping you make progress, but not enough progress. (If HRT is doing *nothing* for you, you might as well discontinue it.) You should have a baseline bone density scan, and repeat it after two years on hormones to gauge your progress. Following your NTX levels will also be helpful. You should see a decrease in the NTX level, and can reasonably expect estrogen to keep your number under 30. Lower

> ### KEEP IT UP
>
> Though up to 85 percent of American women get hot flashes within the first year of menopause, and more than a quarter of women have symptoms lasting five or more years, just 30 percent of women seek medical attention for them. Of all women who leave their doctors' offices with a prescription for hormones in hand (usually in response to complaints about menopausal symptoms), only two-thirds ever fill it. A quarter of all those women stop taking hormones within two years, mostly because they are still afraid of breast cancer or fed up with monthly bleeding or other side effects. All told, less than a quarter of American women take advantage of HRT. Those who feel crummy while taking hormones may be right to rely instead on diet, exercise, and supplements to protect their bones (if changing the type or dose of estrogen does not eliminate unwanted side effects.) But otherwise, anyone who stops taking HRT is missing out on the real benefits. On every point, the best results are seen in those still taking HRT compared to those who have stopped, and those who have taken it for the longest show the biggest benefits.

NTX levels are always better. If you follow healthy eating and exercise guidelines, that is a goal well within your reach.

For women with breast cancer or uterine cancer, or with two close relatives with breast or ovarian cancer, the risks of HRT clearly outweigh the benefits. (Some women with breast cancer can actually be treated with estrogen, but that's another subject altogether.) Women with abnormal vaginal bleeding shouldn't use HRT until the cause is discovered, and those who have had problems with blood clots should also be wary, though there's no proof of increased danger. Anyone with fibrocystic breast disease should be aware that mammograms may be less accurate with that condition, making it difficult to detect breast cancer as early as would be desirable. Uterine fibroids should also make you think twice about taking a drug that can make them grow, or you may wind up needing a hysterectomy you might otherwise avoid.

HORMONES' BENEFITS AND RISKS:
A HEAD-TO-HEAD COMPARISON

BENEFITS

	Prevent Bone Loss	Increase Bone Formation	Estrogen's Benefit to Bone Without Estrogen's Negative Side Effects to Body	Decrease Menopause Symptoms	Restore Sex Drive	Decrease Breast Cancer Risk	Decrease Heart Disease Risk	Decrease risk of Alzheimer's Disease, Colon Cancer, Strokes, Cataracts, Arthritis Symptoms
Estradiol	A	X	n/a	A	X	X	A	A
Estriol	C+	X	A	C	X	X	C	U
Estrone	B	X	B	B	X	X	C	U
Estriol, Estrone, Estradiol combination	A	X	B	A	X	X	B	C+
Estrogen and a progestin	A	A	n/a	A	X	X	A	A
Progesterone	B	B+	B	U	X	X	X	X
Evista	B	X	A	X	X	A	U	U
Testosterone	C+	C+	B	U	A	U	U	U
DHEA	C	C	U	U	U	X	X	X
Ipriflavone	B	B	B	X	X	X	X	X
Isoflavones	B	C−	C	A	X	X	A	U

A = strong, B = moderate, C = weak, U = unknown, X = does not have this effect

With these few exceptions, HRT is the best traditional medicine has to offer when it comes to maintaining bone density, and all women should consider it seriously as they approach menopause. When talking the decision over with a health care professional, keep your bone health in the front of your mind, along with heart disease and cancer risks, and you'll be able to achieve a

RISKS	Possible Increased Risk of Breast Cancer	Increased Risk of Uterine Cancer	Increased Risk of Blood Clots
Estradiol	B	B	A
Estriol	X	X	C−
Estrone	C−	X	C
Estriol, Estrone, Estradiol Combination	C	U	A
Estrogen and a progestin	B	X	A
Progesterone	X	X	X
Evista	X	X	U
Testosterone	X	X	U
DHEA	X	X	X
Ipriflavone	X	X	X
Isoflavones	X	X	X

A = strong, B = moderate, C = weak, U = unknown, X = does not have this effect

healthy balance. The charts above will help you sort through the many types of hormones available to help with bone density and how they affect a range of other health concerns. The "alternative" hormones covered in the next chapter are included here, too, for the sake of comparison, but the highlighted options are the traditional options this chapter covers. If you learn nothing else from this book, I want you to remember that although we tend to use "HRT" to mean estradiol pills, or estradiol/progestin combinations, there are actually a host of choices, each with its own pluses and minuses, and only you can pick *the best one for you*. You should have very specific reasons for taking any hormone, and those hormones should be geared at creating balance within your body. There may be things that can create that balance other than hormones, so when you choose hormones, you want to be clear on the point that this is the best option for you. The current trend of making a blanket recommendation for HRT for every woman at menopause is a mistake. For you as an individual, estrogen may not be the best thing. Or maybe it is. The only way to know is to take into account all the details of your own particular situation.

Chapter 19

"Alternative" Hormones

The party line approach to preventing and treating low bone density—and still the strategy most thoroughly explored and best proven effective—is hormone replacement therapy along the lines of what was presented in the last chapter: synthetic estrogen pills, patches or creams, perhaps with progestins for women with their uteruses. We've seen the many benefits—as well as the potentially serious drawbacks—of these drugs. Often overlooked in the rush to get every woman pushing 50 on a lifetime supply of hormones made by a handful of corporate giants—or just to simplify and settle a troublesome and complex decision about what to take—are several promising nontraditional and natural options well worth considering.

Don't think of hormone replacement as one particular pill or even one type of pill. As you'll see in this chapter, in addition to the many varieties of estrogens commonly prescribed, there are many other approaches to using hormones for bone health.

NATURAL PROGESTERONE

At menopause, estrogen isn't the only hormone taking a nosedive. Progesterone, too, decreases (along with everything else made by the ovaries). In fact, after menopause, the ovaries usually still make a small amount of estrogen, perhaps 10 percent of the pre-menopausal level, but progesterone is entirely cut off (though very small amounts may be made elsewhere in the body). One of pro-gesterone's jobs is to stimulate the osteoblasts to make new bone, and the loss of it contributes to the slowdown in bone formation that leads to low bone density. High levels of progesterone, on the other hand, may also slow down the work of the osteoclasts, help-ing to prevent bone loss.

Synthetic forms of progesterone called progestins are often prescribed in conjunction with estrogen for women with uteruses taking HRT, as we've seen, because it puts the risk of endometrial cancer back to normal (while estrogen alone greatly increases it). There is some question, however, about whether progestins also interfere with the heart-protective effects of estrogen. And progestins definitely come with the potential for several unpleas-ant side effects, including bloating, abnormal vaginal bleeding, weight gain, moodiness, insomnia, unwanted hair growth, and loss of libido. (Those last two can also be signs of testosterone de-ficiency (see page 356), so you should have your hormone levels checked before assuming progestins are to blame.)

Natural progesterone, which has the identical chemical struc-ture to what the body makes and is available without a pre-scription, seems to have all the benefits with none of the side effects. Progestins are actually somewhat different molecules from progesterone—with about as many differences as there are be-tween the structures of progesterone and testosterone. As you can see, small structural changes make huge differences in what effect a substance has on the body! Consider this: synthetic progestins are used in birth control pills, while your body's progesterone aids in conception and is crucial in sustaining a pregnancy.

Dr. John Lee is a leading proponent of natural progesterone. The original study that made Dr. Lee a fan of the hormone fol-lowed 100 women using a progesterone cream. The women were also advised to follow a primarily vegetarian diet and take a range of supplements, including calcium and vitamin D. Sixty-three of the women (those who could afford it) had repeated bone density scans to track their progress. During a time when you would expect to see about a 4.5 percent drop in bone mass, all 63 actually built their bones up. Most improved about 10 percent over the first six months to a year, then 3 to 5 percent a year after that until reaching (and maintaining!) peak density. The average total increase was just over 15 percent over three years, no matter the age of the woman. Most had started out with low bone density, and the women with the weakest bones to begin with showed the biggest gains. None of the women reported side effects, and none suffered fractures (except for the three injured by falling down stairs, being in a car accident, and falling while hiking, and they all healed well) or lost any additional height. Most also reported a renewed sense of energy, increased mobility, and restoration of long-lost sex drive.

Progesterone alone may be enough to prevent or reverse low bone density (though you might still want estrogen for relief of menopausal symptoms). In Dr. Lee's study, women also taking estrogen showed no greater improvement in bone density than women using progesterone alone. That may be because the body can convert progesterone into estrogen as necessary, so you may boost levels of both hormones in your body just by using progesterone. In addition, the balance between the two hormones may be more important than the absolute levels of either. Therefore, when progesterone disappears at menopause, while estrogen is reduced but still present, an imbalance is created. Small amounts of progesterone can restore the balance, even if you don't have as much of either hormone as you did before menopause.

Originally, oral progesterone was thought to be broken down by the liver before it could work in the body, though new forms of "micronized progesterone" seem to be better absorbed. Many experts prefer progesterone creams that are absorbed through the skin because they result in more even and sustained levels of progesterone in the body. Dr. Lee recommends using about ¼ teaspoon of a progesterone cream that is about 3 percent progesterone each night for two to three weeks a month (totaling about 1 ounce a month). You have to choose the cream you use carefully because many products are sold as progesterone cream that actually

TALK WITH YOUR DOCTOR

Progesterone is a powerful hormone, and despite its clean safety record and over-the-counter availability, it is important to discuss it with your health care professional before you start taking it. As with estriol (see below), many doctors may be unaware of this option, but should be willing to at least monitor your progress, and perhaps to investigate it on their own.

contain very little of anything that will help your bones. Be wary of anything labeled "wild yam extract" in particular. Wild yams do contain some progesterone, but almost none of the products claiming to include it have enough progesterone to be biologically active in your body. In general, you'll have to scrutinize labels

Case in Point: Lydia

*L*ydia was afraid to go out for a walk, because even if she made it down the stairs of the building to the front door, the outside steps had no railing, and then the sidewalk into town was downhill and very uneven. Her bone density was so low (45 percent lower in her spine than what you'd expect for her age) by the time she went to see Dr. John Lee that she knew a simple stumble could be disastrous.

Lydia thought 70 was too young to be limited like this, so when Dr. Lee suggested natural progesterone cream, she was ready to try it. She carefully selected a brand with an adequate level of active hormone, and saw immediate improvement. In just six months, she gained 8 percentage points. So she continued with the cream, and diet and exercise strategies similar to those in this book. She got periodic bone scans to monitor her progress, and despite a drop in density after another doctor gave her cortisone injections, over four years her spine was 38 percent denser than before she began using progesterone cream. She's now just 22 percent lower than expected, a gain of 23 percentage points.

and contact the manufacturers if they don't contain adequate information about the levels of active progesterone.

You can use natural progesterone along with any estrogen (though if bone density is your only concern, you may need only the progesterone), and it will moderate the risk of endometrial cancer the same way synthetic progestins do. If "natural" hormones are important to you, you might want to use progesterone with estriol (see section below), if you do use an estrogen. Progesterone cream is available over-the-counter in any health food store. Progesterone, in cream or new pill form, is also available by prescription from some pharmacies.

Even if you've had a bad reaction to synthetic progestins, natural progesterone is less likely to cause any side effects. Progestins may actually reduce your body's production of its own progesterone, so supplements of natural progesterone may be particularly helpful if you're stopping taking progestins. Progesterone is also a promising strategy for counteracting the harmful effect on bones of long-term steroid use.

Progesterone seems to be safer than estrogen, and certainly causes fewer side effects. It may also be even better for your bones. Since there are no large, long-term, carefully designed studies comparing the two yet, you must think carefully about your choices. But if HRT is definitely not for you, for whatever reason, this may be a good alternative. Women with a history or high risk of breast cancer can use it safely. It may also be particularly useful in preventing bone loss in the years just before menopause, before HRT is an option but when your hormones and your bone remodeling processes are both already changing. Dr. Lee's work indicates that older women with frailer bones will see the biggest improvement in bone density from natural progesterone.

ESTRIOL

Estrogen is actually the name for a group of substances, and your body makes three different kinds. The most common prescriptions are synthetic versions of estradiol and estrone. But there is a third type, estriol, which is made in your body and available by

Case in Point: Virginia

*T*hough chemotherapy had pushed her into menopause in her late 30s, Virginia had never taken estrogen, dismissing it as "unnatural." She's been generally healthy in the twenty years since, taking antioxidants and calcium and magnesium supplements (though not getting much in her diet), walking to and from work every day, eating well, and never smoking. Still, as she approached 60, I recommended she have her bone density checked, since early menopause, chemotherapy, and no HRT were all risk factors. Although she had no symptoms and hadn't lost any height, a bone scan showed her spinal bone density was almost 25 percent lower than ideal (though just about what was expected for her age), and her hip was almost 35 percent lower than it would have been at its peak (and close to 20 percent lower than what you would expect at her age). Her NTX level was also relatively high, meaning she needed to take immediate action to avoid a fracture.

Other lab tests pointed out that even with the supplements Virginia took, she wasn't getting enough for her bones, so she increased her dose and backed it up with a range of other nutrients similar to the plan described in Chapter 10. The only change she made in her diet, which was already basically good, was to add more servings of calcium-rich food, which she had been lacking. Her feelings about prescription HRT hadn't changed any, but natural progesterone cream appealed to her, so she started on it right away. She took up some more structured exercise in addition to her daily commute/walk. She decided on strength training focusing on her upper body since it is the lower body that gets more of the impact (and so bone density benefit) of walking.

Virginia's been on the progesterone for a year now, reports no side effects, and says she feels good overall. Her NTX has dropped and in another year a new bone scan should show if her progress has been sufficient to stick with the course, but I'm confident she's stopped losing bone mass and that her body is building some back up.

prescription but is rarely used in this country (because it is not produced by the major drug companies), though it has long been popular in Europe. Estriol was written up in the 1980s in the *Journal of the American Medical Association*, a great bastion of mainstream medicine, as "the forgotten estrogen," but even that good PR didn't raise its profile here significantly.

The greatest benefit of using estriol is that it doesn't cause the changes in the uterus and endometrium that the other estrogens do. Many women taking estrogen experience breakthrough bleeding and abnormal vaginal bleeding, leading to painful diagnostic D & Cs and perhaps unnecessary hysterectomies because of the known increase in cancer risk. Some evidence suggests that estriol may actually *lower* your cancer risk. Estriol also provides a solution for one of the minor annoyances of HRT: you are much less likely to continue (or resume) having periods on estriol than on other estrogens.

Estriol is a prescription medication like any of the other traditional HRT components. Because estriol is much less potent than estradiol, for example, you need higher doses of estriol to see the same level of symptom relief the more usual prescriptions offer: 2–4 mg daily. You may need even more, up to 12 mg a day, for it to have positive effects on bone density. Some women experience nausea at such high doses (though it appears to be otherwise safe), so you might want to consider combining it with other forms of estrogen. Dr. Jonathan Wright is a leading advocate for estriol, and he recommends a mixture of about 80 percent estriol, 10 percent estradiol, and 10 percent estrone. Taking 2.5 mg of this mixture (along with progesterone for part of the cycle) should give you the equivalent effect of the usual dose of estradiol or the higher doses of estriol, but with fewer side effects.

All evidence is that estriol is very safe. In fact, some women with metastatic breast cancer are even being treated with it. One study showed 37 percent of patients taking it went into remission or at least had no further progression—a much better result than would otherwise be expected. At the least, estriol is a good choice for women who need estrogen but who can't take the usual prescriptions because of a history or high risk of breast cancer. But as it becomes more widely used, and studies are conducted to compare the effectiveness of the various kinds of estrogen (I hope!), this promises to be a strong option for every woman who would benefit from estrogen if the risks were reduced: strong enough to prevent osteoporosis and weak enough not to cause cancer. As it stands, it is worth your careful consideration now.

NATURAL ESTROGENS

No matter which estrogen your doctor recommends or you decide to take, natural forms are available. These are the same powerful substances this book describes, and so come with the same risks and side effects, as well as benefits. They surely are no more risky than the prescription alternatives, and may well be safer (though much research awaits before that could be definitively established). We don't have as extensive tests and information available on natural forms as we do synthetic, but the evidence that exists already is compelling, and everything points to at least equal effectiveness. While we wait for hard numbers, I recommend choosing the form closest to nature of anything you buy or take—food, medicine, or otherwise. Seek out natural estrogens for the same reasons you buy fresh produce—and organic whenever you can. It's just better.

Ask your doctor or pharmacist how to get them. Many

Myth: The drop in estrogen is what causes menopausal symptoms, including accelerated bone loss.

Fact: Testosterone levels are low in women to begin with, but the hormone, typically thought of as masculine, performs crucial functions in a woman's body as well. And it drops off by about half at menopause, taking an important role in the changes many women experience at that time. Progesterone, too, drops at menopause, to almost nonexistent levels, another important factor in symptoms. The resulting imbalance between these major hormones—not just a drop in estrogen alone—is at fault for menopausal difficulties.

> **TALK TO YOUR DOCTOR**
>
> Very low doses of testosterone after menopause, combined with standard estrogen replacement therapy, seems to provide even greater benefits to the bones than estrogen alone. If you get too much testosterone, you can have problems with acne and unwanted hair growth. You may have to have a pharmacy compound a low enough dose just for you.

women's health centers and natural pharmacies carry them. If you can't find them locally, Women's International Pharmacy in Madison, Wisconsin, sells them via mail order.

TESTOSTERONE

In men, testosterone is a major hormone involved in regulating bone remodeling. The body's testosterone slows bone breakdown and increases bone building. It plays a part in women's bones, too, though there it joins a larger cast and is generally outshone by estrogen.

For men with lower than normal testosterone levels, supplements of the hormone might be beneficial, particularly for the bones. Low testosterone is a major risk factor for low bone density and osteoporosis in men. Any man who has that should work with his doctor to find the root cause and address it if possible. But consider providing testosterone if the body isn't making enough to protect the bones.

For women, small amounts of testosterone may also be helpful, especially taken together with estrogen (the two together seem to work better than either one alone). This approach is still relatively new, so there is not a lot of clinical data available to pinpoint the best way to take testosterone. One thing we know for sure is that normal ovaries make testosterone, even after menopause. Even if the ovary doesn't produce estrogen, a woman's body can convert testosterone to estrogen. Given the important part it plays in maintaining healthy bones, it is worthwhile to make sure you have enough. Testosterone deficiency in women can cause loss of libido and breast tenderness. If you have these symptoms, especially if they don't clear up if you take estrogen, have your blood tested for testosterone levels. If your levels are low—which can happen even well before menopause, as early as in your 20s or

Case in Point: Barbara

When Barbara first consulted pioneering endocrinologist Ed Klaiber, she was in misery from migraine headaches, depression, reduced sex drive, fibromyalgia, and occasional disturbances in her vision—none of which had bothered her before she had a hysterectomy. She'd had the occasional migraine in the past, but now the headaches were frequent and debilitating. On top of everything else, the bone density scan she'd had just after the surgery showed she already had osteoporosis, even before the accelerated loss you'd expect to see after a drop in estrogen like the one created by a total hysterectomy.

She'd gone under the knife when a fibroid in her uterus grew so big it caused enough bleeding to make her anemic (not to mention the considerable inconvenience). Though her ovaries were fine, her gynecologist recommended having them removed at the same time as the uterus to practically eliminate her risk of ovarian cancer (though she didn't have an elevated risk)—a standard strategy. The ovaries produce most of the body's estrogen, so the surgery threw Barbara into menopause while she was still in her late 30s.

Her gynecologist prescribed hormone replacement therapy to take over the role of the ovaries in the body. When she walked into Dr. Klaiber's office, she'd been taking the standard dose—and struggling with the miserable aftereffects of surgery—for a year and a half. She'd started taking Prozac, too, because she was so depressed, but while that relieved her mood a bit, it made her sex drive disappear altogether and made her unable to reach an orgasm.

Barbara's blood level of estrogen had never been checked, and it turned out that even with the HRT, her body's estrogen levels were very low. She began taking a higher dose, and though her blood levels eventually got into the acceptable range, her symptoms were still just about as bad as they ever had been. An avid horseback rider, Barbara hadn't been able to do that—or any significant physical activity—since her hysterectomy. Even simple things were sometimes problematic. More than once she'd had to pull over to the side of the road and call her husband on the cell phone and have him come pick her up when she felt it wasn't safe for her to drive—when a migraine struck or her vision blurred.

Though Barbara's troubles were particularly dramatic, what happened to her is not uncommon following complete hysterectomies. The ovaries make testosterone as well as estrogen, and though testosterone is always in a woman's body—in relatively low amounts compared to estrogen and progesterone—it drops by up to 50 percent at menopause. Many of the changes in mood, sex drive, and energy levels associated with menopause may come from the loss of testosterone at least as much as the loss of estrogen. Dr. Klaiber suspected Barbara's symptoms, since they didn't respond to estrogen even at a proper dose, might be related to the loss of testosterone.

So she had her testosterone levels checked, another area her gynecologist never looked into. Her estrogen levels had been very low, but her testosterone levels were practically nonexistent. She started taking a very low dose pill along with her estrogen.

At her one-month checkup, Barbara looked like a new woman—though she said it was only her old, presrgery self that was back. "I'm dumbfounded," she said. "After all this time with all these terrible symptoms, now in the first cycle of testosterone everything's turned around. I've had no migraines in a month, a first since the surgery. Last weekend, I rode my horse—for two hours!" She even reported her sex drive seemed to be making a comeback. After checking with her regular doctor, she weaned herself off Prozac and so eliminated its unwanted side effects.

Then, after eight months on testosterone, she had her second bone scan, which showed a 7 percent increase in mass. The biggest change in her life since the surgery was the addition of the testosterone, and she credited it with saving her bones—and her life!

30s—or if you don't have ovaries, you might want to consider supplementation. You should consider low testosterone levels a warning sign of risk of low bone density.

Estratest is a brand that combines estrogen and testosterone so you need only one prescription. Use caution, however: if you get your testosterone levels too high, you could get acne, excess hair growth, and even a deeper voice. Testosterone is not for everyone, but correcting a deficiency will be good for your bones.

DHEA

The hormone known as DHEA (to spare us from pronouncing dehydroepiandrosterone) is similar in structure to estrogen, progesterone, and testosterone—in fact, one of the things the body does with it is convert it into estrogen or testosterone. You can buy it as an over-the-counter supplement in any health food store, and a couple of years ago it got a lot of publicity as some kind of anti-aging miracle cure. Of course, there is never any one magic bullet, especially not when it comes to something diffuse like aging. And DHEA comes with potential side effects and uncertain long-term effects. It does seem to help prevent heart disease and cancer, but it is the effects on bone density I'm most interested in.

DHEA appears to slow bone breakdown, much as estrogen does, as well as stimulate new bone growth and promote calcium absorption. Your body's natural levels of DHEA decrease as you age, and when you hit 70 you have only about a fifth of what you had as a young adult. As with estrogen and progesterone, menopause brings a drop in DHEA levels. The higher your body's levels of DHEA, the higher your bone density is likely to be (though this correlation is not yet proven to be a cause-and-effect relationship). Steroids lower DHEA in your body, which may be one of the reasons they cause low bone density (and raising the question of whether DHEA supplements might reverse or prevent that effect).

Taking DHEA supplements raises the body's levels of estrogen and testosterone, and probably progesterone, too, all of which will be good for your bones. Taking it along with other hormone therapies probably helps your body keep the levels of various hormones in balance, though I'd like to see studies exploring that point.

Although DHEA is available over the counter, as I said, it is a powerful hormone, and you should consult with your health care professional before you start taking it. There are no official guidelines as to dosage, but a common recommendation is 3 to 5 mg a day after menopause, eventually building up to 5 to 15 mg later in life. You may want up to 30 mg for the best bone protection. Such small doses are safe as far as we know, though side effects include acne and unwanted hair growth, especially on your legs and arms. Since this is a relatively new treatment, you should be carefully monitored over the long term by getting your levels of hormones checked periodically. For women, DHEA levels normally change over the course of the monthly cycle, so you may need more than one measurement to be sure your results are reliable.

WHAT *ARE* MY HORMONE LEVELS?

The test I like best to pinpoint a person's hormone levels (given the cyclic variations you'd expect with most of them) is to take saliva samples every few days for a month, to track and plot your levels of all these hormones and their relationship to each other. That's invaluable information unavailable through one-time or one-hormone testing.

IPRIFLAVONE AND PHYTOESTROGENS

Many foods contain chemicals known as phytoestrogens: plant hormones that are similar in structure to estrogen and have similar effects on the human body. Actually, because they are weaker than the estrogens made by the body, phytoestrogens seem to mimic estrogen's effects on bone density, without having any effect on sex organs (and so don't usually cause breast tenderness or endometrial growth). They also augment estrogen (from the body, or from HRT). Many studies are under way to determine which of the various phytoestrogens are the most effective, but until we have more specific answers, upping your intake of phytoestrogens, generally, will be helpful.

The most common source of phytoestrogens is soy. The estrogenlike substances in nearly all soy products (and some other foods) are called isoflavones. (See Chapter 11 on soy foods.) Phytoestrogens come in many other varieties, like the proanthocyanidins and anthocyanidins that give the purplish cast to many berries, including blackberries, blueberries, raspberries, and cherries. Those play a role in strengthening collagen, the key ingredient in bone matrix, which makes them very important to bone density. Citrus peels also have valuable phytoestrogens, as do flaxseeds, obviously a more viable source (see Chapter 11).

You've read about the benefits of incorporating soy foods into your diet in an earlier chapter, but here I'd like to focus on phytoestrogen supplements, of which many, many varieties are available over the counter. As always, getting the nutrients you're after in their most natural form—in food—is the most desirable path. But the reality is that most Americans don't eat a lot of soy. We don't generally eat significant amounts of berries every day, either, and citrus peel is hardly higher on our collective list of favorite foods, so we could use a backup source. Even if your pantry is stocked with tofu and soymilk, supplements of phytoestrogens may still be useful to you. You'll have many to choose from at your friendly neighborhood health food store. The label buzzword most often invoked is *isoflavones*, the group of phytoestrogens in soy. Since soy is already established as beneficial, other phytoestrogens seem to have been assigned second-class status pending more information on the subject.

Most of the clinical research in this area uses one particular kind of phytoestrogen, an isoflavone known as ipriflavone (brand name Osten). It has been in use as an osteoporosis drug in Japan and a few other countries for a decade now, and is available over the counter here. Though it is often sold as a "natural" substance because it is derived from daidzein, a soy phytoestrogen, it is not at all clear it exists outside of what is made in a lab. But don't let the dubious "natural" designation make you overlook the proven benefits. Ipriflavone also has one outstanding advantage in comparison to other phytoestrogens because it works by a slightly different mechanism. Most phytoestrogens work by mimicking estrogen's actions and effects, basically fooling your body into thinking it is getting estrogen. Ipriflavone, on the other hand, has estrogenlike effects (like bone building), but it doesn't attach to estrogen receptor sites, so it does not come with the same side effects as estrogen. It doesn't even have the complete slate of estrogen effects, and therein is the key difference. Ipriflavone works primarily on bone tissue, *not* uterine or breast tissue. That means no increase in risk of uterine or breast cancer, or even of less serious side effects like breast tenderness.

Ipriflavone inhibits bone breakdown *and* stimulates bone building, which makes it and progesterone unique among all other treatment options, all of which work on only one of those pathways. One study showed increases in bone density in the spine and wrist significant enough to lower the risk of fracture. Another study compared ipriflavone and calcitonin—and ipriflavone showed double the gains in bone mass! Gains in all studies were seen in both the hip and the spine. Ipriflavone has also been shown to relieve bone pain. Large and long-term studies of ipriflavone still need to be done, but early results from many, many small studies are promising enough to make supplements a strong option for women and men. Taking ipriflavone may allow women to take lower doses of estrogen, thereby limiting some side effects of HRT while still reaping the full slate of benefits.

RECOMMENDED DOSE

Most of the studies of ipriflavone have used 600 mg a day, in divided doses (200 mg three times a day). Some experts recommend up to twice that amount. Nearly all the studies pair ipriflavone with calcium (1,000 mg in supplements a day), and show results that outpace those of calcium alone. We may have to wait for studies that demonstrate whether it works as well on its own, but in the meantime, don't neglect your calcium!

Case in Point: Rosemary

*A*fter she fought so hard against breast cancer, Rosemary wasn't about to just sign up for HRT as she went into menopause. She simply tolerated the menopausal symptoms she had as best she could, until they subsided after a couple years and she figured her hormonal troubles were over.

But when I sent her for a bone scan when she was in her mid-50s, it showed she had osteoporosis. Fortunately, her NTX was 37, within the normal range, so her fracture risk was still manageably low. I prescribed Miacalcin and she started taking nutritional supplements, including calcium. After a year, however, her NTX levels were up to 57, putting her at higher risk for fracture and indicating an increasing rate of progression of bone loss. For Rosemary, Miacalcin wasn't doing enough.

I had her hormone levels analyzed, and found her estrogen levels were very low. Because of her fear of a breast cancer relapse, Rosemary decided to add the estriol and ipriflavone to the Miacalcin. She felt comfortable with the natural estrogen since it does not increase the risk of breast cancer while still providing some of the benefits of synthetic estrogen. Since estriol has been less studied than other forms of estrogen, and it remains unproven that the bone benefits equal those of synthetic estrogen, Rosemary uses the ipriflavone—with its proven bone benefits—to ensure her bones are covered.

Rosemary pays attention to her diet, and is generally active. She considers herself a spiritual person, and copes with the many stresses in her life with regular meditation. But with her hormones finally in balance, she feels better than she has in a long time, and she now encourages her friends facing menopause to look carefully into alternatives for HRT. If a breast cancer survivor could find a regimen that suited her, she figures, anybody can.

One possible side effect sometimes noted with ipriflavone is gastrointestinal upset, and it clears up on discontinuing the supplement. Ipriflavone may slow down your liver, changing the effects of other drugs you are taking, so it is crucial to discuss this with your health care professional before dosing yourself, and to double-check with your pharmacist about potential interactions.

You should keep an eye out for breaking news as we learn more specifics about how best to use phytoestrogens. There is some controversy about whether phytoestrogens come with some of the same risks as other estrogens, and that's one of the questions new research should resolve—and one of the areas where ipriflavone already has an edge. It's clear from looking at how much lower the rates of major diseases that plague Americans are in cultures that include large amounts of soy in the daily diet that getting phytoestrogens in your diet is safe. If you are worried about potential side effects, rely on diet (see Chapter 11) rather than supplements until we have more information.

I fear natural progesterone, DHEA, and ipriflavone will never be as carefully tested as the standards of mainstream medicine rightfully require. As natural substances, they cannot be patented, so the profit motive will never be strong enough for any company to cough up the huge sums of money for clinical trials that would satisfy the FDA. Testosterone is sold by the big drug companies, and estriol will be as soon as some marketing genius realizes the potential for all the benefits with none of the cancer risk, so I'm a bit more optimistic they will get their due once our national consciousness is raised about them. But on the evidence we have on hand, these seem to be safe and effective products, if used properly and with medical supervision, and should be taken into consideration by anyone concerned about treating low bone density—or avoiding it.

The charts below are the same as the one on pages 347 and 348 in the last chapter, and are included again here for easy reference. This time the "alternatives" explained in this chapter are highlighted. Even if you want to use nontraditional hormones, you still need to carefully consider your individual situation to choose the one that is right for you. These charts give you a starting point to compare the strengths and weaknesses of your options.

HORMONES' BENEFITS AND RISKS: A HEAD-TO-HEAD COMPARISON

BENEFITS

	Prevent Bone Loss	Increase Bone Formation	Estrogen's Benefit to Bone Without Estrogen's Negative Side Effects to Body	Decrease Menopause Symptoms	Restore Sex Drive	Decrease Breast Cancer Risk	Decrease Heart Disease Risk	Decrease risk of Alzheimer's Disease, Colon Cancer, Strokes, Cataracts, Arthritis Symptoms
Estradiol	A	X	n/a	A	X	X	A	A
Estriol	C+	X	A	C	X	X	C	U
Estrone	B	X	B	B	X	X	C	U
Estriol, Estrone, Estradiol combination	A	X	B	A	X	X	B	C+
Estrogen and a progestin	A	A	n/a	A	X	X	A	A
Progesterone	B	B+	B	U	X	X	X	X
Evista	B	X	A	X	X	A	U	U
Testosterone	C+	C+	B	U	A	U	U	U
DHEA	C	C	U	U	U	X	X	X
Ipriflavone	B	B	B	X	X	X	X	X
Isoflavones	B	C−	C	A	X	X	A	U

A = strong, B = moderate, C = weak, U = unknown, X = does not have this effect

❀ ❀ ❀ ❀ ❀ ❀ ❀ ❀ ❀ ❀ ❀ ❀ ❀ ❀ ❀ ❀ ❀ ❀ ❀ ❀

WEEK 5 ACTION PLAN

1. Continue the Bone Density Diet with menus 8 to 14 (with any modifications you planned last week).
2. Follow the first week of the exercise schedule you designed for yourself last week. Make sure it includes at least one yoga workout and two sessions with weights.

RISKS	Possible Increased Risk of Breast Cancer	Increased Risk of Uterine Cancer	Increased Risk of Blood Clots
Estradiol	B	B	A
Estriol	X	X	C−
Estrone	C−	X	C
Estriol, estrone, estradiol combination	C	U	A
Estrogen and a progestin	B	X	A
Progesterone	X	X	X
Evista	X	X	U
Testosterone	X	X	U
DHEA	X	X	X
Ipriflavone	X	X	X
Isoflavones	X	X	X

A = strong, B = moderate, C = weak, U = unknown, X = does
not have this effect

3. If you didn't have your hormone levels checked as part
of your Week 1 checkup, refer to the Decade Planners in
Chapter 7 and get the relevant tests. Ask your doctor to
check the levels in your saliva over the course of a month,
rather than your blood from just one point in time.
(Though if the latter is your only option, go ahead and do
that.)

4. If you are perimenopausal, or have been through menopause, consider HRT from the perspective of your bones. If
you've had a bone screening or know your NTX level, factor the results into your decision. Weigh the relative risks
and benefits for your specific situation. What health risks
do you have that HRT can protect against (particularly

menopausal symptoms, heart health, bone density, and Alzheimer's)? What health risks do you have that suggest HRT may not be for you (mainly elevated cancer risk and blood clots)?

5. If you decide to take HRT, make a plan for which strategies (pill or patch? Progestin or progesterone? natural estrogen or Premarin?) suit you and your lifestyle.

6. If you are already taking HRT, reconfirm your choice of type in light of any new information you picked up here. If you're satisfied where you are, that is OK, but many women would benefit from some fine-tuning to reduce any side effects, increase the likelihood they will stay on the medication, reduce fear of risks, and improve efficacy.

> **WEEK 5 FOCUS**
>
> - Have your hormone levels tested.
> - Consider hormone replacement therapy.
> - Look into alternatives to traditional HRT.
> - Begin your personalized exercise plan.

7. If you are menopausal and *not* taking HRT, reconfirm your decision in light of what you've learned to make sure it is still the right path for you.

8. If you've tried estrogen and progestin, but quit because of side effects, consider trying other forms, combinations, or schedules to find one that won't be uncomfortable.

9. Don't forget your calcium in order to get the maximum benefit from HRT.

10. If you decide to use natural progesterone, do some background research to find a brand that has an appropriate level of active hormone.

11. Consider natural estrogens as part of—or instead of—traditional HRT.

12. Look into testosterone and DHEA as ways to balance your hormones, and talk to your doctor if you think either one may be right for you.

13. Consider using ipriflavone. A phytoestrogen, it has all the

bone-building benefits of soy, without prescription estrogen's negative side effects.

14. Look over the final week's worth of menus for the diet, and make any necessary revisions. Make a shopping list of everything you'll need—and go get it.

❁ ❁ ❁ ❁ ❁ ❁ ❁ ❁ ❁ ❁ ❁ ❁ ❁ ❁ ❁ ❁ ❁ ❁ ❁

EVALUATE TREATMENT AND PREVENTION OPTIONS AND ALTERNATIVE THERAPIES

For people who already have significant bone loss, pharmaceutical options can make a big difference, especially when used in conjunction with diet, exercise, supplements, and hormones. Several excellent options have debuted in the last several years—where almost nothing had existed before—and the rate of discovery shows no sign of slowing as researchers learn more and more about exactly how bone remodeling works. The first chapter of this section presents what you need to know about currently available drugs for treating low bone density, and peeks into the future at some of the emerging frontiers.

On the flip side of the coin, people dealing with low bone density—or interested in preventing it—can learn a great deal from ancient traditions as well as cutting-edge modern science. The second chapter in this section surveys therapies from "alternative" medicine and explores how to use them for maintaining strong bones or in conjunction with mainstream medicine to maximize your results. The Action Plan will help you sort through all the information and choose what is right for you.

Chapter 20

Other Drug Therapies

When bone density is low enough to consider prescription options, hormone replacement therapy is usually the first recommendation for preserving bone density and for osteoporosis treatment. But not everyone can—or wants to—take estrogen or other HRT formulations. Fortunately, the last few years have brought a number of breakthroughs in pharmacological treatment of low bone density, and even more promising medicines are in the pipeline. The good news for anyone who still believes our grandmothers' shrinking and fragility will inevitably be ours is that the new prescription therapies are more effective at countering lowered bone density than the more familiar cholesterol-lowering drugs are at protecting your heart. Numerous rigorous trials of the new medicines show that they can decrease the rate of fractures by up to 50 percent. For those with bone density already so low that supplements, diet, and exercise aren't sufficient protection, that is good news indeed.

Most of these therapies can be combined with hormones for even better results, all work best if supported by a bone-healthy lifestyle, and most are designed to be used at the same time as calcium and vitamin D supplements. Of course, you should discuss all your options with your doctor, but you shouldn't be relying on a medical professional to make your decisions for you. The goal of this chapter is to give you enough information to prepare you to make the discussion an intelligent one, and to allow you to ultimately make a confident, informed decision *together with* a medical professional. No matter how excellent a navigator your doctor may be, you, the patient, must be the captain of the ship. *Your guiding question should be, how can I best help myself?*

My goal for patients taking prescriptions to stop bone loss and protect bone density—in fact, for all my patients concerned about bone density—is to restore them to the levels expected in a healthy 30-year-old. An older person with frailer bones may take longer to attain that goal than a premenopausal woman with only a mild loss of bone density, but it is a goal within reach of anyone. I don't accept osteoporosis as a normal part of aging. As we saw in the chapter on screening, bone density scans give you a pair of results—one score comparing you to ideal levels (for a healthy 30-year-old) and one comparing you to the average for your age and sex. The implication is that different results will raise different levels of alarm, depending on your age. But if we don't accept bone loss in a 30- or 40-year-old, I see no reason why we should accept it in a 60- or 70-year-old, given our current knowledge and available options.

ALENDRONATE (FOSAMAX) AND ETIDRONATE (DIDRONEL)

Alendronate (brand name Fosamax) belongs to the category of drugs known as bisphosphonates, which work by blocking or slowing the breakdown of bone. Your body incorporates bisphosphonates into the bone surface by binding it to the cells where active destruction of bone takes place. The drugs themselves do not stop bone breakdown, but that placement serves to slow down the whole process by limiting the locations where breakdown can occur. That in turn allows a better balance between formation of new bone and destruction of old to be established. Bone density loss will stop, and bone can be built back up. This is why proper diet, exercise, and supplements are so important in combination with medication. When you're doing all you can to alter how bone is built, you also need to provide the best fuel to maximize effectiveness. Drugs alone will never provide optimal results. As we've seen, good cement (or good bones) requires a balance of high-quality materials.

ALENDRONATE (FOSAMAX)

- Dose for treating osteoporosis: 10 mg once daily
- Dose for preventing osteoporosis: 5 mg once daily
- Known drug interactions: none
- Not recommended for people with reflux, chronic indigestion, or kidney failure, or pregnant or nursing women.
- Cost: approximately $55 a month

Take first thing in the morning, on an empty stomach, with plenty of water, and remain upright for 30 minutes. Do not eat or drink (except water) until half an hour after taking medication.

Alendronate is used for both prevention of bone density loss and treatment of osteoporosis. For anyone who can't—or doesn't want to—use hormone replacement therapy, it can be the best pharmacological option. Like all bisphosphonates, it works by inhibiting bone breakdown, so bone density increases (or at the very least stops decreasing). The rate of fractures is reduced, and so are deformities in the spine and loss of height.

Eighty-six percent of patients using alendronate preventively, and 96 percent using it to treat osteoporosis, have increases in bone density. You can expect 6 percent increases the first year, with 2 percent gains per year after that. Studies show reductions in all types of fractures of about 50 percent independent of the specific bone density results. That is, even if your bone density doesn't increase, or doesn't increase much, on alendronate, you will still gain significant protection from fractures. And that is,

My Story: Jackie

I'm five foot nothing, and don't weigh a hundred pounds soaking wet. I went into menopause on the early side, at 45, and when I did, I got my first bone scan. I know now that it showed I had a 17 percent loss of bone density in my spine and 15 percent in my hip, but my doctor at the time considered these results normal, and she never even called to give them to me.

So a whole year went by where I had no period, no estrogen, and no information. The next year, when my annual scan showed 23 percent bone loss in my spine and 16 percent in my hip, my doctor diagnosed me with osteopenia. She still said it was no big deal, and not to worry about it. She suggested I take calcium, but she didn't breathe a word about vitamin D or magnesium or exercise or anything else I could do to help myself.

I've always been health-conscious. I'm a runner. I teach nutrition. So when I found out I wasn't as healthy as I thought I was, I freaked out. I also knew there had to be a role for improved nutrition in keeping my bones strong. So I calmed down and got proactive. I started to get myself informed. I read every book I could find with sections on bone density. I searched the Internet. I checked out mainstream and alternative sources. The more I read, the more confused I got, and it started to seem that every new thing I read contradicted the last one. I went to a naturopath, and also to a mainstream doctor at a rehab center who specialized in exercise. That doctor asked for the results of both bone scans I'd had, and he was the one who told me about how much I had lost even at the time of my first scan. Then he told me I had the spine of an 81-year-old woman. I hit the roof. Of course, I've never gone back to my original doctor who neglected to alert me to the loss. But I can never get back that year when I could have been doing all the things I've since learned to do to prevent any further loss.

I really like my rehab doctor. He is a big believer in HRT, particularly for the first few years of menopause, but I have a knee-jerk reaction against the hormones even though I have no family history of breast cancer. So he listens to all my beefs and works with what I'm prepared to do. The naturopath, on the other hand, was hysterical at the mention of

HRT. Even though I can relate to that, I wanted a more balanced, open-minded perspective. With all the information coming at you, in the end, you just have to go with your gut.

So I did start taking Fosamax. I increased my running to three times a week. I added in some exercises with hand weights. I take calcium supplements regularly, and other supplements—expensive trace minerals and extra vitamin D—with a bit less devotion. I have alfalfa and some Chinese herbs, and I started using a natural progesterone cream a year ago after I found out the "wild yam" stuff I was using doesn't have enough active hormone to make any difference.

My diet is totally focused on calcium and my bones. I have a calcium chart stuck on my refrigerator, and I know spinach isn't as good a source as kale, and so on. I eat tofu every single day. I buy extra-firm, not the jiggly, wiggly stuff, slice it thin, marinate it in soy sauce, ginger, and garlic, and pan-fry or grill it. It keeps in the fridge for a week, and I eat some plain for lunch every day. When my students make faces at the thought of tofu, this is what I bring in to let them try—anything marinated this way will taste good—and they always love it. I eat at least one can of salmon every week, bones and all, and broccoli, sesame seeds, fortified soymilk, leafy greens, and so on often enough that I get about half of the 1,500 mg of calcium I aim for each day in my food, without relying too heavily on dairy products.

It's all paying off. It's been a year since that second scan threw me into action, so I just had my third bone density scan. It shows I stopped the loss, and recovered everything I'd lost in the year between my first and second scans. I'm back down to 17 percent low from average peak density.

My doctor recommends staying on Fosamax indefinitely. But he knows I can't stand taking all this stuff, even supplements, even though I haven't had side effects from any of it. My goal is to maintain my bone density through diet and exercise. So our compromise is that after another year, assuming I'll be pretty close to normal density by then, I'll stop the Fosamax, keep up with my diet and weight lifting, and increase my running to five days a week. I'll get another scan after a year of that to make sure I'm still on the right track.

after all, the main goal of any therapy for low bone density. The drug also results in fewer spine deformities and significantly lessened height loss. Alendronate also reduces disability and lessened activity due to vertebral fractures, and reduces the hospitalization rate for osteoporosis-related injuries—and staying out of the hospital is one of the key goals in managing osteoporosis. Better still, of course, is to preserve your bone density in the first place, which alendronate can help you do.

Alendronate is nonhormonal, so it is good for women who do not use hormone replacement therapy. It provides bone benefits equivalent to those of estrogen. It does not protect the heart the way estrogen does, but it also does not increase cancer risks. The combination of estrogen and alendronate is even better than either one alone.

Alendronate is generally the first choice of drug therapy for men, since men don't have the same hormonal issues as women do. It is FDA approved for treatment of bone loss caused by steroids, which is also a separate problem from the usual hormonal issues men or women face.

Pregnant women should not take alendronate. And unless your bone scan shows your density to be at least two standard deviations below peak (in the lowest 20 to 30 percent for people your age) you should give diet, exercise, and supplements a serious try before considering drug treatment. However, if your N-telopeptide level is high—indicating a high fracture risk and rapid progression—you may need the additional protection of drugs regardless of your bone density.

The most common—though still unlikely—side effect of alendronate is stomach acid reflux. Others are nausea, indigestion, abdominal pain, constipation, and diarrhea. The risk of stomach problems increases when used with NSAIDs like aspirin, which can cause similar symptoms, and increases as you get older. The most serious—though uncommon—side effect is irritation and inflammation of the esophagus, leading, in the most extreme cases, to ulcers in the esophagus. A reformulated coating on Fosamax capsules has greatly reduced the incidence of this side effect by moving the medicine through the esophagus more quickly.

If you do have a problem with reflux, careful dosing may help. Just 5 mg daily is the usual dose for prevention, and 10 mg a day is for treatment of established osteoporosis. The lower the dose, the less likely you are to experience side effects. Take alendronate with a large cup of water first thing in the morning, and wait at least half an hour before having anything else to eat or drink or taking any other medication. That allows it to be well absorbed and helps limit any effects on your digestive tract. Staying upright for that half hour also helps. Ask your doctor to start you off by slowly increasing your dose to the level right for you, to give your body a chance to adjust to the drug and, again, limit side effects. Don't be tempted to divide tablets, as that may increase irritation.

New studies have shown the effectiveness of "pulsing" alendronate—taking larger doses less often. Your doctor might recommend, for example, seven pills once a week, rather than one every day. For people who do experience side effects, having them only once a week, rather than every day, may make using the drug much more agreeable.

The very long-term effects of alendronate are still unclear, though experts are satisfied with the safety and effectiveness overall. Beneficial results may last after you stop taking it, but generally it is a prescription you should stay on as long as your bones are benefiting. As with any drug therapy, your doctor should monitor your progress closely.

A new bisphosphonate released after the first publication of this book is **risedronate** (brand name Actonel). Actually an older medication reformatted for osteoporosis, risedronate is at least as effective—if not more so—than alendronate (Fosamax), and is more user-friendly. Packaged with a new coating that makes it move through the esophagus more quickly, avoiding the reflux problems some patients experience with alendronate. It is also given in much smaller doses. I'm not changing anything for my patients currently using alendronate with no side effects, but in new cases I now prefer risedronate.

The first form of bisphosphonate used for prevention of osteoporosis, *etidronate* (brand name Didronel), is no longer commonly used. Originally, it was developed for a bone disease and for bone cancer, and for many years was the only recourse against osteoporosis. But while etidronate does prevent bone loss by slowing breakdown of old bone, the preserved bone was increasingly made of old or damaged cells. And etidronate also interferes with formation of new bone. On this drug, your bones will be denser, but also perhaps more brittle, exposing you to a higher fracture risk. The long-term effects of taking the drug remain unknown, and studies show that the benefits may wear off after about two years.

Etidronate remains a relatively inexpensive drug and has few side effects. But because of the threat of its creating osteomalacia (soft bones) over the long term, it is rarely used now that more effective options are available. If it is used, it should be taken cyclically (two weeks on, twelve weeks off) to minimize the problems with new bone formation. And it should always be used in conjunction with calcium supplements. But I'd recommend you steer clear of it altogether.

THE WHOLE IS GREATER THAN THE SUM OF THE PARTS

To maximize the effectiveness of any prescription aimed at increasing bone density, you should always be taking, in addition, supplements of calcium and vitamin D—and possibly the trace minerals—at the levels recommended in earlier chapters. Most of the studies done on the effectiveness of these drugs actually test them in combination with calcium or calcium and vitamin D supplements.

CALCITONIN (MIACALCIN)

The second major medication for preserving and increasing bone density is *calcitonin* (brand name Miacalcin). Calcitonin is a natural hormone made by the thyroid gland that limits the release of calcium from bones into the blood. Levels in the body generally decrease with age, and estrogen stimulates the secretion of it;

CALCITONIN (MIACALCIN)

- Dose: 1 spray in one nostril daily (200 U)
- Known drug interactions: none
- Not recommended for people with recurrent nosebleeds, or pregnant or nursing women
- Cost: approximately $60 a month

Alternate nostrils each day.

---

menopause, with markedly decreased levels of estrogen, causes even lower levels. Low bodily calcitonin does *not* indicate low bone density, but prescription calcitonin can help protect bones. What you get in a prescription, though, is actually from salmon because it is fifty to a hundred times stronger than human calcitonin. Like estrogen and bisphosphonates, calcitonin acts to slow bone breakdown.

Case in Point: Maya

One patient I recommended calcitonin to was a Middle Eastern woman just reaching menopause. A DEXA scan showed Maya's bone density to already be 15 percent below ideal levels in her spine and 12 percent lower than I would have liked to see at the hip. Her NTX level was still in the normal range, but at the high end of it (41), indicating a risk of fracture mildly higher than her bone density alone would predict. She was an avid exerciser, and was glad to learn how much that contributed to protecting bones. She was determined to go through menopause as "naturally" as possible, and didn't want HRT for this reason. But she was concerned enough about her bones to consider other prescription treatments if she could avoid side effects and not raise her risk of any other condition. Calcitonin appealed to her since it is "natural" in the sense that the pills are made from salmon; the substance is also *produced in the human body and has no known side effects other than nasal irritation in one in ten people who use it (it comes in a nasal spray).*

To aid and abet calcitonin to the best of her ability, Maya adopted a diet rich in plant estrogens, upping the amount of tofu and other soy products she ate (see Chapter 11). She started taking the recommended doses of calcium and vitamin D supplements, along with a multivitamin and other supplements similar to those described in Chapter 6. She kept up her regular exercise program, with a renewed focus on strength training.

One year later, her bone scan showed her vertebrae to now be 13 percent above expected, though her hip was still 4 percent below ideal levels. She was among the fortunate 90 percent of patients who experience no side effects from calcitonin, so she continues to take it every day. I expect that when she comes back for her next scan in about two years, she'll have rebuilt all her bones to the level of a healthy 30-year-old woman—or even better!

Over three-quarters of the patients who use calcitonin will see increases in their bone density. Studies show gains of over 3 percent a year in bone density after two years of taking calcitonin, in most—but not all—patients, and a 40 percent reduction in risk of fractures in the spine. So my patient was ahead of the curve—a plug for adopting a healthy lifestyle to maximize the results of drug treatment. Even if there is no gain but there is also no loss, calcitonin is beneficial. It works best in men, and women more than five years after menopause and hence no longer in the accelerated phase of bone loss, and it may be more effective in the spine than other parts of the skeleton. (Although I'm convinced we'll eventually find out that it is equally effective all over the body, and I use it as if it is.) Calcitonin is not yet proven to decrease the rate of fractures.

Calcitonin is the best choice for those who do not take estrogen and who cannot tolerate alendronate. Calcitonin, unlike other treatment options, can help control bone pain, although we don't know why. So it may also be the best choice for those in pain from vertebral fractures. *More studies have been done on alendronate than on calcitonin, so it is most doctors' first recommendation. But*

Case in Point: Madeleine

*S*evere back pain is what prompted Madeleine to come see me. At 75, Madeleine had normal bone density readings (for her age), but an NTX of 90 and arthritis, which can sometimes interfere with the results of a bone density scan. The diagnosis: compression fracture of the spine.

She began taking Miacalcin, and after a year her NTX dropped to 34, greatly lowering her risk of fracture. A second bone scan showed no change in her bones' density—but while there was no gain, at her age, no additional loss is definitely a positive result. More important, the Miacalcin relieved her bone pain, and she's been symptom free, which has allowed her to start a moderate exercise program that will help build her bones and won't bother her back.

given the safety record of and lack of side effects associated with calcitonin, I usually recommend starting with that. I'm betting that as more studies are completed, calcitonin will be shown to equal or even surpass alendronate in overall effectiveness, especially in women not taking HRT. My stance is slightly against the current, but I'm a believer in giving calcitonin a chance to work as long as there is time to play with, because it is the safest and most physiologically natural choice when a prescription is required.

For years, the only way to get calcitonin was by injection several times a week, but now a nasal spray makes using it much simpler (not to mention more appealing). The usual dose is 200

TALK TO YOUR DOCTOR

Calcitonin (Miacalcin) is the only prescription treatment option that can reduce or eliminate the pain sometimes associated with osteoporosis as well as improve bone density and decrease risk of fractures.

FOSAMAX OR MIACALCIN?

Fosamax is the most common prescription to counter low bone density, though as I said, I favor Miacalcin, at least to begin with, for patients who don't need urgent care. Both are excellent choices, alone or together, but here are some instances where you should choose Miacalcin:

- You have bone pain.
- You prefer a natural product.
- You have side effects from Fosamax.
- You can't take Fosamax because you have GERD (gastro-esophageal reflux disease).
- Fosamax's dosing routine is too inconvenient for you.

IU, sprayed in alternating nostrils daily. About 10 percent of patients experience nasal dryness and irritation. Calcitonin must be kept refrigerated. You should take supplements of calcium and vitamin D to maximize the effectiveness. Calcitonin is considered very safe, since it has been used (in the injectable form) for over twenty years to treat bone disease without any significant problems.

Case in Point: Laurie

When Laurie had her first bone scan last year, at 52, she felt confident about her bone density, since she'd been taking hormone replacement therapy (Estrace micronized estradiol and Provera progestin) every day for over two years, took calcium supplements, and was an avid biker, runner, and boater—and took her dogs for long walks every day. But the results came back with severe osteopenia in the hip and borderline osteoporosis in the spine.

Her vitamin D and thyroid levels were normal, as were her other hormones. With her NTX an alarming 112, indicating a real and immediate risk of fracture, Laurie wanted reasonably aggressive intervention.

From the options I described, she chose Miacalcin, and to maximize the benefit to her bones, she overhauled her diet. She increased how much calcium she ate, added more beans and soy, and started to use flaxseeds regularly. I recommended adding a supplement of trace minerals to her usual routine with calcium supplements.

Laurie now regrets the year after menopause she waited before starting HRT, because she blames the delay for exposing her bones to accelerated rates of loss of mass. She was also perimenopausal for an unusually long time—at least ten years—and suspects her estrogen dropped enough during that time, but before her periods stopped altogether, to make a big difference.

In just six months on Miacalcin and a new way of eating, Laurie's NTX was down to 68, at the top of the range considered normal. Estrogen, which had been her first plan of attack, maintains bone metabolism, but it can't reverse bone loss, so it didn't do everything Laurie wanted from a medication. Miacalcin slows bone loss, and the combination—more bone building and less bone loss—moved Laurie out of the danger zone so she can continue the high-energy lifestyle she's used to without compromise.

My Story: Frances

I took estrogen for twenty years, but had to stop after I developed a serious blood clot. After that, the trouble started. I broke bones a few times from doing nothing in particular. I kept cracking vertebrae, and was in excruciating pain. I was crippled from it. I could hardly walk. I know I would have been in a wheelchair by now if I hadn't found a way to make improvement.

A bone scan confirmed I had severe osteoporosis, and my doctor recommended Fosamax. A year later, a scan showed I had 5 percent improvement. The doctor was pleased, but I thought the process was very slow. So the doctor started me on Miacalcin nasal spray, too, and in an-

*other year I gained another 6 percent. The improvements were in my
back and hip.*

*I take 1,000–1,200 mg of calcium a day, and I try to get as much
calcium in my diet as I can. I haven't had any more breaks since I started
on the prescriptions, and though I still need my pain medication when I
go out, I don't use it as constantly as I used to.*

*I am so much better than I was three years ago. I feel better. Going
up and down stairs is still hard because I have arthritis in my hip—I am
over 80, you know—but I get around and do things around the house
just fine. I'm going out and having a bit of fun, rather than just sitting in
my house.*

RALOXIFENE (EVISTA)

The newest pharmaceutical option for protecting bone density is
raloxifene (brand name Evista). Raloxifene is a selective estrogen receptor modulator (SERM), which, simply stated, means it has a
chemical structure similar to estrogen and attaches itself to molecules in the body where estrogen would otherwise attach. It prevents
bone loss by reducing breakdown of bone much the way estrogen
replacement therapy does. Post-menopausal women can expect
about a 3 percent increase in bone density in the first year of taking
raloxifene and 1 to 2 percent per year after that. This brings a 40 to
50 percent reduction of risk of fracture in the spine. Less than 60 percent of women will see increases in bone density with raloxifene, a markedly lower response
rate than with the options described earlier, including estrogen.
Raloxifene is sometimes given with a progesterone, which might improve your chances of benefiting, as well as the magnitude of your
results, though there is no hard evidence of that yet.

Since raloxifene blocks estrogen, it is the best choice for

> **THINGS TO THINK ABOUT**
>
> Any drug treatment will be most
> useful for women during the
> first years of menopause, when
> the rate of bone loss peaks to
> such high levels.

postmenopausal women who can't take estrogen, especially those fearing an increase in breast cancer risk. It is *not* an option for men. Although it isn't quite as effective as other prescription options in protecting bone at the hip, and is only about half as effective in the spine, it doesn't increase the risk of uterine cancer (as estrogen does) and may actually *protect* against breast cancer. (Raloxifene is very similar to tamoxifen, which has gotten a lot of press as preventing breast cancer.) It doesn't cause breast soreness or uterine bleeding, as estrogen can.

If you can take estrogen but are hesitant to, and are wondering if this is a better alternative, note that raloxifene does not offer some of the benefits that estrogen does. Raloxifene's effect on the heart is still unclear. Though it appears to lower cholesterol levels, it is unknown as yet whether that translates into protection against heart disease and heart attacks equivalent to estrogen's. Raloxifene does not relieve menopausal symptoms, and can even *cause* or increase hot flashes. No studies have yet been completed on raloxifene's effect

> **TALK TO YOUR DOCTOR**
>
> Raloxifene, the drug generating excitement as a "safe" estrogen, with no increase in cancer risk—and even a *protective* effect— will do nothing to relieve menopausal symptoms.

> **TALK TO YOUR DOCTOR**
>
> Raloxifene (Evista) and tamoxifen are closely related, and I think you probably get bone benefits when taking tamoxifen for preventing breast cancer recurrence. But none of the research on that drug has looked into the question, so you shouldn't rely on it. If you are taking tamoxifen, I'd suggest adding ipriflavone (see Chapter 19) to your routine, to cover your bones just in case.

RALOXIFENE (EVISTA)

- Dose: 60 mg once daily
- Known drug interactions: Coumadin (you'll need your medication monitored if you're taking a blood thinner), cholestyramine (this cholesterol-lowering drug, sometimes given after gallbladder surgery, too, makes you unable to absorb Evista), Valium, and NSAIDs (if you use ibuprofen, Alleve, or aspirin for pain or inflammation, you'll need to watch for side effects).
- Not recommended for use with estrogen, people with prolonged immobilization, liver disease, or pregnant or nursing women
- Cost: approximately $60 a month

on colon cancer or Alzheimer's disease, but estrogen is known to offer protection against both. Finally, raloxifene has one of the same potential side effects as estrogen: dangerous blood clots.

TAKE YOUR CALCIUM

Almost three quarters of women taking the most commonly prescribed bone density medications do *not* take calcium. Yet all those treatments require optimal levels of calcium (and vitamin D and all the other nutrients) in the body to provide their full benefits. Taking a prescription drug doesn't let you off the hook in terms of nourishing your bones! Imagine if you had a general contractor and bunch of subcontractors remodeling your home—but no materials for them to work with. Even with all the right workers in place, the project will never get done without the proper supplies. Building and maintaining your bones works the same way.

The usual dose for prevention is 60 mg a day. You have a bit more flexibility when you take your pill, since it doesn't matter whether you take it with food. Be sure to take calcium and vitamin D supplements, especially if your diet isn't up to par, to get the best results.

DO YOU NEED DRUG THERAPY?

If a bone scan shows you have bone loss—osteopenia or osteoporosis—you should consider drug therapy. The following recommendations assume you are using diet and exercise to protect your bones, that you're using the right supplements, and that you have an individualized plan about using hormones if you are in perimenopause or menopause. If your periods are stopping (or have stopped), HRT is strongly recommended—with variations and "alternatives" recommended if you don't want or can't take standard traditional HRT. Remember, though the specific way to do it will vary from person to person or over a lifetime, the goal is always the same: to improve bone formation and slow bone loss.

- *If you have not reached perimenopause or menopause yet*, significant bone loss most likely indicates another problem, like hyperthyroidism, or use of corticosteroids, or some other metabolic disorder. Get to the heart of that matter first, and treat what's treatable and compensate for whatever can't be eliminated. With that corrected, you may not need anything else. But if you've had enough loss, or the rate of progress is rapid enough, you may want to take one of these prescriptions just until you get back to normal density. The greater the extent of the bone loss you've had, the more aggressive your approach should be.
- If you are menopausal or perimenopausal, and have *osteopenia but an NTX under 50*, so the progression of your bone loss is slow, you may want to give diet, exercise,

and supplements a chance to work before you start a prescription. Some of the complementary strategies described in Chapter 21 may support your progress, or you may want to consider one of the gentle natural hormonal options for bone health, like natural progesterone, ipriflavone, or isoflavones, just as a few examples (which you may be able to use together with HRT).

- If you are menopausal or perimenopausal, and have *osteoporosis but an NTX under 50*, so the progression of your bone loss is slow and your fracture risk manageable, again, you have time on your side. You have enough loss that you should seriously consider Fosamax or Miacalcin, or Evista if you are not taking HRT, or some combination thereof. You could also consider working first with just diet, exercise, supplements, and "alternatives," including natural hormones. To build your bones that way, you'll have to take an aggressive approach to all these things, really buckling down to the exercise, calcium foods, and tofu and using high-quality supplements religiously. Have your bones checked again in six months to a year to make sure you're making improvements, and if you're not, you should try a drug therapy.

- If you are menopausal or perimenopausal, and have *osteopenia and an NTX over 50*, the progression of loss is rapid and the risk of fracture is higher, so you should carefully consider Fosamax, Miacalcin, or, if you're not taking HRT, Evista—or some combination of those, in addition to the strategies above.

- If you are menopausal or perimenopausal, and have *osteoporosis and an NTX over 50*, the progression of loss is rapid enough and the risk of fracture is high enough that a drug treatment is strongly recommended in combination with HRT. If you are not taking traditional HRT, then it would be important to use Evista or one of the alternative hormones.

MIX WELL FOR BEST RESULTS

Combination therapy (particularly Fosamax and Miacalcin) might be right for you if:

- A single therapy isn't giving you the desired results
- Your NTX is very high (over 100) so your fracture risk is very high
- You have a condition, like hyperthyroidism, that accelerates bone loss
- You have to use a medication, like steroids, that accelerates bone loss
- You have side effects when you take Fosamax daily

In this last case, ask your doctor to "pulse" Fosamax so you don't take it every day, and combine this with Miacalcin used daily. You may avoid Fosamax's side effects this way, and the combination will be more effective than Miacalcin alone.

You can (and most people should) combine Fosamax and/or Miacalcin with HRT (or the alternatives to the traditional hormones), or with Evista if you are not taking other hormones.

Case in Point: Cheryl

*C*heryl had no family history of osteoporosis, but was 50 and peri-menopausal, so I recommended she get a bone density scan to see just where she stood. As it turned out, her spine was 19 percent below normal and her hip 8 percent below. Her NTX levels (142) indicated rapid progression of bone loss and a very real risk of fractures.

Even so, she didn't want to take HRT—my first recommendation—but agreed she needed something more quickly than what diet and exercise could provide. She chose a combination of Evista and Fosamax, and one year later had dropped her NTX to just 29, well within the normal range. She had gained five percentage points in her spine and three in her hip in just that first year, so she continued with the drugs—as well as good diet and exercise habits, and calcium supplements—with her sights set on regaining the bone density of a young adult.

BONE FORMATION AND BREAKDOWN BY AGE

As in the previous chapter, you should bear in mind the stage your body is in when choosing a treatment.

	Bone Formation	Bone Breakdown
Childhood	↑ ↑ ↑ ↑	↓
Adolescence	↑ ↑ ↑	↓
Age 30	↑ ↑	↓
Age 40	↑	↓ ↓
Age 50/menopause	↑	↓ ↓
Age 60	↑	↓ ↓ ↓
Age 70	↑	↓ ↓ ↓ ↓

FLUORIDE

I used to prescribe *sodium fluoride* because it stimulates bone formation. But the bone formed turned out not to be of high quality—and sometimes even abnormal—resulting in dense, but fragile, bones and *increases* in the rate of fractures. Side effects include gastrointestinal problems and joint and/or bone pain, and it is potentially toxic in high doses. With newer, far better options, the benefits no longer outweigh the drawbacks, so my advice is to avoid it.

However, studies are under way on lower doses in special slow-release formulations that may build bone and *decrease* fractures, as well as reduce or eliminate side effects. Low doses (45 to 75 mg daily) are already used in Europe, with apparently satisfactory results, but haven't been approved by the FDA here as of yet. More study is needed, but perhaps lower doses that keep fluoride safe and effective will bring this drug back into favor. It should be a relatively inexpensive option if it does prove useful in the future. If it does make a comeback, you may want to take it along with calcium and vitamin D supplements, and possibly another medicine that blocks bone breakdown.

EXPERIMENTAL TREATMENTS

Several breakthroughs since the first publication of this book are already pointing out new directions for overcoming low bone density.

A class of drugs known as **statins**, which are FDA approved for lowering cholesterol levels, turn out to *stimulate* bone growth. It is too early to say if taking statins specifically to treat low bone density is advisable, but for now they should certainly be considered by anyone needing cholesterol medication who also has concerns about bone density. And if you are, for example, taking estrogen only because you have high cholesterol, it may turn out that you'd be better off using a statin to lower cholesterol, since you'll reap the bone benefits that way, too.

The statin drugs, including Pravachol, Zocor and Mevacor, are now made in a lab, but were originally derived from Chinese red rice bran. **Red rice bran** is now sold as Cholestin, and this natural statin may be worth trying for high cholesterol (especially when bone density is a factor).

Another drug originally used for another purpose has turned out to have benefits in treating low bone density. **Aredia** has been used to tame the side effects of cancer therapies that create calcium metabolism problems. New results show that it can be a useful treatment for osteoporosis when very aggressive intervention is necessary—for example, in someone already experiencing painful fractures. I have patients who have taken it via IV once every six months with results that outpace Fosamax over the same time period.

Several more options are currently being studied, though for all the treatments named below there is not enough information available right now to be able to recommend them. Developments in this area have been coming fast and furious in the last few years—after decades of almost no options—and your doctor should apprise you of the availability of better choices as they are proven.

Trials are currently under way on two bisphosphonates: *tiludronate* and *pamidronate*.

Testosterone seems to increase bone density. It is already FDA-approved for treatment of menopausal symptoms (see Chapter 18), though not for osteoporosis, and may turn out to work well in conjunction with estrogen, with the combination having an edge over estrogen alone. For men with low testosterone levels, who are at increased risk for loss of bone density, testosterone supplements may prevent bone loss. The benefits will have to be weighed against the potential to exacerbate prostate problems and heart risks.

Low-dose injections of *parathyroid hormone* stimulates bone formation, though high levels in the body can trigger bone breakdown. Some advocates suggest using it in conjunction with estrogen, androgens (male hormones), or calcitonin. The parathyroid gland helps calcium to be absorbed, which may be the secret of this hormone's success.

Research into *other things* that might stimulate bone growth (since current available options work by blocking bone breakdown) are putting a spotlight on growth hormone, growth hormone-releasing hormone, transforming growth factor beta, platelet-derived growth factor, insulinlike growth factor, fibroblast growth factors, IGF-I, IGF-II, and zeolite. Some clinical trials are already under way, and some animal studies have shown encouraging results, so one or more may eventually find its way to your local pharmacy's shelves.

Though it isn't specifically a treatment for bone density, one more promising development is worth mentioning here. One study showed that *aspirin* given after surgery to repair a hip fracture reduced the risk of dying while in the hospital by 75 percent, probably because most deaths following hip fractures are actually heart-related. We'll need more information before we know if this simple step should be routine.

I'm not a psychic or a biochemist, so I don't know which of the above will prove useful. But whatever happens, the important thing to note is that we are getting a lot better at this. Ten years ago we had no wonderful options for treating low bone density (combined with a poor understanding of how to prevent it). The last few years have brought a relative explosion of options, with more choices surely on the way. I'm looking forward to choices that equal the results from HRT, without the attendant trade-offs. But the biggest breakthrough will be in alternatives that make healthy bone, as opposed to current treatments that simply block destruction of bone.

Chapter 21

Other Alternatives

While there is little in the way of placebo-controlled, double-blind studies to document exactly what effect any of the approaches in this chapter have on your bones, these techniques—whether ancient or modern—are valuable additions to your defense strategies. The prescription options covered in the last chapter are strong medicine, which may be just the ticket if your bones are already weakened. But they come with too many downsides to take them "just in case." Here are some choices more geared to prevention or use as adjuncts to conventional therapies, though some may also help in more advanced cases. And certainly if you can't tolerate any of the drugs described, but need help with your bones, these are all good avenues to explore (in conjunction, as always, with good diet and exercise habits and smart supplementation). As mainstream medicine investigates these options more closely, and we develop experience in using them, we will be able to target bones more and more specifically. In the meantime, these are natural, gentle strategies (though some require professional guidance) to keep your bones healthy.

HERB SOURCES OF PHYTOESTROGENS

Black cohosh
Chastetree (Vitex)
Dong quai
Elder
False unicorn root
Fennel
Fenugreek
Ginseng
Lady's slipper
Licorice
Liferoot
Passionflower
Sarsaparilla
Sassafras
Unicorn root
Wild yam root bark

HERBS

Herbalists do not claim to cure or reverse osteoporosis with herbs, but they can help your body slow bone loss and maximize bone growth. Herbs are also useful for symptom relief. Any herbs that help with joint or muscle pain, or that reduce inflammation, will help relieve related osteoporosis symptoms. Some herbs are excellent sources of calcium or other nutrients crucial for healthy bones, and some herbs work something like estrogen does, including supporting bone density.

The herbs recommended for menopausal symptoms (or any low-estrogen condition) or PMS are good choices to protect bone health as well, because they are usually rich in phytoestrogens. (As we saw in Chapter 11, phytoestrogens boost the effects of estrogen when body levels are low, and block excess estrogen when levels are high.) Using any one of these (see above), or any combination, will help relieve symptoms of menopause and probably benefit your bones. Black cohosh probably has the best scientific evidence behind its ability to work in the body much in the way HRT does: women who took black cohosh in a German study reported the same level of relief from menopausal symptoms as women taking HRT. The dose being studied was the equivalent of 10 to 15 drops of tincture once or twice a day, or between 50 and 500 mg a day of dried, powdered herb, or two tablets twice a day of prepared pills. The goal is to get about 1 mg of the active ingredient known as deoxyacteine.

Chastetree (also known as Vitex) boosts the body's production of progesterone and other hormones. Try 20 mg of extract a day. Nettle (which contains many important minerals), alfalfa, and slippery elm are all good for building and maintaining healthy bones. Burdock, yellow dock, and dandelion help maximize the effects of estrogen in the body after menopause by supporting the liver. Fennel and anise can increase estrogen production.

For osteoporosis, David L. Hoffman, past president of the American Herbalist Guild, has recommended mixing tinctures of chastetree, horsetail, black cohosh, oat straw, and alfalfa (with twice as much chastetree as each of the other ingredients), and taking 1 teaspoon three times a day. Or use 2 teaspoons of the mixed dried herbs per cup of water to make tea, and drink three cups a day. Look for similar premade preparations in your health food store. For menopausal symptoms (and by extension bone density), Dr. Andrew Weil has recommended using dong quai, chastetree, and damiana, taking two capsules, or one dropperful of tincture mixed in warm water, of each once a day.

Many herbs are rich in calcium (see below), making them an excellent addition to a bone density program. Pigweed, for example, has about 1,500 mg of calcium per ounce of fresh leaves. You might have to grow your own, or seek out a specialized organic or herb farm to get it fresh, but once you find it you can take care of a whole day's calcium requirement in one shot (or one salad, as the case may be). Just use it as you would spinach (steam it, put it in a salad, dress up a sandwich). Dandelion is rich in boron and silicon, too, making it a well-rounded package for promoting healthy bones. You can prepare fresh dandelion greens the same way you

CALCIUM-RICH HERBS

Chaya
Comfrey
Dandelion
Horsetail
Mugwort
Oatstraw
Pigweed
Plaintain leaves
Purslane
Raspberry leaves
Red clover
Sage
Stinging nettle
Yellow dock

would any bitter green. Purslane provides calcium and magnesium in roughly equal proportions, which is ideal, and has heart-healthy omega-3 fatty acids (like fish oils) and other antioxidants besides. You can eat it raw or steamed—this is another one much like spinach. Horsetail is rich in other minerals, too, particularly the crucial magnesium and silicon you need for strong bones. It

DRINK YOUR CALCIUM

Try making a tea with 3 tablespoons of dried calcium-rich herbs in a quart of boiling water. Cover and steep for at least 15 minutes. Drink three cups a day.

Or make soup stock. Start with bones (fish or chicken) simmered in water (with a good splash of vinegar to help pull out the calcium). Add bone-healthy fresh or dried herbs and cook until they are soft. Enjoy it as is or puréed, as soup, or use it as stock for a more substantial soup. You'll get a host of other nutrients along with your calcium boost.

THE DENSITY DOZEN: HERBS FOR BONE HEALTH

Alfalfa
Anise
Bayberry bark
Black currant seed
Oil blessed thistle
Blue cohosh
Burdock root
Cramp bark
Damiana
Motherwort
Pennyroyal
Slippery elm

---

has some estrogenic substances as well. Use it in making soup, or steep it into a tea. Oatstraw is also a good source of silicon. Stinging nettle is also a great source of magnesium, silicon, boron, zinc, and vitamin D, among other minerals, making it a great overall herb for bone health. You can eat it fresh as you would any greens, or use the dried herb to make tea.

Herbs are powerful chemicals, so don't let their "naturalness" fool you into thinking you can treat them offhandedly. Herbal medicines are also most effective when carefully matched to the individual, so your best bet if you are interested in herbal remedies would be to consult a professional. I'm not an herbalist, so don't rely solely on me regarding what to take and how to take it. You should do some research on your own. *Herbs of Choice* by Varro E. Tyler, Ph.D., *Prescription for Natural Healing* by James Balch and Phyllis Balch, and *Natural Health, Natural Medicine* by Andrew Weil, M.D., among others, are all good references for laypeople.

The most reliable standards nonexperts like me have in judging herbs are the ones laid down by Germany's Commission E. Commission E functions something like the FDA does in this country, but is devoted to the science of herbs. It is the best medical authority on the subject we have, so you should focus on herbs approved by Commission E as effective and safe. Look for the new *Physician's Desk Reference for Herbal Medicines* at your library. It is based on Commission E recommendations, and though intended for doctors, is accessible enough for laypeople to refer to. It is also available for sale (though more expensive than a standard book) through PDR in Des Moines.

TRADITIONAL CHINESE MEDICINE

In traditional Chinese medicine, bone health is believed to be inextricably linked to the health of the kidneys. So any treatment recommended for strengthening the kidneys (increasing their "energy") would be good for your bones as well. The kidneys are also thought to be related to aging in general. Chinese medicine has long been used to relieve the symptoms of a difficult menopause with much success, so low bone density might also be improved along with more overt signs of a drop in hormone levels.

An expert in Chinese medicine will generally recommend a combination of diet, herbs, acupuncture, and exercise, particularly tai chi and qi gong, or a similar type of movement. I'm a fan of this kind of exercise, as described earlier in the book, since it builds bone mass and develops strength and balance, and at the same time reduces stress, so that's one of the appeals of TCM to me. Acupuncture has some of the best science behind it of any other "alternative" therapy. But the key thing about traditional Chinese medicine is that it uses a *combination* of tactics that are greater than the sum of their parts. You can use just one strand, if necessary, but weaving them together results in a stronger whole cloth.

Acupuncture is an excellent way to relieve pain, including pain from osteoporosis or low bone density. The Kidney 3, Kidney 10, and Spleen 6 points for acupuncture—or acupressure, if you want to try this at home—are important for preventing and treating low bone density and the pain that can result. (If you don't get results with self-administered acupressure, don't throw the baby out with the bathwater. Working with a properly trained acupuncture professional could well make all the difference.) If done properly, it can also alter the body's metabolism and biochemistry in ways Western science does not yet fully understand to actually stimulate bone growth and retard loss. It is generally acknowledged that acupuncture points have more nerves and increased blood flow than the areas around them, so stimulating them produces changes in nerve conduction and releases serotonin and endorphins, which improve mood and decrease pain throughout the body, among other things.

I read an anecdote in an alternative medicine reference book from a leader of a school of traditional Chinese medicine who treated a woman whose bone density was 30 percent below desirable. After two and a half months of acupuncture and herbs (and no other intervention), she had no more pain and her bone density had increased 50 percent. Blood tests showed her hormone levels had increased. The expert in traditional Chinese medicine I work with doesn't have his clients get bone scans, but reports his patients with suspected low bone density find balance and strength with the practice of traditional medicine, with little in the way of menopausal complaints.

For a shot at such remarkable results, consult a specialist in Eastern medicine, not someone with just the few months' training required to hang out a shingle. Only a few hundred people in this country have taken the four- to five-year formal medical training available to become experts, and the number of people with the less intense training is growing by leaps and bounds. (A good acupuncturist should be able to help you with symptom relief, at least, even with the more rapid training course.)

Chinese herbs are usually given in combination and treat your body's unique energy. So again you should seek professional guidance to find the mix that is best for you. Good herbologists won't give generic recommendations for particular conditions. Rather, they treat each individual by working to restore balance to the body overall. If you want to experiment yourself, eycinnuam dipsaci is a common recommendation. Dong quai contains phytoestrogens $1/400$ as strong as estrogen, but with some of the same effects on the body. (Do not take dong quai if you are pregnant.) Two

Immortals Decoction and Eight Flavor Rehmannia formulas are generally good choices for women looking to protect their bones. Six Flavor Rehmannia supports the kidney, as do shou wu, dong quai, and ginseng, which are often used in combination (including a drink called Shou Wu Chih) for easing the aging process. Ginseng has a lot of beneficial phytoestrogens, but use it carefully, as high levels can cause high blood pressure, anxiety, and insomnia. Ox knee root and three-edge root have estrogenic effects, which should support healthy bones. In an animal study, tochu bark extract was proven to help the body absorb calcium, and was shown to increase bone density and muscle mass. In humans, licorice (gan cao) and peony (bau shao and chi shao) have been shown to increase the ratio of estrogen to testosterone, following animal studies that revealed the herbs helped convert testosterone into estrogen, raising overall estrogen levels. Liu wei di huang tang formula can increase estrogen levels and estrogen receptors after menopause. Dan shen also increased estrogen levels in another study in animals.

Be aware that using these herbs off-the-rack, without consulting with an expert, isn't really traditional Chinese medicine (though it may or may not work for you). Simply substituting another chemical ("natural" though they may be, herbs work because they are sources of potent chemicals) for a prescription won't get you any closer to optimal health or bone density.

AYURVEDIC HERBS

In this ancient Indian tradition, the herb shatavari is used as a "rejuvenative" for women, and so would be good for balancing hormones and therefore bone density. Boswella, or the extract boswellin, is used for bone and joint pain. The herb amla is often recommended for osteoporosis. Use any or all as directed on the package.

HOMEOPATHY

Homeopathy is often confused with herbal medicine, but its guiding principle is quite distinct. Homeopathy views any symptom as the result of some injury to or imbalance in the body, and holds that substances that elicit the same symptoms, when taken at microscopically small dilutions, will paradoxically help relieve them by restoring balance (the hair of the dog that bit you). Many homeopathic preparations are marketed for relief of menopausal symptoms, including hot flashes and night sweats, moodiness, and nausea. Since the same hormonal imbalance that produces those signs forces decreases in bone density, relieving the overt symptoms might also mean improving your bones. Classical homeopathy doesn't offer treatments specifically for low bone density, though it offers some remedies to address symptoms of osteoporosis. But new homeopathic remedies from outside the orthodoxy, like blends including Silica, Chamomilla, and/or Mercurius, are aimed directly at promoting healthy, dense bones.

One of my patients, a woman with a thyroid disorder, already had dangerously low bone density in her 50s. She didn't want to take HRT and opted for diet, exercise, and supplements, including isoflavones (see Chapter 11) instead. She also then began a homeopathic regimen because she felt her density was low enough to merit direct intervention. She had a low NTX level, indicating a low fracture risk, so she had time to experiment with this kind of treatment before considering less gentle and more aggressive options. When she comes back for another bone density screening, I expect to see improvement. If I don't, we'll consider changing tactics.

Two common homeopathic prescriptions for imbalances along the lines of menopausal symptoms (one of which would be bone loss) are calcarea carbonica and calcarea phosphorica. Once again, you'd do well to consult a professional, as homeopathy is always carefully geared to the individual and her particular symptoms. There is not a lot of science backing up homeopathy for low bone density, but at the very least it will cause no harm. If homeopathy appeals to you, I think it is well worth investigating.

TOP 6 HOMEOPATHIC REMEDIES FOR STRONG BONES

Asa Hershoff, N.D., D.C., a naturopath and chiropractor and author of *Homeopathy for Musculoskeletal Healing*, points out that homeopathic remedies are meant to be individualized to the person taking them and her particular symptoms. Working with a professional is the best way to get the best results, but in general he recommends the following remedies for various aspects of bone health:

- Calc Carb optimizes the function of calcium in the body.
- Homeopathic Comfrey (symphytum) accelerates bone healing.
- Homeopathic Silica (silicea) improves bone nutrition and growth.
- Calc Fluor (calcium fluoride) strengthens brittle bones.
- Lycopodium addresses complaints of aging, longevity.
- Sepia (from ink of cuttlefish) helps with hormone deficiency.

MIND-BODY MEDICINE

Holistic medicine means paying attention to the mind and spirit as well as the body. Stress reduction, meditation, and faith or spiritual focus are all proven risk-factor reducers for a range of health concerns, and despite a lack of specific studies on the topic, I see no reason why bone density wouldn't be among them. One study showed that women in their 40s (when they should still be near peak bone mass) with clinical depression had bones that looked like they belonged to 70-year-olds. It was a small study, but the dramatic results at least hint at the powerful interconnection between your bones and your brain. It should be no surprise, after all we've learned about the role of emotions, stress, social support, faith, prayer, beliefs, and attitude toward heart disease and cancer, and a host of other disorders. Bones are no different from any other part of your body when it comes to being affected by whatever is going on anywhere in the body.

Case in Point: Lillian

One of my colleagues told me about one patient taking only Fos-amax. A small woman in her early 70s, Lillian eats a fairly average American diet, has difficulty walking (and in fact uses a walker), and so gets little exercise and refuses to take calcium or any other supplements. Despite being about 30 percent low in bone density in her hip and spine, Lillian generally feels fine and is always happy and peppy when she comes into the doctor's office. But the scan results did convince her she needed something to protect her bones if she didn't want to fracture her hip or suffer from compression fractures in the spine, so she decided on Fosamax. In two years, she's had over 6 percent gains in her back and almost 11 percent in her hip, impressive results given the fact that the medicine wasn't getting support from the recommended lifestyle changes. In Lillian's case, a positive attitude seemed to be the best medicine.

Stress triggers the release of stressor hormones that (among other things) greatly accelerate bone loss. The unrelenting nature of chronic stress makes it particularly important to reduce the constant stresses we've come to think of as almost normal, as well as the intermittent, specific stresses that are bound to come into your life. The emotions stirred up by your car's breaking down, for example, are stressful, and you'll feel better in general if you find a way to manage them effectively. But constant worry about whether your old clunker will make it all the way to the office each morning, and about how you'll pay the bill next time it does give out, are more serious in the long run. By all means, switch to public transportation or get a more reliable car if you can, and set aside some money out of each paycheck to cover any necessary repairs to try to set your mind at ease. But beyond that, try some of the techniques here to ease the inevitable stresses of day-to-day living. Do away with as many sources of stress as you can, but learn how to manage what does come your way.

THE MENOPAUSE ALTERNATIVE

In other cultures, women experience few, if any, of the symptoms commonly associated with menopause in the United States. There may be medical reasons for that, but attitude also plays a significant role. Where older women are respected for their wisdom and experience, and accepted, physically, for who they are, menopause tends not to be a difficult experience. In our youth-oriented culture, older people in general—and women in particular—are too easily dismissed as irrelevant and/or unattractive. A little-discussed menopausal remedy would be to honor aging, rather than fear or ignore it.

On average, an American woman spends a third of her life postmenopausal, so an attitude adjustment has plenty of time to pay off. You may not be able to change the way everyone else thinks, but let it begin with you. I can't guarantee you that you'll improve your bone density and the other symptoms of menopause, but as powerful as the mind-body connection is, I wouldn't be a bit surprised.

You (and in all likelihood your bones) will benefit from guided imagery, meditation, focused walking, and anything that elicits "the relaxation response"—the term coined by Harvard scientist Herbert Benson, M.D., to describe the calm state of the body without the rush of "fight or flight" messages stress-crazed Americans seem to subsist on. Stress raises hormone levels that can interfere with bone remodeling, so lowering stress takes one more obstacle out of the way of healthy bones. (Exercise is another excellent way to reduce stress, so any technique described in Chapter 15, and in particular yoga, tai chi, and qi gong, will have that additional benefit.)

The simplest approach is simply *being present in the moment.* Unless you are a Zen monk, you'll probably find this difficult to do in the midst of your daily life (though that is the ultimate goal), so start by taking some time out specifically to practice it.

Case in Point: Gail

Gail's personal mantra seemed to be "it's just killing me." Just about anything she mentioned about her life (job, marriage, home) had those words tacked on somewhere. She was unhappy with her life situation, and the constant stress of dissatisfaction decreased the quality of her life emotionally and physically. She came to see me seeking relief for digestive trouble, skin problems, abnormal heart rate, headaches, and muscle aches that were . . . well, killing her. It was worse than menopause, she said.

That was how it came about that just as events in Gail's personal life were reaching a breaking point (divorce), she had a bone density screening test that revealed she was already osteoporotic. She didn't want to start on traditional hormone replacement therapy, so she began using natural progesterone cream. She began taking nutritional supplements along the lines of what is recommended in Chapter 10.

Gail also began meditating every day. With practice, she learned that healing comes from inside. She didn't alter the reality of her life: she was still going through a messy divorce and coping with a frightening new piece of information about her health. But by grounding herself and not being taken prisoner by her emotions, she allowed her body to function more as Mother Nature designed it—naturally and efficiently. She began to feel better about herself and about her life. Her body was no longer at war with itself and she felt well. Actually, she felt good, a feeling that had escaped her for far too long. Her newfound tranquillity should allow the progesterone and supplements to do their work, and in another year she'll have another bone scan to monitor her physical progress. I'm not psychic, so I don't know what that will show, but Gail is clearly a much healthier person in all respects now than when I first met her, and I expect the data we eventually get back to reflect that.

Relax in a comfortable position, breathing slowly and quietly. As you listen to your breath go in and out, pay attention to your inner self as well as your immediate surroundings. Focus on how you feel. If you notice tension anywhere in the body, focus on it and what it represents. Focus your breath and thoughts in the tense area, maintaining your focus until you can let the tension go. Relax and breathe and focus on any other tense spots. Keep going until you find no more tension. End quietly.

Benson provides a simple two-step process to help you achieve the *relaxation response*. First, select a word, short phrase, or sound, and repeat it to yourself. Choosing something meaningful to you is a good idea. For example, you might pick one line of a favorite prayer ("the Lord is my shepherd"), or something from an affirmation you've used ("I am healing"), or just a positive thought ("peace"). (For believers, prayers seem to be an especially powerful entrée to the relaxation response, and spiritual feelings on their own have been associated with being healthier overall.) Even just repeating a number (like "one") will work. Dr. Benson jokes that some of his studies were done with Harvard medical students who couldn't handle anything more complicated than that! A repetitive physical activity, including walking or even knitting, can serve a similar purpose, on its own or together with a repetitive phrase. The second step is to determinedly let go of any other thoughts trying to horn in on your quiet mind, going back to focusing on your repetition. Pausing once or twice a day to do this for ten to twenty minutes will undo the harmful effects of essentially living in a constant state of "fight or flight" arousal. Even five minutes will help, so don't discard this idea if you feel you don't have enough time. The continual presence of stress-induced hormones is itself a stressor, and one we would all be better off without.

Focused walking, also known as prayer walking or walking meditation, is a concept rapidly gaining in popularity, and an excellent practice for mind, body, and spirit all in one. It may be finally the vehicle that brings meditation into the mainstream, since Americans already recognize the importance of exercise and like the feeling of being busy—not "just sitting there." Here the benefit to your bones is more obvious: if meditation doesn't help you out, you can be sure walking does.

This is basically the relaxation response in motion. Walking outdoors is ideal, as it gives you more immediate access to a sense of the divine than, say, a treadmill facing a blank wall in the gym with the television blaring. As you walk, notice your breath, counting how many steps fill the time of each inhalation and exhalation. Label them with numbers or phrases ("one, two, three" or "breathe, breathe, breathe," for example) to keep time. As you get more advanced, you'll be able to use any calming, repetitive phrase you like, as above, but keep it simple for starters. Again, your goal is to stay in the present moment and let any intruding thoughts of the past or future slip right on by. Keep breathing consciously, even if you pause to admire the scenery. As long as you feel calm and centered, you're doing it right.

❀ ❀ ❀ ❀ ❀ ❀ ❀ ❀ ❀ ❀ ❀ ❀ ❀ ❀ ❀ ❀ ❀ ❀ ❀ ❀

WEEK 6 ACTION PLAN

1. Continue the Bone Density Diet with menus 15 to 21 (with any modifications you planned last week).

2. Continue to follow the exercise schedule you designed for yourself last week. Make sure it includes at least one yoga workout and two sessions with weights.

3. Evaluate whether, in addition to the basic lifestyle measures of diet, exercise, and supplements and whatever hormones you've decided to use, if any, your bones need more aggressive intervention.

4. If you do decide to use a drug therapy, remember that medication is just one part of a total plan for quality health and long life. All the other strategies in this program will maximize the results of any drug, so don't take on a "magic bullet" mentality, thinking that all you need to do is swallow a pill every day.

5. Talk with your doctor about the medications you think might be right for you, and about possible combinations of therapies.

6. If you are nearing (or newly in) menopause, recognize this as a crucial window for drug treatment, just as it is for hormone replacement therapy, because of the way bone loss accelerates for the first several years after your periods stop. This is especially true if you are not using hormones

and if a bone scan shows you're already below peak density. In any case, if you haven't already done so, talk with your doctor about your options.

7. If you are taking hormones, but also have bone loss on your screening test, consider combining another prescription bone density treatment with your HRT for more dramatic results.

8. If you have a personal objection to HRT, or if you *can't* take hormones, consider raloxifene as a strong alternative.

9. Find a way to keep up with health news. Developments in the area of bone health are fast-breaking, and you can expect new and improved treatments to be available in the near future—but you'll have to know about them in order to use them. Subscribing to a good health newsletter or magazine (or following the new issues at your local library), finding an authoritative Web site and checking it regularly, following the health column in your local newspaper, or joining a newsgroup on the Internet are all good ways to stay ahead of the curve.

> ## WEEK 6 FOCUS
>
> - Evaluate if you need more aggressive drug therapy in addition to lifestyle changes.
> - Choose a medication, if necessary.
> - Investigate what "alternative" health systems have to offer for supporting strong bones and slowing bone loss.

10. Even if your bone density is still good, experiment with some of the gentle, natural approaches to supporting bone density to see which make you feel good.

11. Try getting at least some of your supplemental calcium from herbs, since that way it comes automatically packaged with a range of complementary nutrients.

12. Pursue whichever "alternative" health system appeals to you. Most are geared not to a particular problem or disease, like osteoporosis, or even to prevention of specific

conditions, but rather to building and maintaining overall wellness. We can all benefit from this shift in mind-set.

13. Check your personal beliefs about menopause, your health in general, and aging. What you experience is closely tied to what you *think*, so make sure the images you rely on are positive ones you would like to be central in your life.

❀ ❀

Going Forward:
Your Personal Plan

Congratulations! You've finished the full six-week program for bone health. Of course, you're not just done after these 42 days. Bone density isn't a thing you can get perfect one time that lasts forever. Bone is a dynamic, living organism, and keeping it in good shape requires a lifetime plan. You've got all the pieces in place now, but you have to keep using what you've learned if you want your bones to stay strong for as long as you're using them. The good news is, this program *works*. With these basic steps, you'll keep your bones at maximum density. Anyone can do it.

The same areas you've been focusing on still apply as you move forward: diet, exercise, supplements, hormones, and, if necessary, medication. To help you stay on top of all the progress you've made these six weeks, here's one last Action Plan to help you organize your strategy for the rest of your life:

❁ ❁ ❁ ❁ ❁ ❁ ❁ ❁ ❁ ❁ ❁ ❁ ❁ ❁ ❁ ❁ ❁ ❁ ❁ ❁

1. Continue on the Bone Density Diet, either going through the cycle of menus provided or picking and choosing from the menus the meals you like and want to use and filling in with your own creations and combinations beyond that.

2. Continue with the exercise plan you've made for yourself, increasing duration, frequency, variety, and/or difficulty as you get more and more fit. Keep scheduling exercise specifically into your calendar at least a month in advance.

3. Keep up with your supplements, making any necessary adjustments if your circumstances change (e.g., you develop lactose intolerance and stop drinking milk, or you discover calcium carbonate upsets your stomach).

4. Continue taking whichever hormones, if any, you decided upon, and reevaluate your choice as your situation changes (e.g., you enter menopause, or you develop a health problem affected by hormones, or new research gives you a different perspective). Reevaluating after five years on menopausal HRT is a must.

5. Keep taking any drug therapies you decided on, and consider adjusting them according to the results of later bone scans. Whether or not you choose a prescription to start with, and no matter which one or ones you use now, reevaluate your plan if your circumstances change (e.g., you go into menopause or start taking a medication that can change bone density).

6. Check back with your regular doctor about any and all changes you are making to keep him or her up-to-date, and coordinate between the doctor and any other health care professionals you may be working with (nutritionist, physical therapist or personal trainer, endocrinologist, herbalist, etc.). Get follow-up bone scans and NTX measurements as necessary to track your progress.

7. Keep a diary of all that you are doing—food, exercises, supplements—and review it at the end of two weeks to see if you are meeting your goals. Make any necessary adjustments.

8. Stay strong and live long!

❁ ❁ ❁ ❁ ❁ ❁ ❁ ❁ ❁ ❁ ❁ ❁ ❁ ❁ ❁ ❁ ❁ ❁ ❁ ❁

Index

About the Authors

GEORGE J. KESSLER, D.O., P.C., is an attending physician at The New York Hospital Cornell Medical Center, clinical instructor in medicine at The Albert Einstein College of Medicine, and an adjunct clinical assistant professor at The New York College of Osteopathic Medicine. He is a diplomate and member of the American Academy of Pain Management and the American Osteopathic Board of Family Practice. He has a private practice in general and complementary medicine, and pain management in New York City.

COLLEEN KAPKLEIN is a freelance editor and writer specializing in health, psychology, and alternative medicine. She is the author of *Take Two* and the writer for *Plato Not Prozac!*